CLINICAL

SKILLBUILDERS™

Crisis Drugs

Springhouse Corporation
Springhouse, Pennsylvania

STAFF

Executive Director, Editorial
Stanley Loeb

Editorial Director
Matthew Cahill

Clinical Director
Barbara F. McVan, RN

Art Director
John Hubbard

Senior Editor
William J. Kelly

Clinical Project Editor
Joanne Patzek DaCunha, RN, BS

Drug Information Editor
George J. Blake, RPh, MS

Editors
Barbara Delp, Margaret Eckman, Kevin Law, Elizabeth Mauro

Clinical Editor
Beverly Ann Tscheschlog, RN

Copy Editors
Jane V. Cray (supervisor), Traci A. Ginnona, Nancy Papsin, Doris Weinstock

Designers
Stephanie Peters (associate art director), Matie Patterson (senior designer), Linda Franklin

Illustrators
David E. Cook, Robert Neumann

Art Production
Robert Perry (manager), Anna Brindisi, Donald Knauss, Thomas Robbins, Robert Wieder

Typography
David Kosten (director), Diane Paluba (manager), Elizabeth Bergman, Joyce Rossi Biletz, Phyllis Marron, Robin Rantz, Valerie Rosenberger

Manufacturing
Deborah Meiris (manager), T.A. Landis, Jennifer Suter

Production Coordination
Colleen M. Hayman

Editorial Assistants
Maree DeRosa, Beverly Lane, Mary Madden

The clinical procedures described and recommended in this publication are based on research and consultation with nursing, medical, and legal authorities. To the best of our knowledge, these procedures reflect currently accepted practice; nevertheless, they can't be considered absolute and universal recommendations. For individual application, all recommendations must be considered in light of the patient's clinical condition and, before administration of new or infrequently used drugs, in light of the latest package-insert information. The authors and the publisher disclaim responsibility for any adverse effects resulting directly or indirectly from the suggested procedures, from any undetected errors, or from the reader's misunderstanding of the text.

Printed in the United States of America.

CS8-010991

Library of Congress Cataloging-in-Publication Data
Crisis drugs.
p. cm. – (Clinical Skillbuilders™)
Includes bibliographical references and index.
1. Drugs – Handbooks, manuals, etc.
2. Emergency nursing – Handbooks, manuals, etc.
I. Springhouse Corporation.
II. Series. [DNLM: 1. Drugs – administration & dosage – handbooks. 2. Drugs – administration & dosage – nurses' instruction. QV 39 C832]
RM301.12.C75 1991
615'.1 – dc20
DNLM/DLC 91-4890
ISBN 0-87434-385-2

CONTENTS

ADVISORY BOARD AND CONTRIBUTORS

At the time of publication, the advisors held the following positions.

Sandra G. Crandall, RN,C, MSN, CRNP
Director
Center for Nursing Excellence
Newtown, Pa.

Ellen Eggland, RN, MN
Vice President
Healthcare Personnel, Inc.
Naples, Fla.

Terry Matthew Foster, RN, BSN, CEN, CCRN
Clinical Director, Nursing Administration
Mercy Hospital—Anderson
Cincinnati
Staff Nurse, Emergency Department
St. Elizabeth Medical Center
Covington, Ky.

Sandra K. Goodnough-Hanneman, RN, PhD
Critical Care Nursing Consultant
Houston

Doris A. Millam, RN, MS, CRNI
I.V. Therapy Clinician
Holy Family Hospital
Des Plaines, Ill.

Deborah Panozzo Nelson, RN, MS, CCRN
Cardiovascular Clinical Specialist
Visiting Assistant Professor
EMS Nursing Education
Purdue University, Calumet Campus
Hammond, Ind.

Sally S. Russell, RN, MN, CS
Instructor
Clinical Specialist
St. Elizabeth Hospital Medical Center
Lafayette, Ind.

Marilyn Sawyer Sommers, RN, PhD, CCRN
Nurse Consultant
Instructor
College of Nursing and Health
University of Cincinnati

At the time of publication, the contributors held the following positions.

Bruce M. Frey, RPh, BS, PharmD
Clinical Pharmacist in Pediatrics and Neonatology
Thomas Jefferson University Hospital
Philadelphia

Diane Foley Osbourne, RN, CEN
Staff Nurse
McLeod Regional Medical Center
Florence, S.C.

FOREWORD

When a patient needs a drug in a crisis, you have to act fast—often within seconds. You don't have time to page through a drug textbook for the right dosage or route. You need a resource that puts such essential information at your fingertips.

Crisis Drugs, the latest volume in the Clinical Skillbuilders series, does just that. This compact manual provides easily accessible, up-to-date information on the most frequently used crisis drugs. It includes drugs used for obvious crises, like cardiac arrest, as well as for any acute changes in a patient's condition that require rapid intervention.

To help you find information quickly, this alphabetically arranged book uses the same format for each drug. First, you'll find an introduction that briefly covers the drug's indications, mechanism of action, and pharmacokinetics. Then come sections on contraindications and cautions, drug preparation, incompatibilities, and drug administration. The next section covers adverse reactions. For your convenience, the life-threatening reactions appear separately, and the common reactions are highlighted with ***bold italic*** type. Following a section on drug interactions, you'll find the special considerations you need to administer the drug safely and to care for your patient during and after therapy.

Throughout the book, special graphic devices called logos alert you to key information. For every drug, you'll see a *Dosage finder* logo that directs you to a brief listing of indications and dosage recommendations. A *Mechanism of action* logo calls your attention to a fully illustrated explanation of how a drug works—for instance, how cimetidine reduces gastric acid. And when you see an *Emergency intervention* logo, you'll find the steps to take when a patient experiences an overdose. As an added feature, the book also gives you drip rate conversion charts for several drugs, so you don't have to calculate the rate before the infusion.

After the last drug, you'll find a self-test. The multiple-choice questions and answers will help you evaluate and further build your knowledge and skills. After the self-test comes a helpful appendix—a chart on antidotes to drug overdoses and poisons, with a special emphasis on nursing considerations.

With all this information in a portable, quick-reference manual, *Crisis Drugs* will prove indispensable for nurses today. No matter where you work or how long you've practiced, you need an up-to-date book on the drugs you must give in a crisis. Quite simply, *Crisis Drugs* is the best available.

Carol A. Higgins, RN, MSN, CCRN
Clinical Nurse Specialist, Critical Care
McLaren Regional Medical Center
Flint, Michigan

INTRODUCTION

Any drug that you must administer in a clinically urgent situation or an emergency can be considered a crisis drug. Of course, crisis drugs include those you'd give in life-threatening conditions—for example, lidocaine for a cardiac arrest. But they also include drugs you'd give for acute changes in a patient's condition, such as an exacerbation of a chronic disorder. Thus, furosemide becomes a crisis drug when given for acute symptoms of congestive heart failure.

In this book, you'll find the information you need to administer more than 60 common crisis drugs quickly and safely. But before you turn to the information on individual drugs, review the following general considerations for all crisis drugs.

Contraindications and cautions

Every drug poses certain risks. In some cases, the risks are so great that the drug is contraindicated even in an emergency. For instance, despite the benefits of epinephrine, you would never give it to a patient who's in cardiogenic shock. But in many cases, the risks don't completely outweigh the benefits of the drug. In such cases, you'll administer the drug but have to monitor the patient carefully for adverse reactions. For example, you may give epinephrine to a patient with a sulfite allergy, but you'll need to be alert for complications, such as paradoxical worsening of respiratory function.

Pregnancy risk categories. Weighing the risks and benefits of a drug becomes particularly important when the patient is pregnant. To help you assess the risks, the Food and Drug Administration (FDA) classifies all drugs as Category A, B, C, D, or X, based on their potential to cause birth defects or fetal death.

- *Category A.* Controlled studies show no risk to the fetus. Adequate studies in pregnant women have failed to demonstrate a risk to the fetus.
- *Category B.* Evidence shows no risk to humans. Either animal studies show risk and human studies don't, or adequate human studies haven't been done and animal studies have proven negative.
- *Category C.* The potential for risk can't be ruled out. Adequate human studies don't exist, and animal studies either lack data or indicate fetal risk. Despite the risk, the drug may be useful for pregnant women.
- *Category D.* Evidence of risk to the fetus exists. But in some cases, the benefits may still outweigh the risks.
- *Category X.* Animal or human studies indicate a fetal risk that clearly outweighs any benefits. The drug is contraindicated for pregnant patients.

Potential for abuse. The FDA also classifies certain drugs according to their potential for abuse. Schedule I drugs have the highest potential for abuse; schedule V, the lowest. You'll never administer Schedule I drugs because they have no acceptable medical use. When you must administer a schedule II, III, IV, or V drug, assess the patient's risk for developing a dependence.

Drug preparation and incompatibilities

Typically, in a crisis you'll be responsible for preparing the drugs. This may include reconstituting an I.V. drug from powder as well as further diluting the drug solution in a large volume. Before mixing a drug and a diluent, make sure they're compatible.

An incompatibility may cause a precipitate to form or a change in the drug's potency, color, or chemistry. Such problems may develop either immediately or after some time. If you know that the incompatibility will be delayed, you may be able to mix the drug and diluent and give the solution immediately. Such solutions must be discarded after a certain length of time if they haven't been used.

Label all solutions with the amount of drug and the time it was prepared. If you're not administering the drug immediately, store it appropriately, based on the potential effects of temperature and light.

To avoid a potential incompatibility, don't administer two drugs through the same I.V. line at the same time, if possible. When giving a drug intermittently or by direct injection, first flush the primary tubing or heparin lock with a compatible solution—0.9% sodium chloride or dextrose 5% in water (D_5W), for instance. Administer the drug, then flush the tubing again.

In a crisis—when a patient may need several drugs—you may have to alter your technique. For instance, you may piggyback a drug into an existing I.V. line. If you do, make sure the drugs and the solutions are compatible. In some cases of delayed incompatibility, you can even administer two incompatible drugs simultaneously. But you must know how much time you have and make sure one drug will be delivered before an incompatibility can occur. If you have questions about incompatibilities, ask your hospital pharmacist.

Narcotic precautions

When you handle narcotics, you need to take some additional precautions.

- Sign the narcotics form when you take a drug from the cabinet. Always relock the cabinet.
- Never leave a narcotic unattended.
- If you must waste a controlled substance, do so in the presence of another nurse. Both of you should note the waste on the narcotics form.
- With another nurse present, take an inventory of the narcotics at the end of your shift.

Administration routes

Depending on the drug and the situation, you may use the following routes in a crisis: I.V., I.M., S.C., oral, sublingual, buccal, endotracheal, intracardiac, inhalation, and intraosseous.

I.V. administration. Usually the preferred route in a crisis, I.V. administration provides immediate and predictable therapeutic effects. This route allows accurate titration and enables you to stop the infusion immediately should an adverse reaction occur. However, the I.V. route also has certain drawbacks. Incompatibility problems and adverse reactions may develop more quickly and more severely than with other routes. And gaining vascular access isn't always a simple matter.

Direct injection. With this method, the drug rapidly achieves its therapeutic blood level. Before giving the drug, you'll usually dilute it in 10 ml of solution; you shouldn't use more than 25 ml. Typically, you'll administer a direct injection through a heparin lock or through the Y-site of a free-flowing I.V. line. Or you may inject a drug directly into a vein. To maintain the blood level of a short-acting drug, you may follow a direct injection with a continuous infusion.

Adverse reactions occur more often with direct injection because of the high drug concentration. And, because this method exerts more pressure on the vein, the risk of infiltration in patients with fragile veins increases.

Intermittent infusion. The most common I.V. method, an intermittent infusion delivers medication over short periods at varying intervals. The resulting peak and trough levels produce the maximum therapeutic effectiveness.

You'll dilute the drug in a small volume of fluid (25 to 250 ml) and infuse it over a period of several minutes to a few hours. Because the patient receives a lower concentration of drug, this method helps reduce the risk of severe adverse reactions.

Continuous infusion. With a continuous infusion, the patient receives a regulated dose delivered over a prolonged period. Sometimes you'll give an initial loading dose to quickly achieve peak blood levels. Once this occurs, a continuous infusion can maintain the therapeutic level.

I.M. and S.C. injections. Drugs given by I.M. or S.C. injection must be absorbed through blood vessels in the muscle or subcutaneous tissue before they act. This can cause a significant delay during a crisis. However, when venous access isn't possible, the I.M. or S.C. route may be an appropriate choice. Some drugs can't be given I.M. or S.C. because they cause tissue damage.

Oral administration. You'll administer few crisis drugs orally because the absorption time delays the drug's action. However, in some situations, you'll administer an I.V. loading dose first, then give oral doses to maintain the therapeutic level. Also, antidotes to ingested poisons can be given orally because absorption isn't necessary for the drug to act.

Sublingual and buccal administration. You'll place certain drugs sublingually (under the tongue) or in the buccal pouch (between the teeth and cheek or the gum and cheek). These routes produce a rapid absorption and onset of action. Nitroglycerin serves as a good example of a crisis drug given via this route.

Endotracheal administration. During cardiac or respiratory arrest, certain drugs can be instilled into the lungs through the endotracheal tube. After instillation, you'll deliver a few breaths with a hand-held resuscitation bag to force the drug into the alveoli. The drug then passes through the capillary membrane and into the circulatory system. Used when venous access isn't available, this route works only with certain drugs.

Intracardiac injection. During cardiac arrest, a doctor can administer certain drugs directly into the heart. Then chest compressions can be given to circulate the drug. Because this route can cause ventricular rupture or arrhythmias, a doctor will use it only as a last resort.

Inhalation and nebulization. Some drugs can be administered directly to the lungs by having the patient inhale small particles in solution. This route allows quick drug action and limits the amount of drug needed to achieve a therapeutic effect. Because this route avoids systemic absorption, the risk of adverse reactions is reduced.

Intraosseous administration. When you can't obtain I.V. access in a pediatric emergency, intraosseous administration may be necessary. The anteromedial surface of the proximal tibia about 1" (2.5 cm) below the tibial tuberosity provides the best infusion site. The bone marrow serves as a noncollapsible vein, and the drug enters systemic circulation via an extensive network of venous sinusoids. Drug absorption and effectiveness are the same as with the I.V. route.

Adverse reactions

Any crisis drug may cause adverse reactions. In this book, you'll find life-threatening adverse reactions listed separately for quick reference. Also, the most common adverse reactions appear in ***bold italic*** type so you can see them at a glance.

Interactions

When a patient receives two or more drugs, an undesirable interaction may occur. A synergistic interaction produces an exaggerated effect. For instance, when a patient receives both haloperidol and a central nervous system depressant, the result may be excessive sedation, respiratory depression, and hypotension.

An antagonistic interaction has just the opposite effect, with one or both drugs becoming less effective. If a patient receives both labetalol and an anti-inflammatory drug, for example, the effects of labetalol will be diminished.

Quick, safe administration

This introduction forms the foundation for using this book effectively. The specific information that follows will guide you in a crisis, telling you how to prepare and administer the drugs, how to monitor the patient, and when and how to treat him for an overdose. Following these guidelines carefully will help you build your confidence and skills—and help you administer these important drugs quickly and safely.

CRISIS DRUGS

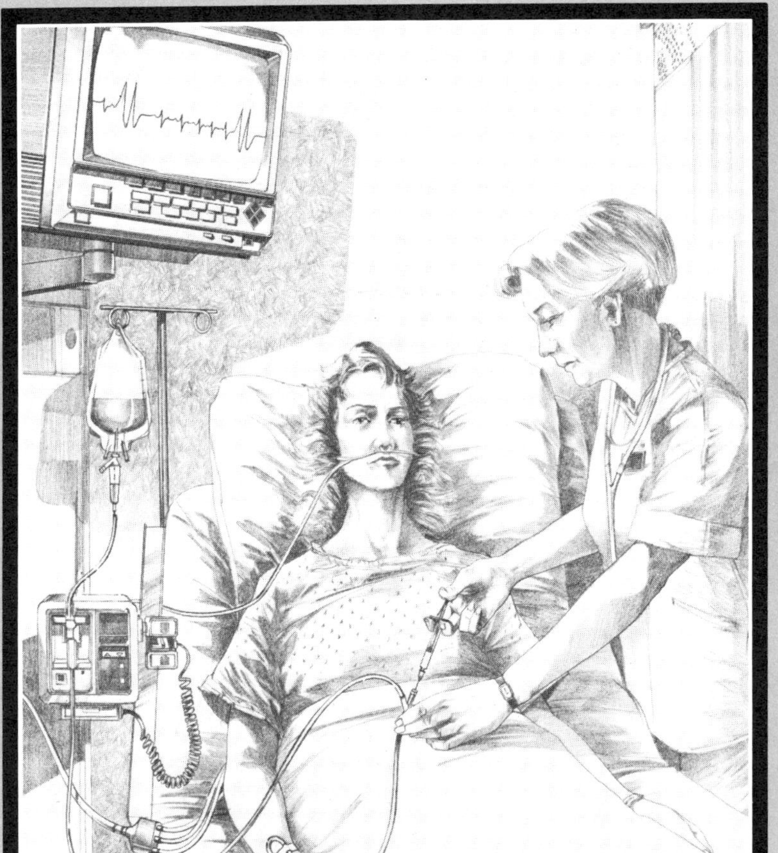

Alteplase
(Activase)

A tissue plasminogen activator produced by recombinant deoxyribonucleic acid (DNA) technology, alteplase helps restore perfusion in occluded coronary and pulmonary arteries by destroying thrombi. The drug works by binding to the fibrin-plasminogen complex within a thrombus and converting it into plasmin, which then dissolves the thrombus (see *How alteplase helps restore perfusion*).

Ideally, treatment of an acute myocardial infarction should begin within 6 hours of the onset of the patient's symptoms. Early treatment decreases the infarct's size, improves ventricular function, and reduces the risk of congestive heart failure and death. Treatment of a pulmonary embolism should begin within 5 to 7 days.

Administered by continuous I.V. infusion, alteplase is distributed in about 4 minutes. The drug is rapidly metabolized in the liver. About 80% of alteplase is excreted as metabolites in the urine within 18 hours. (See *Alteplase: Indications and dosages.*)

Contraindications and cautions

Because alteplase increases the risk of bleeding, it shouldn't be administered to a patient with internal bleeding, an aneurysm, an arteriovenous malformation, or bleeding diathesis. For the same reason, the drug shouldn't be given to a patient with a history of central nervous system surgery or trauma in the past 2 months, a cerebrovascular accident, or a brain tumor. The drug is also contraindicated for patients with systolic pressure above 179 mm Hg or diastolic pressure above 109 mm Hg.

Use alteplase cautiously in patients at risk for a thrombus on the left side of the heart (someone who has mitral stenosis and atrial fibrillation, for instance) and in those with acute pericarditis, cerebrovascular disease, diabetic hemorrhagic retinopathy, significant hepatic disease, marked hypertension, subacute bacterial endocarditis, septic thrombophlebitis, or an occluded arteriovenous cannula at an infected site. Also, use caution when giving the drug to patients over age 75, those receiving oral anticoagulants, those who've experienced GI or gen-

DOSAGE FINDER

Alteplase: Indications and dosages

Lysis of thrombi obstructing coronary arteries in acute myocardial infarction

▶ For adults 143 pounds (65 kg) or more, give 100 mg over 3 hours.

In the first hour, give 60 mg – 6 to 10 mg as a bolus in the first 1 to 2 minutes, and the rest as a diluted continuous infusion over the rest of the hour. Then administer 20 mg/hour as a continuous infusion for the next 2 hours. Don't exceed the recommended dosage of 100 mg over 3 hours; higher dosages may lead to intracranial bleeding.

▶ For adults under 143 pounds, give 1.25 mg/kg over 3 hours.

In the first hour, give 60% of the total dose – 10% as a bolus in the first 1 to 2 minutes and the rest as a diluted continuous infusion. Then give the remaining 40% of the total dose over the next 2 hours, 20% each hour.

Lysis of pulmonary emboli

▶ For adults, give 100 mg as a diluted continuous infusion over 2 hours.

MECHANISM OF ACTION

How alteplase helps restore perfusion

When a thrombus forms in an artery, it obstructs the blood supply, causing ischemia and necrosis. Alteplase can dissolve a thrombus in either the coronary or pulmonary artery, restoring the blood supply to the area beyond the blockage.

OBSTRUCTED ARTERY

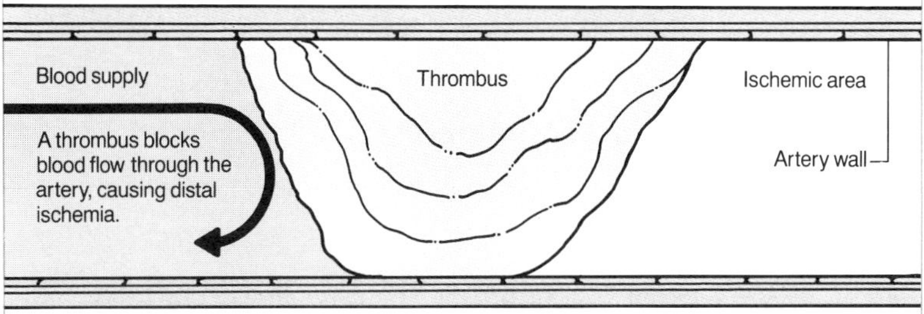

A thrombus blocks blood flow through the artery, causing distal ischemia.
Artery wall

INSIDE THE THROMBUS

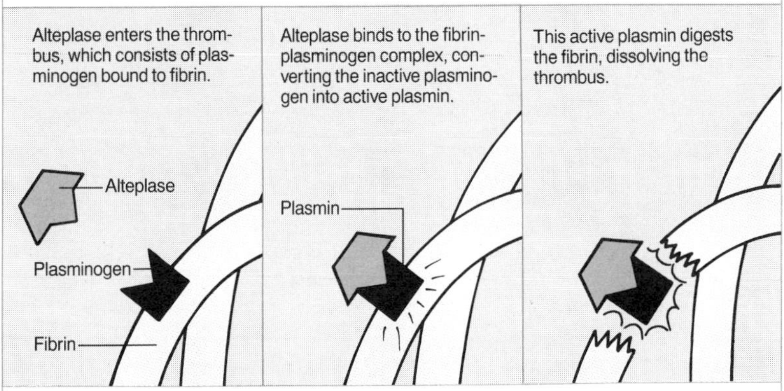

Alteplase enters the thrombus, which consists of plasminogen bound to fibrin.
Alteplase
Plasminogen
Fibrin
Alteplase binds to the fibrin-plasminogen complex, converting the inactive plasminogen into active plasmin.
Plasmin
This active plasmin digests the fibrin, dissolving the thrombus.

RESTORED BLOOD FLOW

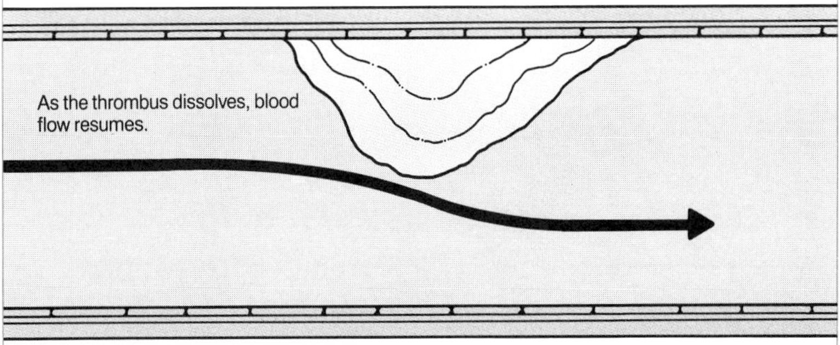

itourinary bleeding or trauma, and those who've undergone major surgery or given birth within the last 10 days.

Because alteplase is a pregnancy risk category C drug, it should be given cautiously to pregnant patients. Safety and efficacy guidelines for children haven't been established.

Preparation

Alteplase is available as a lyophilized powder in 20- and 50-mg vials. Reconstitute it using a large-bore needle (18G, for example) and either a 20- or 50-ml syringe filled with sterile water for injection. (You'll use a 20-ml syringe with a 20-mg vial and a 50-ml syringe with a 50-mg vial.) Add the diluent to the vial, directing the stream into the lyophilized cake, which may foam slightly. Then mix the drug by gently rolling and tilting the vial—not by shaking it. Use the reconstituted drug within 8 hours to avoid contamination.

Never reconstitute alteplase with bacteriostatic water for injection or other diluents that contain preservatives because they may interact with the drug. Dispose of the alteplase if the vial vacuum isn't intact, if the drug becomes discolored, or if protein coagulates in the vial.

If you need to dilute the reconstituted drug, mix it with 0.9% sodium chloride injection or dextrose 5% in water in a polyvinylchloride bag or glass bottle. You can dilute the drug to a concentration as low as 0.5 mg/ml. Use the diluted drug at once.

Incompatibilities

Because compatibility studies aren't complete, you shouldn't combine alteplase with any other product. Use one I.V. line exclusively for the alteplase.

Administration

- *Direct injection:* Give the recommended portion of the first dose over a 1- to 2-minute period.
- *Continuous infusion:* Administer the diluted solution at the recommended rate.

Adverse reactions

- *Life-threatening:* uncontrolled bleeding.
- *Other:* allergic reaction, fever, hypotension, nausea, ***oozing or bleeding from wounds or gums,*** vomiting.

Interactions

- *Drugs that alter platelet function (aspirin, dipyridamole):* increased risk of bleeding.

Special considerations

Before infusing alteplase, establish a separate I.V. line for emergency drugs in case of bleeding. Cover any recent puncture sites with pressure dressings, sandbags, or ice packs to prevent bleeding.

Check the dose before administering alteplase. A dose of 150 mg or more increases the patient's risk of intracranial bleeding. (See *Managing an alteplase overdose.*)

During the infusion, make sure the patient stays in bed to minimize the risk of an injury that might cause bleeding. Move him only if necessary, and, if possible, avoid invasive procedures, including I.M. injections and arterial punctures. If you must perform an arterial puncture during the infusion, select a site on the arm distal to the infusion site and apply pressure to that site for 30 minutes after the puncture.

Monitor the patient's cardiac rhythm strip for transient arrhythmias caused by reperfusion after coronary thrombolysis. Keep atropine or lidocaine on hand. If the patient is receiving alteplase for

EMERGENCY INTERVENTION

Managing an alteplase overdose

An overdose of alteplase can cause uncontrollable bleeding. If this occurs, take the following steps:
- Stop the alteplase infusion immediately.
- If necessary, administer a fibrinolytic.
- Replace lost blood with fresh whole blood, packed red blood cells, cryoprecipitate, or fresh frozen plasma, as needed. If you must use a plasma expander, avoid dextran because it inhibits platelet aggregation.
- Monitor the patient for signs of intracranial bleeding.
- Apply pressure to any bleeding sites.

pulmonary embolism, monitor him for signs of reembolization. Alteplase can cause the lysis of underlying deep vein thrombi, which can result in reembolization.

During or after the infusion, administer heparin as ordered to prevent the formation of new clots. For the treatment of coronary artery occlusion, the patient should receive concurrent heparin and alteplase therapy to reduce the risk of new thrombus formation and reocclusion. Start aspirin or dipyridamole therapy during or after the heparin therapy, as ordered. For the treatment of pulmonary embolism, start heparin therapy near the end of or right after alteplase therapy, when the partial thromboplastin or thrombin time returns to twice the normal rate or less.

Keep in mind that alteplase alters the results of coagulation and fibrinolytic tests.

Aminophylline

(Aminophyllin Injection, Somophyllin)

A water-soluble salt of theophylline, aminophylline helps relieve acute bronchial asthma and reversible bronchospasm associated with chronic bronchitis and emphysema. The pharmacologic effects of this bronchodilator are produced by the theophylline. Although the mechanism of action isn't fully understood, the theophylline appears to act as an adenosine receptor antagonist, inhibiting phosphodiesterase, the enzyme that degrades cyclic adenosine monophosphate. This, in turn, alters intracellular calcium levels, relaxing bronchial smooth muscles and pulmonary vessels. The theophylline also causes coronary vasodilation, diuresis, and cardiac, cerebral, and skeletal muscle stimulation.

When taken orally, aminophylline releases free theophylline in the stomach and starts working in 1 to 2 hours. An I.V. dose starts working as soon as adequate serum levels are achieved. The duration of action varies with the patient's age, sex, and activities. The serum half-life varies, ranging from 3 to 12 hours in nonsmoking asthmatic adults to 1½ to 9½ hours in children.

Aminophylline is quickly dispersed throughout extracellular fluids and body tissues and rapidly dissociates to theophylline, which crosses the placenta and partially penetrates red blood cells. The drug

DOSAGE FINDER

Aminophylline: Indications and dosages

Symptomatic relief of bronchospasm in patients not receiving theophylline

▶ For adults and children, administer a slow I.V. loading dose of 6 mg/kg (equivalent to 4.7 mg/kg of anhydrous theophylline) at a rate of no more than 25 mg/minute. Follow this with a maintenance infusion. (Or give an oral dose of 5 to 6 mg/kg of anhydrous aminophylline tablets or solution.)

▶ For nonsmoking adults, the maintenance rate is 0.7 mg/kg/hour for 12 hours, then 0.5 mg/kg/hour.

▶ For otherwise healthy adult smokers, the maintenance rate is 1 mg/kg/hour for 12 hours, then 0.18 mg/kg/hour.

▶ For older patients and adults with cor pulmonale, the maintenance rate is 0.6 mg/kg/hour for 12 hours, then 0.3 mg/kg/hour.

▶ For adults with congestive heart failure or liver disease, the maintenance rate is 0.5 mg/kg/hour for 12 hours, then 0.1 to 0.2 mg/kg/hour.

▶ For children between ages 9 and 16, the maintenance rate is 1 mg/kg/hour for 12 hours, then 0.8 mg/kg/hour.

▶ For children ages 6 months to 9 years, the maintenance rate is 1.2 mg/kg/hour for 12 hours, then 1 mg/kg/hour.

Symptomatic relief of bronchospasm in patients receiving theophylline

▶ For adults and children, give an infusion of 0.63 mg/kg (equivalent to 0.5 mg/kg anhydrous theophylline) to increase plasma levels of theophylline by 1 mcg/ml. Some clinicians recommend a dose of 3.1 mg/kg (equivalent to 2.5 mg/kg anhydrous theophylline) if the patient doesn't show any obvious signs of theophylline toxicity.

is metabolized in the liver and excreted mainly in urine, although a small amount passes unchanged in the feces. Theophylline also appears in breast milk at about 70% of serum levels. (See *Aminophylline: Indications and dosages.*)

Contraindications and cautions

This drug shouldn't be given to patients with a hypersensitivity to aminophylline or other xanthine compounds or ethylenediamine. It's also contraindicated for patients with preexisting cardiac arrhythmias—especially tachyarrhythmias.

Use the drug cautiously in young children and in elderly patients with congestive heart failure or other types of cardiac or circulatory impairment, cor pulmonale, or hepatic disease. Also give the drug cautiously to patients with active peptic ulcers because it may increase the volume and acidity of gastric secretions, and to those with hyperthyroidism or diabetes mellitus.

Aminophylline is a pregnancy risk category C drug and should be given cautiously to pregnant women.

Preparation

Oral forms of the drug include 105 mg of anhydrous aminophylline in a 5-ml solution and 100- and 200-mg anhydrous aminophylline tablets.

Injectable aminophylline comes in several forms, including 250 mg/10 ml, 500 mg/20 ml, 500 mg/2 ml, 100 mg/100 ml in 0.45% sodium chloride solution, and 200 mg/100 ml in 0.45% sodium chloride solution. You can use the drug undiluted or mixed with 0.9% sodium chloride solution or dextrose 5% in water.

Store containers of aminophylline at room temperature and protect them from freezing and light. Before administering any liquid form of the drug, inspect it for precipitate and discoloration. Discard any abnormal liquid.

Incompatibilities

I.V. forms of aminophylline are incompatible with ascorbic acid, chlorpromazine, codeine phosphate, corticotropin, dimenhydrinate, epinephrine, erythromycin gluceptate, hydralazine, hydroxyzine, insulin, levorphanol, meperidine hydrochloride, methadone, methicillin, morphine sulfate, norepinephrine, oxytetracycline, papaverine, penicillin G potassium, phenobarbital, phenytoin, prochlorperazine, promazine, promethazine, tetracycline, vancomycin, vitamin B complex with C, and any strong acidic solution.

Administration

- *Direct injection:* Administer an undiluted loading dose (usually 25 mg/ml) slowly, making sure you don't exceed 25 mg/minute because a rapid injection can cause a fatal reaction. For the same reason, don't give an injection through a central venous catheter.
- *Continuous infusion:* Dilute the drug in 250, 500, or 1,000 ml of a compatible solution and infuse it at the prescribed rate.
- *Oral:* Give the drug with a full glass of water, preferably when the patient's stomach is empty.

Adverse reactions

- *Life-threatening:* bradycardia, cardiac arrest, circulatory collapse, confusion, generalized tonic-clonic seizures, hypotension, ventricular fibrillation.
- *Other:* albuminuria, ***anorexia,*** arrhythmias, diarrhea, ***dizziness,*** epigastric pain, flushing, headache, hematemesis, hyperglycemia, ***insomnia,*** irritability, light-headedness, muscle twitching, ***nausea, palpitations,*** precordial pain, ***reflex hyperexcitability,*** restlessness, syncope, syndrome of inappropriate antidiuretic hormone secretion, tinnitus, vomiting.

Interactions

- *Adrenergic bronchodilators and other xanthines:* additive toxicity.
- *Alkali-sensitive drugs:* reduced theophylline activity. (Don't add these drugs to I.V. fluids containing aminophylline.)
- *Barbiturates, phenytoin, and rifampin:* increased metabolism and decreased theophylline blood levels.
- *Beta-adrenergic blockers:* antagonism. (Propranolol and nadolol in particular may cause bronchospasm in sensitive patients.)
- *Central nervous system (CNS) stimulants:* additional CNS stimulation.
- *Cimetidine, erythromycin, influenza virus vaccine, oral contraceptives, ranitidine, and troleandomycin:* decreased hepatic clearance of theophylline and increased serum concentration.
- *Ciprofloxacin and possibly other fluoroquinolones, diltiazem, and verapamil:* increased serum theophylline concentration and possible CNS toxicity.
- *Hydrocarbon inhalation anesthetics:* increased risk of cardiac arrhythmias.
- *Lithium:* decreased lithium effect.

Special considerations

Before giving aminophylline, check the order carefully. Don't confuse aminophylline with theophylline. Aminophylline USP, made up of

EMERGENCY INTERVENTION

Managing an aminophylline overdose

An overdose of aminophylline causes signs and symptoms of theophylline toxicity. The patient may experience anorexia, apnea, confusion or behavior changes, diarrhea, dizziness, facial flushing, headache, hyperthermia, hypotension, irritability, insomnia, lightheadedness, muscle twitching, nausea, polyuria, severe vomiting, stomach cramps, tachycardia, tachypnea, or trembling. If you note these signs and symptoms, take the following actions:

- Stop the aminophylline infusion.
- Treat the symptoms as ordered. Give lidocaine for atrial arrhythmias and I.V. fluids for dehydration, acid-base imbalance, and hypotension. For severe hypotension, give a vasopressor. Use a tepid bath or hypothermia blanket to treat hyperthermia, and initiate mechanical ventilation for apnea.
- Monitor the patient's serum theophylline levels. When they exceed 60 mcg/ml, he may need charcoal hemoperfusion, even if he's asymptomatic.

79% to 86% theophylline, also contains ethylenediamine. Question the patient closely about other drugs he's taking. Ask about over-the-counter drugs that may contain ephedrine and theophylline salts. If he's taking such a drug, aminophylline may cause excessive stimulation.

Before giving a loading dose, make sure the patient hasn't had theophylline therapy recently.

Base your dosage calculation on the patient's lean body weight and his serum theophylline level. Expect to give a smaller dosage to neonates and elderly patients and to those with chronic obstructive pulmonary disease, active influenza, or cardiac, renal, or hepatic dysfunction because they'll have a decreased theophylline clearance. You may also need to increase the dosage for smokers because they have an accelerated plasma clearance of theophylline.

If the patient complains of vein irritation and burning when he receives a direct injection of aminophylline, dilute it with a compatible solution.

Throughout therapy, monitor the patient's trough and peak serum levels of theophylline to maintain the optimal therapeutic level and avoid toxicity (see *Managing an aminophylline overdose*). Optimal levels range from 10 to 20 mcg/ml.

Monitor the patient's vital signs during therapy. You should see an improvement in both his pulse and respirations. Also monitor his cardiac rhythm strip for arrhythmias, particularly if he's prone to them. Record his fluid intake and output.

When switching the patient from a continuous infusion to an oral preparation, discontinue the I.V. drug and give him the extended-release oral preparation. Start him on the immediate-release form of the drug 4 to 6 hours later.

Keep in mind that serum uric acid tests using the Bittner or colorimetric methods will show falsely elevated levels.

Amrinone lactate

(Inocor)

Amrinone lactate, a bipyridine derivative, treats congestive heart failure (CHF) by increasing myocardial contractility in patients who haven't responded adequately to cardiac glycosides, diuretics, and vasodilators. And it does so without causing the ventricular irritability or other signs of digitalis toxicity associated with cardiac glycosides.

This cardiac inotropic agent works by inhibiting phosphodiesterase, which raises cellular levels of cyclic adenosine monophosphate. That, in turn, increases the strength of muscular contractions. A noncatecholamine, nonglycoside, cardiotonic drug, amrinone also acts as a vasodilator, reducing central venous pressure, pulmonary capillary wedge pressure, systemic and peripheral vascular resistance, and preload and afterload. Amrinone also increases atrioventricular conduction slightly.

With rapid administration, the onset of action occurs in 2 to 5 minutes and peak levels occur in 10 minutes. The duration of action ranges from 30 minutes to 2 hours. The serum half-life of the drug averages almost 4 hours, although, with a controlled infusion, it increases to about 6 hours.

The drug is thought to be distributed throughout body tissues, with 10% to 49% binding to plasma proteins. Whether the drug crosses the placenta or blood-brain barrier isn't known. Amrinone is metabolized in the liver into several metabolites—probably undergoing acetylation, glucuronidation, and glutathione addition. The drug is then excreted primarily in urine, with 10% to 40% passing unchanged in the first 24 hours. Whether or not the drug passes into breast milk isn't known. (See *Amrinone: Indication and dosages.*)

DOSAGE FINDER

Amrinone: Indication and dosages

Short-term management of congestive heart failure in patients unresponsive to cardiac glycosides, diuretics, and vasodilators

▶ For adults and children, give 0.75 mg/kg I.V. over 2 to 3 minutes. Follow this with a continuous infusion of 200 mg of amrinone in 250 ml of sodium chloride solution, delivered at a rate of 5 to 10 mcg/kg/minute. Adjust the dosage according to the patient's clinical response. If necessary, give him a bolus of 0.75 mg/kg 30 minutes after therapy starts.

The daily dosage shouldn't exceed 10 mg/kg, although some patients have received up to 18 mg/kg a day for short durations. The patient should maintain a steady state plasma level of 3 mcg/ml.

Contraindications and cautions

Amrinone is contraindicated for patients with a hypersensitivity to it or to sulfites, as well as for those with an acute myocardial infarction or ischemic coronary artery disease without CHF. Patients with severe aortic or pulmonary valve disease shouldn't receive the drug; surgery is needed to relieve the obstruction. The drug may aggravate outflow tract obstruction in those with hypertrophic subaortic stenosis.

The safety and efficacy of amrinone in children haven't been established. Amrinone is a pregnancy risk category C drug.

Preparation

Amrinone comes in 20-ml ampules of a clear yellow solution. Each ampule contains 5 mg/ml. Protect the ampules from light and store them at room temperature.

To give the drug as an I.V. infusion, dilute 200 mg in 250 ml of 0.45% or 0.9% sodium chloride solution for a concentration of 0.8 mg/ml. If you note discoloration or a

Drip rates for amrinone infusions

This chart shows you the drip rates to use to achieve prescribed infusion rates for a solution of 200 mg of amrinone in 250 ml of 0.9% sodium chloride solution (a concentration of 0.8 mg/ml).

DRIP RATE (MICRODROPS/ MINUTE)	INFUSION RATE
75	1 mg/minute
150	2 mg/minute

precipitate, discard the solution. Use the diluted solution within 24 hours.

Incompatibilities
Amrinone is incompatible with furosemide, bicarbonate, and dextrose. Avoid using dextrose as a diluent because amrinone interacts chemically with it. But because this reaction occurs slowly, you can infuse or inject the drug into an I.V. line of a free-flowing dextrose solution.

Administration
- *Direct injection:* Administer the diluted or undiluted drug into a vein or an I.V. line of a free-flowing, compatible solution over 2 to 3 minutes. If you inject the drug into an I.V. line, flush the line and cannula with 0.9% sodium chloride solution.
- *Continuous infusion:* Infuse the diluted amrinone at a rate of 5 to 10 mcg/kg/minute, using a pump to maintain the rate. You can piggyback the drug into an I.V. line with a free-flowing, compatible solution, using a Y-connector close to the insertion site. (See *Drip rates for amrinone infusions.*)

Adverse reactions
- *Life-threatening:* anaphylaxis, arrhythmias, thrombocytopenia.
- *Other:* abdominal pain, anorexia, burning at injection site, chest pain, diarrhea, fever, hepatotoxicity, hypotension, nausea, vomiting.

Interactions
- *Cardiac glycosides:* increased inotropic effect.
- *Disopyramide:* excessive hypotension.

Special considerations
Before administering amrinone to a patient who has undergone vigorous diuretic therapy, administer fluid and electrolyte replacements as ordered. He'll need them to raise his cardiac filling pressure, so he can respond to amrinone.

Because amrinone increases the ventricular response rate, a patient with atrial fibrillation or flutter may need concomitant cardiac glycoside therapy to slow the atrial impulse.

During the infusion, closely monitor the patient's fluid and electrolyte levels, hepatic and renal function, and platelet count. If his platelet count drops below 150,000/mm^3, expect to decrease the dosage. Monitor his cardiac rhythm strip for arrhythmias. Also check his vital signs every 5 to 15 minutes. If his blood pressure drops, slow or stop the infusion and notify the doctor. Provide symptomatic treatment.

Amrinone shouldn't affect the results of any diagnostic tests.

Anistreplase
(Eminase)

When given within 6 hours of the onset of symptoms of a myocardial infarction (MI), anistreplase can destroy a thrombus blocking a coronary artery, allowing reperfusion of the ischemic area of the myocardium. Formerly called anisoylated plasminogen-streptokinase activator complex (APSAC), anistreplase is derived from Lys-plasminogen and streptokinase. The drug consists of a fibrinolytic enzyme-activator complex with the activator temporarily blocked by an anisoyl group. Once anistreplase is in the body, a nonenzymatic process removes the anisoyl group, activating the drug.

The activated drug causes plasminogen to form plasmin in the bloodstream or the clot itself. The reaction works more efficiently within the clot, but wherever the plasmin forms, it will degrade the fibrin clot.

The drug causes reperfusion in 45 minutes and has a half-life of 94 minutes. The distribution, metabolism, and excretion of anistreplase aren't fully understood. (See *Anistreplase: Indication and dosage.*)

DOSAGE FINDER

Anistreplase: Indication and dosage

Lysis of coronary artery thrombi after acute myocardial infarction

▶ For adults, give 30 units I.V. over 2 to 5 minutes within 6 hours of the onset of symptoms.

Contraindications and cautions

Anistreplase shouldn't be given to patients with a known allergy to the drug, or to those with internal bleeding, an aneurysm, arteriovenous malformation, intracranial neoplasm, or bleeding diathesis. The drug is also contraindicated for patients who've had intraspinal or intracranial surgery or trauma in the past 2 months and for those who've had a cerebrovascular accident.

Give this drug cautiously to patients who've experienced major surgery, trauma (including cardiopulmonary resuscitation), or GI or genitourinary bleeding within the past 10 days. Also use caution in patients with cerebrovascular disease, hypertension (systolic pressure at or above 180 mm Hg, diastolic pressure at or above 110 mm Hg, or both), acute pericarditis, subacute bacterial endocarditis, septic thrombophlebitis, or diabetic hemorrhagic retinopathy. Give the drug carefully to patients with mitral stenosis, atrial fibrillation, or any other condition that could lead to a thrombus in the left side of the heart. Use caution too when administering the drug to patients receiving anticoagulants and those over age 75.

A pregnancy risk category C drug, anistreplase should be used cautiously in pregnant patients.

Preparation

Anistreplase comes in 30-unit vials. Refrigerate the drug at 36° to 46° F (2° to 8° C).

To reconstitute anistreplase, slowly add 5 ml of sterile water for injection. Make sure you direct the stream against the side of the vial, not at the drug itself. Then gently roll the vial to mix the dry powder and water. Don't shake the vial, or the drug will foam. The reconstituted drug should look colorless or pale yellow without any particles.

Use the reconstituted drug within 30 minutes. Don't dilute it.

Incompatibilities

Don't mix anistreplase with any

other drug because its compatibility with other drugs hasn't yet been determined.

Administration

• *Direct injection:* Inject the reconstituted drug into an I.V. line or vein over 2 to 5 minutes.

Adverse reactions

• *Life threatening:* anaphylactoid reactions (rare), ***arrhythmias,*** intracranial hemorrhage.
• *Other:* **bleeding, conduction disorders,** delayed purpuric rash (2 weeks after therapy), flushing, GI bleeding, hematoma, hematuria, hemoptysis, hemorrhaging in mouth and gums, hypotension, itching, urticaria.

Interactions

• *Heparin, oral anticoagulants, and drugs that alter platelet function (including aspirin and dipyridamole):* increased risk of bleeding.

Special considerations

For anistreplase to be effective, the patient must receive it within 6 hours of the onset of symptoms.

During therapy, carefully monitor the patient's cardiac rhythm strip. You may see arrhythmias such as those caused by an acute MI, including sinus bradycardia, accelerated idioventricular rhythm, ventricular tachycardia, and premature ventricular contractions—all signs of successful thrombolysis. Keep emergency equipment nearby to treat bradycardia or ventricular irritability.

Monitor the patient for bleeding, the most common adverse reaction to anistreplase. Use pressure dressings, sandbags, or ice packs on recent punctures sites to prevent bleeding, and move the patient as little as possible. Avoid I.M. injections, venipunctures, and arterial punctures. If you must perform an arterial puncture, choose a site (such as the arm) where you can apply pressure for 30 minutes afterward.

After treatment, the doctor may order heparin therapy to decrease the risk of new thrombus formation. Teach the patient to watch for signs of internal bleeding, including hematemesis, hematuria, and black, tarry stools. He should report such signs at once. Also teach him about proper dental care to prevent gum trauma.

Although anistreplase is made from human plasma, the manufacturing process is designed to purify it. No cases of hepatitis or human immunodeficiency virus infection have been reported.

Keep in mind that anistreplase alters coagulation tests. Adding aprotinin (2,000 to 3,000 kallikrein-inhibiting units/ml) to blood samples can counteract this effect.

Atropine sulfate

Used to treat symptomatic bradycardia, this anticholinergic binds to postganglionic receptors and blocks acetylcholine. By suppressing acetylcholine's vagal effect on the sinoatrial (SA) node, atropine sulfate increases the heart rate.

When used in advanced cardiac life support, atropine can be given I.V. or endotracheally to restore normal heart rate and blood pressure in patients with severe hypotension associated with sinus bradycardia, junctional bradycardia, third-degree atrioventricular (AV) block, or second-degree AV block (Mobitz Types I and II). The drug

DOSAGE FINDER

Atropine: Indications and dosages

Treatment of symptomatic bradycardia during advanced cardiac life support (ACLS)

▶ For adults, give 0.5 mg I.V. or 1 to 2 mg endotracheally every 5 minutes until the heart rate increases to the desired rate (usually 80 beats/minute). Don't exceed a total dose of 2 mg.

Treatment of ventricular asystole during ACLS

▶ For adults, give 1 mg I.V. every 5 minutes or 1 to 2 mg endotracheally.

▶ For children and adolescents, give 0.02 mg/kg I.V. every 5 minutes as needed. Don't give a child more than 1 mg or an adolescent more than 2 mg per dose.

Blocking of muscarinic effects of anticholinesterase agents

▶ For adults, give 0.6 to 1.2 mg I.V. or I.M. for each 0.5 to 2.5 mg of neostigmine methylsulfate or 10 to 20 mg of pyridostigmine bromide.

▶ For children, give 10 mcg/kg S.C. every 4 to 6 hours. Don't exceed a total dose of 400 mcg.

▶ For neonates, give 0.02 mg/kg S.C. for each 0.04 mg/kg of neostigmine methylsulfate.

Antidote to anticholinesterase toxicity

▶ For adults, start with 1 to 2 mg I.V. or I.M. Then give 2 mg every 5 to 60 minutes until signs and symptoms subside. In severe cases, start with 2 to 6 mg. Then repeat the dose every 5 to 60 minutes, as needed.

▶ For children, start with 1 mg I.V. or I.M. Then give 0.5 to 1 mg every 5 to 10 minutes, until either the signs and symptoms disappear or the signs of atropine toxicity occur.

can also be used to treat vagally-mediated bradycardia resulting from an attempted intubation.

Because the drug increases impulse conduction through the AV node, it can be given to restore a pulse in a patient with ventricular asystole. And atropine may be ordered to block the muscarinic effects of anticholinesterase agents or to act as an antidote to anticholinesterase toxicity.

The onset of action occurs within 2 to 4 minutes of administration, and the drug has a duration of 4 to 6 hours. Its serum half-life ranges from 2 to 3 hours.

Atropine is distributed throughout the body tissues and across the blood-brain barrier and placenta. The drug is metabolized in the liver into several metabolites, including tropine acids and esters. About 18% of the drug binds to serum albumin. Atropine is excreted mainly in urine, although feces and expired air also contain small amounts. Trace amounts pass into breast milk. (See *Atropine: Indications and dosages.*)

Contraindications and cautions

Don't give atropine to patients hypersensitive to the drug or to other belladonna alkaloids or salicylates. Also, patients with asymptomatic bradycardia or bradycardia without significant ventricular ectopy usually won't receive atropine. That's because the drug suppresses vagal stimulation and may lead to sympathetic hyperactivity and severe ventricular arrhythmias.

Atropine is contraindicated for patients with glaucoma because it may raise intraocular pressure (IOP). (The exception: a patient with open-angle glaucoma who's being treated with miotics.) The drug is also contraindicated for patients with myasthenia gravis, obstructive uropathy, and unstable cardiovascular status caused by acute hemorrhage.

Administer atropine carefully to patients with benign prostatic hyperplasia or other obstructive uropathies, or autonomic neuropathy because the drug may cause urine retention. Also give the drug carefully to those with obstructive GI disease, intestinal atony, paralytic ileus, or ulcerative colitis because it may impair intestinal motility.

Use atropine cautiously in patients with reflux esophagitis because it increases reflux; those with fever because it can suppress sweat gland secretions; those with hypertension, including pregnancy-induced hypertension, because it can aggravate the condition; and those with hyperthyroidism because it increases the risk of severe tachycardia. Also, give the drug cautiously when tachycardia threatens to cause cardiac decompensation.

Patients with hepatic or renal impairment may be unable to metabolize or excrete atropine easily, and, in those with xerostomia, it may further decrease salivary flow.

Use atropine cautiously in children with brain damage because it can exacerbate central nervous system (CNS) effects and in those with Down's syndrome because it can cause abnormal pupillary dilation and tachycardia.

Atropine is a pregnancy risk category C drug. An I.V. injection may cause fetal tachycardia.

Preparation

Atropine comes in single-dose ampules of 0.4 mg/ml, 0.5 mg/ml, and 0.4 mg/0.5 ml; in single-dose vials of 0.4 mg/ml, 1 mg/ml, and 1.2 mg/ml; in multidose, 20-ml vials of 0.4 mg/ml; and in prefilled syringes that contain 0.5 mg or 1 mg of the drug. Store the drug at room temperature.

To prepare the drug for endotracheal administration, mix it with 10 ml of sterile water for injection or 0.9% sodium chloride solution.

Incompatibilities

Atropine is incompatible with alkalies, bromides, iodides, isoproterenol, metaraminol, methohexital, norepinephrine, phenobarbital sodium, and sodium bicarbonate.

Administration

- *Direct injection:* Administer the prescribed amount of undiluted drug into a vein or I.V. tubing slowly over 1 to 2 minutes.
- *Endotracheal administration:* Before administering the drug, give the patient several deep breaths of oxygen with a manual resuscitation bag. Then instill the drug (mixed with sterile water for injection or 0.9% sodium chloride solution) deep into the endotracheal tube. Follow this with several more deep breaths from the resuscitation bag to distribute the drug into the alveoli for absorption.
- *I.M. injection:* Inject the prescribed dose into any I.M. injection site.
- *S.C. injection:* Inject the prescribed dose into any S.C. injection site.

Adverse reactions

- *Life-threatening:* aggravated AV block, anaphylaxis, ventricular fibrillation, ventricular tachycardia.
- *Other:* abdominal distention, anhidrosis, ataxia, bloating, ***blurred vision,*** coma, confusion, ***constipation,*** cycloplegia, delirium, dizziness, drowsiness, ***dry mouth,*** flushing,

hallucinations, ***headache,*** hyperpyrexia, increased IOP, insomnia, light-headedness, local irritation at the injection site, ***mydriasis,*** nausea, nervousness, photophobia, rash, ***restlessness,*** tachycardia, urinary hesitancy, urine retention, urticaria, vomiting, weakness.

Interactions

- *Alphaprodine, antihistamines, antiparkinsonian drugs, buclizine, disopyramide, meperidine, orphenadrine, and quinidine:* intensified antimuscarinic effects.
- *Antimyasthenics:* possible further reduction in intestinal motility.
- *Antipsychotics, benzodiazepines, glutethimide, phenothiazines, and tricyclic antidepressants:* intensified antimuscarinic effects.
- *Cholinesterase inhibitors:* blocked miosis.
- *Cyclopropane:* increased risk of ventricular arrhythmias.
- *Digoxin:* elevated serum digoxin levels resulting from decreased GI motility.
- *Ketoconazole:* reduced ketoconazole absorption.
- *Methotrimeprazine:* possible extrapyramidal effects.
- *Monoamine oxidase inhibitors:* intensified atropine action and blocked detoxification.
- *Opioids:* increased risk of severe constipation and paralytic ileus.
- *Potassium chloride (wax-matrix preparations):* increased risk of GI lesions.
- *Urinary alkalinizers:* delayed excretion of atropine.

Special considerations

Make sure you don't administer atropine too slowly. A small dose (one that's less than 0.5 mg) or a dose that's given too slowly can cause transient paradoxical slowing of the patient's heart rate, possibly leading to ventricular arrhythmias.

During therapy, monitor the patient's blood pressure closely to evaluate his tolerance of the drug. Also monitor the cardiac rhythm strip of a patient receiving atropine for bradycardia or heart block. If it shows a heart rate above 100 beats/minute, increased premature ventricular contractions, or ventricular tachycardia, notify the doctor at once (see *Managing an atropine overdose*).

When a patient receives a large

EMERGENCY INTERVENTION

Managing an atropine overdose

An overdose of atropine can cause many adverse reactions. These include blurred vision, coma, confusion, delirium, difficulty swallowing, dilated pupils, drowsiness, flushed and dry skin, muscle weakness, nausea, photophobia, psychotic behavior, restlessness, seizures, stupor, and vomiting. An overdose can also produce hypertension or hypotension, palpitations, a rapid pulse and respirations, respiratory depression, tachycardia with a weak pulse, and vasodilation—all indications of circulatory collapse.

If you detect signs and symptoms of an atropine overdose, provide the following treatment as ordered:

- For shock, give the patient I.V. fluids.
- If he has severe hypotension, start an infusion of either norepinephrine or metaraminol.
- For an anticholinergic reaction, give physostigmine by slow I.V. infusion.
- For central nervous system irritability, administer diazepam, a short-acting barbiturate, I.V. thiopental sodium, or a rectal infusion of chloral hydrate.
- For hyperpyrexia, use cooling measures.
- To prevent urine retention, catheterize the patient.

dose, monitor his fluid intake and output and palpate his bladder every 4 hours to check for urine retention. A large dose of the drug can inhibit parasympathetic control of the bladder. Because such a dose can also decrease intestinal tone and motility, auscultate the patient's bowel sounds and observe the amount and quality of his stool to assess for paralytic ileus or obstruction.

After the patient receives the drug, encourage him to drink fluids because atropine decreases his mucous membrane secretions. Provide mouth care as necessary, and assess him for mucus plugs blocking his airway.

When assessing pupil dilation in a patient with CNS trauma, remember that atropine also causes this effect.

Keep in mind that atropine antagonizes pentagastrin and histamine action in gastric acid secretion tests.

Biperiden lactate

(Akineton)

Biperiden lactate helps relieve the extrapyramidal effects caused by antidopaminergic drugs such as reserpine, phenothiazines, dibenzoxazepines, thioxanthines, and butyrophenones. Such effects include shaking limbs; involuntary swinging of the arms; rapid, dancing motions (chorea); and slow, writhing, snakelike movements (athetosis). Biperiden acts by blocking cholinergic receptors, thus restoring the balance between dopaminergic and cholinergic activity in the basal ganglia. (See *How biperiden relieves extrapyramidal symptoms.*) The drug also relaxes smooth muscle, dilates pupils, and diminishes GI, bronchial, and sweat-gland secretions.

Biperiden's onset and duration of action aren't known. The drug's distribution isn't fully understood either, but biperiden is probably dispersed throughout most body tissues, metabolized in the liver, then excreted unchanged or as metabolites in urine. Whether the drug appears in breast milk isn't known. (See *Biperiden: Indication and dosages,* page 18.)

Contraindications and cautions

Don't give this drug to patients with a known hypersensitivity to biperiden.

Use the drug cautiously in patients with closed-angle glaucoma to prevent increased intraocular pressure and in those with prostate disorders to prevent urine retention. Also use caution when giving biperiden to patients with fever or those exposed to heat because the drug decreases the ability to sweat. In debilitated patients or those with tachycardia, biperiden can cause thyrotoxicosis or decreased cardiac output. It can also increase the risk of further arrhythmias in patients with cardiac instability and existing arrhythmias.

Use biperiden cautiously in patients with hypertension or tardive dyskinesia because it can aggravate these conditions; those with a history of extrapyramidal reactions because it can worsen symptoms; those with intestinal obstruction because it decreases GI motility and tone; and those with myasthenia gravis because it causes increased weakness. Patients with renal impairment run a greater risk of biperiden toxicity, and confused or elderly patients may experience euphoria, confusion, and agitation from taking the drug.

MECHANISM OF ACTION

How biperiden relieves extrapyramidal symptoms

At the basal ganglia cell, an antidopaminergic drug blocks postsynaptic dopaminergic receptors, decreasing inhibitory (dopaminergic) activity. This blockade alters the balance between inhibitory and excitatory (cholinergic) activity, causing extrapyramidal symptoms.

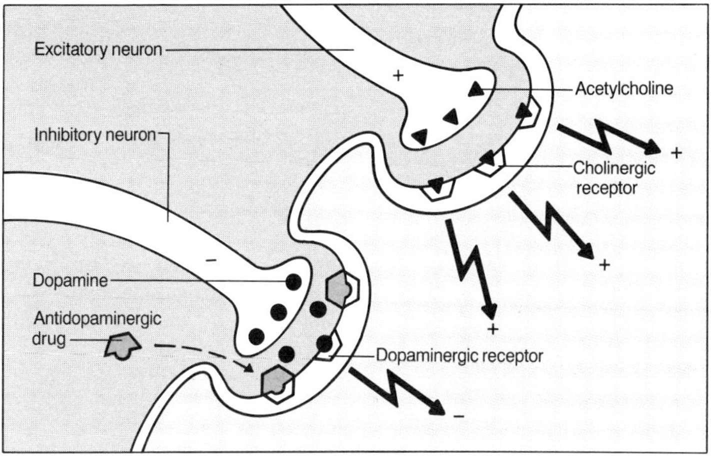

Biperiden blocks the cholinergic receptors at the basal ganglia cell, restoring the balance between inhibitory and excitatory activity. With the inhibitory and excitatory neurons equally blocked, the extrapyramidal symptoms are relieved.

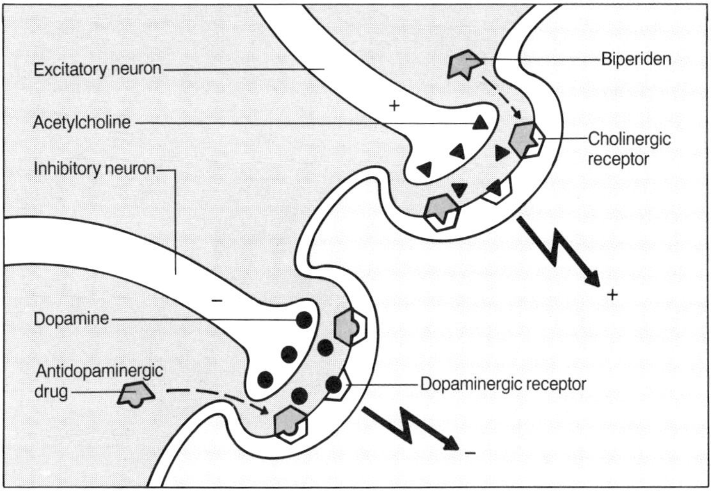

DOSAGE FINDER

Biperiden: Indication and dosages

Treatment of drug-induced extrapyramidal disorders

▶ For adults, give 2 mg (0.4 ml) I.V. or I.M. initially. Repeat the dose every 30 minutes until symptoms subside. Don't exceed four doses (or 8 mg) in 24 hours.

▶ For children, give 40 mcg/kg (0.04 mg), or 1.2 mg/m² I.M. initially. Repeat the dose every 30 minutes as necessary, up to four doses per day.

Use this pregnancy risk category C drug cautiously in pregnant women.

Preparation
Biperiden comes in 1-ml ampules that contain 5 mg of the drug. Stable at room temperature, the drug needs protection from light and freezing.

Incompatibilities
No incompatibilities have been reported.

Administration
- *Direct injection:* Using a 21G or 23G needle, inject the drug over at least a 1-minute period into a vein or into I.V. tubing that contains a free-flowing solution.
- *I.M. injection:* Inject the ordered dose into any I.M. injection site.

Adverse reactions
- *Life-threatening:* orthostatic hypotension.
- *Other:* agitation, blurred vision, ***constipation,*** disorientation, dizziness, drowsiness, ***dry mouth,*** euphoria, hematuria, hyperpyrexia, impaired coordination, photophobia, tachycardia, transient psychotic reactions, urine retention.

Interactions
- *Anticholinesterase drugs:* reduced efficacy of these drugs.
- *Antihistamines, meperidine, phenothiazines, quinidine, and tricyclic antidepressants:* enhanced anticholinergic effects.
- *Central nervous system depressants:* deepened sedation.

Special considerations
Before administering biperiden, obtain the patient's baseline blood pressure and heart rate. During and after administration, monitor him for hypotension and tachycardia. (See *Managing a biperiden overdose.*) Keep him in bed until his blood pressure stabilizes, and warn him to change positions slowly. After administration, monitor his bladder and bowel functions for urine retention and constipation. Expect the doctor to switch the patient to an oral form of the drug as soon as possible.

If the patient complains of photophobia after receiving the drug, darken his room. Take steps to keep him safe if he becomes confused or disoriented, and provide frequent mouth care if he has a dry mouth.

Biperiden doesn't have any known effects on diagnostic tests.

Bretylium tosylate
(Bretylate, Bretylol)

A Class III antiarrhythmic, bretylium tosylate suppresses ventricular fibrillation and tachycardia as well as other ventricular arrhythmias. Though the mechanism of action isn't fully understood, the drug

EMERGENCY INTERVENTION

Managing a biperiden overdose

An overdose of biperiden can cause severe anticholinergic effects—clumsiness or unsteadiness; severe dryness of the mouth, nose, and throat; shortness of breath; tachycardia; and warm, dry, flushed skin. An overdose can also produce central nervous system (CNS) depression (extreme drowsiness) or stimulation (hallucinations, insomnia, and seizures) as well as toxic psychosis (mood or mental changes).

To treat an overdose, take the following actions:

- Give the patient a vasopressor for persistent hypotension, as ordered.
- Provide respiratory support, and administer an antipyretic and fluids, as ordered.
- To help manage CNS stimulation, administer a short-acting barbiturate, as ordered. You shouldn't administer a phenothiazine because it could cause coma.
- If the overdose becomes life-threatening, give physostigmine as ordered to reverse toxic cardiovascular and CNS effects.

seems to increase the threshold for ventricular fibrillation by prolonging repolarization, possibly by blocking postganglionic sympathetic neurons or depleting catecholamines. Bretylium's direct effect on the myocardial cell membrane rapidly suppresses ventricular fibrillation.

The drug's subsequent adrenergic blocking action also prolongs repolarization, probably contributing to the suppression of ventricular tachycardia. The duration of the action potential and the effective refractory period are also increased. Other possible effects of bretylium include vasodilation, cardiostimulation, and weak local anesthesia.

When the drug is used to treat ventricular fibrillation, the onset of action occurs in 5 to 10 minutes if given I.V. and in 20 to 60 minutes if given I.M. When the drug is used to treat ventricular tachycardia, the onset of action can occur anywhere from 20 minutes to 2 hours after I.V. or I.M. administration. The duration of action ranges from 6 to 24 hours. Bretylium's serum half-life averages 5 to 10 hours but can extend up to 4 days in patients with renal impairment (those with a creatinine clearance of less than 30 ml/minute).

Bretylium is distributed to tissues that have high adrenergic innervation, including the sympathetic ganglia, heart, and spleen. Traces of the drug concentrate in the adrenal glands. Between 1% and 10% of the drug binds to plasma proteins. Bretylium doesn't cross the blood-brain barrier. Whether it crosses the placenta isn't known. The body doesn't metabolize the drug but excretes it unchanged in urine. It's not known if the drug passes into breast milk. (See *Bretylium: Indications and dosages,* page 20.)

Contraindications and cautions

Bretylium is contraindicated for digitalis-induced arrhythmias, unless they're life-threatening.

Use the drug cautiously in patients with impaired cardiac output because it can trigger severe hypotension. A pregnancy risk category

DOSAGE FINDER

Bretylium: Indications and dosages

Treatment of ventricular fibrillation
▶ For adults, give 5 mg/kg of undiluted bretylium as a rapid I.V. bolus. Then infuse 10 mg/kg every 15 to 30 minutes as needed. Don't exceed 30 mg/kg/day.

Treatment of ventricular tachycardia and other ventricular arrhythmias
▶ For adults, give an infusion of 5 to 10 mg/kg over 10 to 30 minutes. If needed, repeat the infusion after 1 or 2 hours. Administer a maintenance dosage of 5 to 10 mg/kg infused over 10 to 30 minutes every 6 hours, or a continuous infusion of 1 to 2 mg/minute.

As an alternative, administer 5 to 10 mg/kg of undiluted drug I.M. Repeat the dose after 1 to 2 hours if necessary, and give the same dose every 6 to 8 hours.

C drug, bretylium should be given cautiously to pregnant women.

Preparation
Bretylium comes in single-dose, 10-ml ampules that contain 500 mg of the drug. Store the drug at 59° to 86° F (15° to 30° C).

To infuse bretylium, dilute it with at least 50 ml of dextrose 5% in water or 0.9% sodium chloride solution. The diluted drug will remain stable for 48 hours at room temperature and for 7 days if refrigerated.

Bretylium also comes in prediluted, commercially prepared solutions for infusion.

Incompatibilities
Bretylium is incompatible with dobutamine, nitroglycerin, phenytoin, and procainamide.

Administration
- *Direct injection:* Using a 20G to 22G needle, inject the undiluted drug over a 1-minute period into a vein or an I.V. line of a free-flowing, compatible solution.
- *Intermittent infusion:* Administer the diluted solution over 10 to 30 minutes.
- *Continuous infusion:* Administer the diluted solution at a rate of 1 to 2 mg/minute. (For more information, see *Drip rates for continuous bretylium infusions.*)
- *I.M. injection:* Administer no more than 5 ml of undiluted bretylium at each injection site. Rotate sites to avoid tissue destruction.

Adverse reactions
- *Life-threatening:* severe postural and supine hypotension.
- *Other:* abdominal pain, ache in legs, angina, anorexia, anxiety, bradycardia, chest pressure, confusion, conjunctivitis, depression, diaphoresis, ***dizziness,*** dyspnea, emotional lability, facial flushing, frequent bowel movements, generalized tenderness, headache, lethargy, ***lightheadedness,*** nausea, paranoid psychosis, rash, renal dysfunction, ***syncope,*** transient hypertension, ***vertigo,*** vomiting.

Interactions
- *Cardiac glycosides:* increased toxicity of these drugs.
- *Lidocaine, procainamide, propranolol, and quinidine:* neutralized inotropic effect and potentiated hypotension.

Special considerations
Because of the high risk of toxicity, reduce the dosage for a patient with renal impairment.

During therapy, closely monitor the patient's cardiac rhythm strip, heart rate, pulse, and blood pres-

Drip rates for continuous bretylium infusions

This chart shows you appropriate drip rates, based on the drug concentration and the prescribed infusion rate.

CONCENTRATION	DRIP RATE (MICRODROPS/MIN) TO DELIVER 1 MG/MIN	DRIP RATE (MICRODROPS/MIN) TO DELIVER 2 MG/MIN
500 mg in 500 ml (1 mg/ml)	60	120
1,000 mg in 500 ml (2 mg/ml)	30	60
1,000 mg in 250 ml (4 mg/ml)	15	30

sure. If ordered, use norepinephrine, dopamine, dobutamine, or volume expanders to raise his blood pressure. Closely observe a patient who's susceptible to angina for signs of pain.

After the patient receives the drug, keep him supine until he develops a tolerance to hypotension. This may take several days. Remember that even subtherapeutic doses of bretylium may produce hypotension.

Keep in mind that hemodialysis can remove the drug.

Bretylium doesn't have any known effects on diagnostic tests.

Bumetanide

(Bumex)

This sulfonamide-type loop diuretic reduces the edema associated with congestive heart failure and acute pulmonary edema. Bumetanide is also used as an adjunct to enhance the elimination of toxins or toxic drug levels. The precise mechanism of action isn't known, but the drug appears to inhibit sodium, potassium, and chloride reabsorption, mainly in the ascending limb of the loop of Henle. (See *How bumetanide produces diuresis,* page 23.)

The onset of action occurs within a few minutes. Peak levels are achieved in 5 to 30 minutes, and the duration of action lasts 2 to 3 hours. The drug has an elimination half-life of 60 to 90 minutes.

The distribution of bumetanide isn't fully understood, but the highest concentrations seem to occur in the kidneys, liver, and plasma; the lowest, in the heart, lungs, muscle, and adipose tissue. It probably crosses the placenta. The drug is partially metabolized in the liver into at least five metabolites. About 80% of the drug is excreted in urine unchanged or as metabolites by glomerular filtration and possibly by renal tubular secretion. From 10% to 20% is excreted in feces and bile, almost entirely as metabolites. Whether bumetanide passes into breast milk isn't known. (See *Bumetanide: Indications and dosages,* page 22.)

Contraindications and cautions

Don't give bumetanide to patients hypersensitive to it. The drug is

DOSAGE FINDER

Bumetanide: Indications and dosages

Treatment of edema associated with congestive heart failure and acute pulmonary edema

▶ For adults, give 0.5 to 2 mg I.V. or I.M. or as an I.V. infusion over 30 minutes. If needed, repeat every 2 to 3 hours up to a maximum daily dose of 10 mg.

Adjunctive treatment to enhance drug or toxin elimination

▶ For adults, the dosage varies depending on the desired response. Never exceed 10 mg a day.

also contraindicated for patients with hepatic impairment or severe electrolyte depletion because it increases the risk of dehydration and electrolyte imbalance, possibly leading to hepatic coma and death. The drug is also contraindicated for patients with severe renal impairment because of the risk of toxicity.

Give bumetanide cautiously to patients sensitive to sulfonamides because they may have an increased sensitivity to the drug. Also give bumetanide cautiously to patients at increased risk for hypokalemia and to those with a history of ventricular arrhythmias. The drug can also raise serum uric acid levels in patients with gout or hyperuricemia and may cause excessive diuresis in patients with acute myocardial infarction, leading to shock.

Bumetanide is a pregnancy risk category C drug.

Preparation

Bumetanide comes premixed with a preservative in 2-ml ampules and 2-, 4-, and 10-ml vials that contain 0.25 mg/ml. Protect the drug from light to avoid discoloration.

To dilute the drug further, mix it in a glass or polyvinylchloride container with dextrose 5% in water, 0.9% sodium chloride solution, or lactated Ringer's solution. Use the diluted drug within 24 hours.

When preparing a large dose, use vials instead of glass ampules to avoid the risk of glass particles in the solution. If you must use ampules, add a filter to the I.V. tubing.

Incompatibility

Bumetanide is incompatible with dobutamine.

Administration

- *Direct injection:* Using a 21G or 23G needle, inject the prescribed dose over 1 to 2 minutes.
- *Intermittent infusion:* Administer the diluted drug through an intermittent infusion device, or piggyback it into a running I.V. line of a compatible solution. Infuse the drug at the prescribed rate.
- *I.M. injection:* Inject the ordered dose into any I.M. injection site.

Adverse reactions

- *Life-threatening:* acute fluid depletion, circulatory collapse, ***electrolyte depletion,*** embolism, hypovolemia, vascular thrombosis.
- *Other:* abdominal pain, anorexia, arthritic pain, asterixis, chest pain, confusion, cramps, dehydration, diaphoresis, diarrhea, dizziness, dry mouth, earache, electrocardiogram changes, hearing loss, hyperventilation, hypotension, lethargy, leukopenia, musculoskeletal pain, nausea, paresthesia, pruritus, thirst, thrombocytopenia, urticaria, vomiting, weakness.

Interactions

- *Aminoglycosides and other oto-*

MECHANISM OF ACTION

How bumetanide produces diuresis

Bumetanide acts mainly in the ascending limb of the loop of Henle where it inhibits the transport of sodium (Na^+), potassium (K^+), and chloride (Cl^-) ions into the tubular epithelium.

Normally, the tubular filtrate is dilute in the ascending limb. A cotransporter moves sodium, potassium, and chloride ions out of the tubular filtrate and into the tubular epithelium; water follows the ions. From there, the cotransporter moves the ions first to the intracellular space and then to the peritubular capillaries in the vascular space.

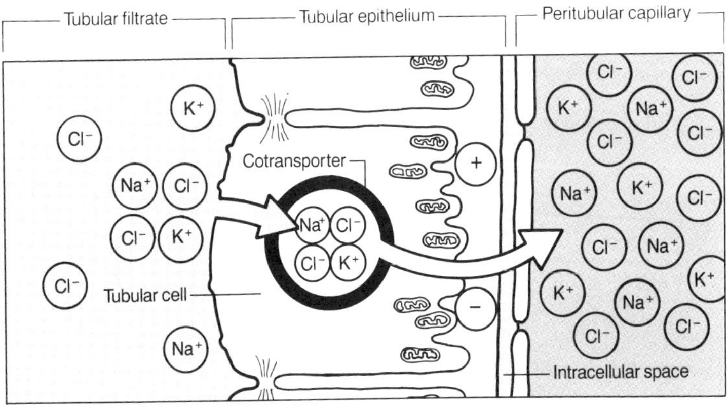

Bumetanide blocks the passage of ions into the tubular epithelium, thereby preventing their reabsorption. This results in a hyperosmolar filtrate. When the filtrate reaches the distal convoluted tubule, less water than usual will be absorbed. Thus, urine output increases.

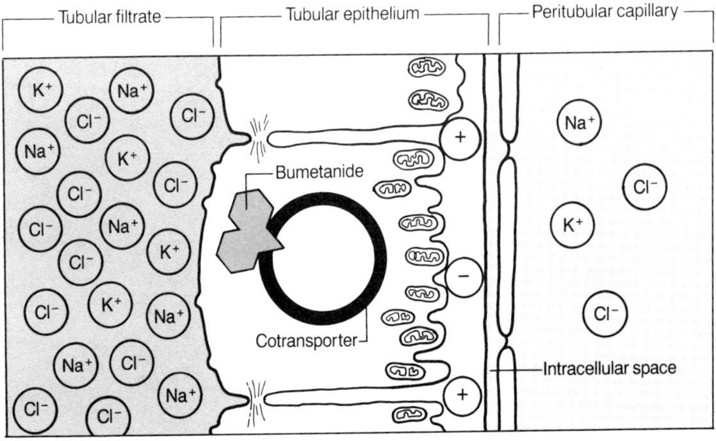

toxic drugs: increased risk of ototoxicity.
- *Amphotericin B:* increased risk of hypokalemia and ototoxicity.
- *Antihistamines, loxapine, phenothiazines, thioxanthines, and trimethobenzamide:* masked signs of ototoxicity.
- *Antihypertensives:* potentiated hypotensive effects.
- *Cardiac glycosides:* hypokalemia and an increased risk of digitalis toxicity.
- *Corticosteroids and corticotropin:* increased risk of hypokalemia.
- *Dopamine:* increased diuresis.
- *Estrogens and sympathomimetics:* reduced antihypertensive effects.
- *Indomethacin and probenecid:* reduced diuresis.
- *Lithium:* toxicity from reduced renal clearance of lithium.
- *Nephrotoxic drugs:* increased risk of nephrotoxicity.
- *Nondepolarizing neuromuscular blocking drugs:* prolonged effects of these drugs.
- *Sodium bicarbonate:* increased risk of hypochloremic alkalosis.

Special considerations

Keep in mind that bumetanide may contain benzyl alcohol. During therapy, monitor the patient's serum electrolyte levels and observe him for signs of hypokalemia—weakness, dizziness, confusion, anorexia, lethargy, vomiting, and cramps. Also monitor his vital signs and cardiac rhythm strip, noting hypotension, tachycardia, and arrhythmias.

An overdose of bumetanide can cause extreme volume depletion, dehydration, and hypotension. To treat these effects quickly, start fluid volume and electrolyte replacement. Continue monitoring the patient's cardiac rhythm strip carefully because electrolyte depletion can trigger life-threatening arrhythmias.

Keep in mind that the drug can cause hypochloremic metabolic alkalemia. It also causes potassium loss, so administer potassium replacements as needed.

The I.V. route allows a rapid onset of action, but the patient should be switched to an oral form of the drug as soon possible.

Bumetanide affects several laboratory tests. It increases blood urea nitrogen levels, as well as serum levels of creatinine, uric acid, alkaline phosphatase, bilirubin, lactate dehydrogenase, aspartate aminotransferase (AST), formerly SGOT, alanine aminotransferase (ALT), formerly SGPT, hematocrit, and hemoglobin. The drug also prolongs prothrombin time and may decrease serum calcium, magnesium, potassium, and sodium levels. Bumetanide may either increase or decrease serum cholesterol levels. What's more, bumetanide may alter white blood cell (WBC) count and WBC differential and increase urine phosphate levels.

Calcium chloride
Calcium gluceptate
Calcium gluconate

(Kalcinate)

The calcium salts—chloride, gluceptate, and gluconate—have several emergency applications. They replace depleted serum calcium in life-threatening hypocalcemia—including hypocalcemic tetany—and hypocalcemia associated with secondary cardiac toxicity. They also strengthen myocardial contractions during a cardiac arrest; for instance, they may be given following defibrillation or when a patient doesn't respond to catecholamine therapy. And these drugs help alleviate central nervous system (CNS) depression in magnesium toxicity. Plus, they help prevent hypocalcemia associated with the rapid transfusion of citrated blood. (See *Calcium: Indications and dosages.*)

Severe calcium deficiency may produce paresthesia, hyperreflexia, tonic-clonic seizures, muscle weakness, cramping, tetany, and skeletal abnormalities, including osteoporosis. But these three calcium salts can provide the calcium necessary to maintain a patient's nervous system integrity, muscular function, and skeletal integrity. (See *Calcium's role in muscle activity,* pages 26 and 27.)

Calcium's onset of action begins immediately after infusion. The duration of action lasts between 30 minutes and 2 hours.

Calcium salts are distributed throughout the extracellular fluid, after which 99% of the calcium is rapidly incorporated into bone. The remaining 1% is divided between intracellular and extracellular fluid, with 45% of serum calcium binding to plasma proteins. Calcium crosses the placenta, reaching even higher levels in fetal blood than in maternal blood.

Calcium isn't metabolized. Unabsorbed calcium is excreted mainly in

DOSAGE FINDER

Calcium: Indications and dosages

Emergency treatment of hypocalcemia

▶ For adults, administer 7 to 14 mEq I.V. Repeat this dose every 1 to 3 days as needed.

▶ For children, administer 1 to 7 mEq I.V. Repeat this dose every 1 to 3 days as needed.

▶ For infants, administer less than 1 mEq I.V. Repeat this dose every 1 to 3 days as needed.

Treatment of hypocalcemic tetany

▶ For adults, administer 4.5 to 16 mEq I.V.

▶ For children, administer 0.5 to 0.7 mEq/kg I.V. three or four times a day or until the tetany is controlled.

▶ For infants, administer 2.4 mEq/kg I.V. daily in divided doses.

Treatment of hypocalcemia associated with secondary cardiac toxicity

▶ For adults, administer 2.25 to 14 mEq I.V. while monitoring the cardiac rhythm strip. Dose may be repeated after 1 to 2 minutes, if necessary.

Treatment of cardiac arrest in advanced cardiac life support

▶ For adults, give an I.V. dose of 2.7 mEq of calcium chloride, 4.5 to 6.3 mEq of calcium gluceptate, or 2.3 to 3.7 mEq of calcium gluconate. Repeat the dose as necessary. Or, the doctor may administer 2.7 to 5.4 mEq of calcium chloride intracardially.

▶ For children, give 0.27 mEq/kg I.V. of calcium chloride. Repeat the dose in 10 minutes if necessary.

Treatment of magnesium toxicity

▶ For adults, give 7 mEq I.V. Base further doses on the patient's response. When I.V. administration isn't possible, give adults 2 to 5 mEq of calcium gluceptate I.M.

Transfusion of citrated blood

▶ For adults, give 1.35 mEq/dl of citrated blood.

▶ For neonates, give 0.45 mEq/dl of citrated blood.

MECHANISM OF ACTION

Calcium's role in muscle activity

If serum calcium levels drop enough to diminish muscle contractility, such drugs as calcium chloride, calcium gluceptate, and calcium gluconate can replenish depleted stores in the sarcoplasmic reticulum located in muscle cells. The reticulum can then release the calcium ions needed to start a muscle contraction. Once released, the calcium ions diffuse to adjacent myofibrils (which are composed of myosin and actin filaments). Here the ions elicit a muscle contraction then they return to the reticulum, allowing the muscle to relax until another release of ions triggers another contraction.

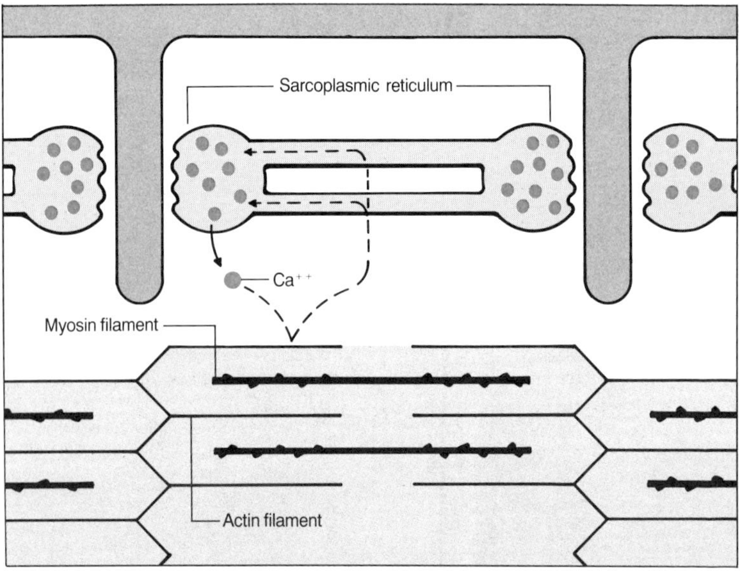

feces or as part of bile and pancreatic juices. The renal glomeruli filter calcium, but the loop of Henle and the convoluted tubules reabsorb it. Small amounts of calcium can pass from the body in urine, breast milk, and sweat.

Contraindications and cautions

Don't give calcium salts to patients with digitalis toxicity or ventricular fibrillation because calcium increases the risk of arrhythmias. Calcium is also contraindicated for patients with hypercalciuria, calcium renal calculi, or hypercalcemia because it can exacerbate these conditions, and for patients with sarcoidosis because it can potentiate hypercalcemia.

Use calcium salts cautiously in patients with renal impairment, dehydration, or electrolyte imbalance because of the increased risk of hypercalcemia and in those with cardiac disease because of the risk of

These two close-up views of a myofibril show muscle relaxation and contraction.

In this illustration, the calcium ion isn't bound to the tropomyosin-troponin complex. Thus, this complex blocks the active binding site, preventing the contractile proteins actin and myosin from interacting. The result: muscle relaxation.

MUSCLE RELAXATION

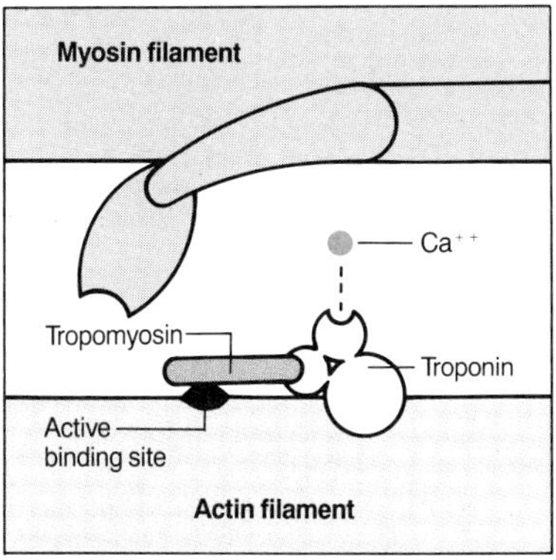

In this illustration, the calcium ion binds with the tropomyosin-troponin complex. This activates the enzyme adenosine triphosphatase (ATPase) – which, along with adenosine triphosphate (ATP), is found in muscle cells. Once activated, ATPase breaks down ATP into adenosine diphosphate (ADP), releasing energy that frees the active binding site. When the site is free, myosin and actin interact. The result: a muscle contraction.

MUSCLE CONTRACTION

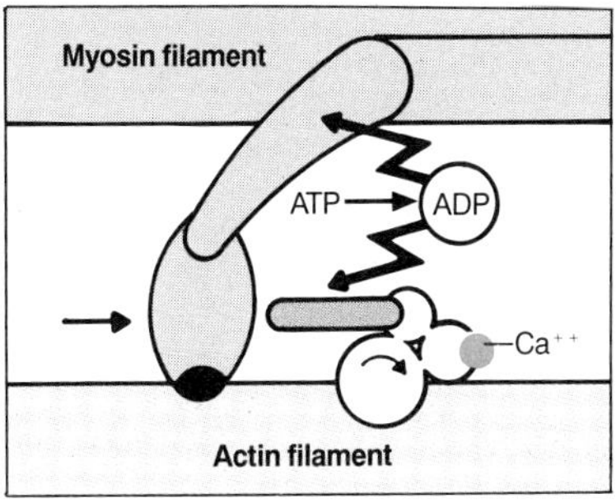

arrhythmias. Use calcium chloride carefully in patients with cor pulmonale, respiratory acidosis, renal disease, or respiratory failure because of its acidifying effects.

Use calcium, a pregnancy risk category C drug, cautiously in pregnant women.

Preparation

Calcium chloride comes in 10-ml ampules, vials, and syringes of a 10% solution containing 1.36 mEq calcium/ml; calcium gluceptate, in 5-ml ampules and 50- and 100-ml bulk containers of a 22% solution containing 0.9 mEq calcium/ml; and calcium gluconate, in 10-ml ampules and vials and 20-ml vials of a 10% solution containing 0.472 mEq calcium/ml.

Before infusion, dilute the calcium salt by mixing it with a compatible solution. You can use most total parenteral nutrition solutions. Use the drug only if it looks clear. If you see crystals in calcium gluceptate, discard it. You can dissolve crystals in calcium gluconate by warming the solution to between 86° and 104° F (30° to 40° C). Store the drug between 59° and 86° F (15° and 30° C), unless otherwise specified by the manufacturer.

Incompatibilities

The three calcium salts form precipitates when mixed with bicarbonates, carbonates, phosphates, sulfates, or tartrates. Chelation occurs when the salts are mixed with tetracyclines. They're also incompatible with cephalothin sodium and magnesium sulfate.

Each salt also has its own incompatibilities. Calcium chloride is incompatible with amphotericin B, chlorpheniramine maleate, and dobutamine; calcium gluceptate, with cefamandole nafate, prednisolone sodium phosphate, and prochlorperazine edisylate; and calcium gluconate, with amphotericin B, cefamandole nafate, dobutamine, methylprednisolone sodium succinate, and prochlorperazine edisylate.

Administration

- *Direct injection:* Slowly inject the drug through a small-gauge needle into either a large vein or an I.V. line of a free-flowing, compatible solution. Don't inject more than 1 ml/minute (1.36 mEq/minute) of calcium chloride, 2 ml/minute (1.8 mEq/minute) of calcium gluceptate, or 5 ml/minute (2.36 mEq/minute) of calcium gluconate. You shouldn't inject the drug into a scalp vein of a child.
- *Intermittent infusion:* Give the diluted solution through an I.V. line of a compatible solution. Don't infuse more than 200 mg/minute of calcium gluceptate or calcium gluconate.
- *Continuous infusion:* Administer the drug in a large volume of fluid. Don't infuse more than 200 mg/minute of calcium gluceptate or calcium gluconate.
- *I.M. injection:* Inject calcium gluceptate into the gluteal region in adults, the lateral thigh in infants, and either area in children. Use this route only if an I.V. route isn't available.
- *Intracardiac injection:* Using an intracardiac needle, the doctor will inject the drug directly into the ventricular cavity, making sure he avoids the cardiac muscle.

Adverse reactions

- *Life-threatening:* arrhythmias, bradycardia, cardiac arrest, hypotension, syncope, vasodilation (all from rapid I.V. injection).
- *Other:* cellulitis, chalky taste, dizziness, drowsiness, hot flashes, irregular heartbeat, nausea, paresthesia, soft tissue calcification, sweating, ***venous irritation,*** vomiting.

Interactions

- *Cardiac glycosides:* arrhythmias from potentiated inotropic and toxic glycoside effects.
- *Nondepolarizing neuromuscular blocking drugs:* reversed effects of these drugs.
- *Parenteral magnesium sulfate:* neutralized effects of magnesium.
- *Potassium supplements:* arrhythmias.
- *Thiazide diuretics:* reduced calcium excretion, possibly resulting in hypercalcemia.

Special considerations

If you have time before administering calcium, review the results of any renal function tests that the patient has undergone. If he has impaired renal function, you should expect to administer a lower dose.

Make sure you have the right form of the drug. If the order calls for an I.M injection, for instance, you must use calcium gluceptate—the only form of calcium that can be given I.M. And you'll rarely see calcium chloride ordered for a child because it causes more tissue irritation than the other forms. Make sure you get the ordered form of the drug when you take a calcium salt from a crash cart because the cart usually contains both calcium chloride and calcium gluconate.

During therapy, monitor the patient for a moderate drop in blood pressure. You may see a hypertensive or elderly patient's blood pressure rise briefly. Also monitor the patient's serum calcium levels and his cardiac rhythm strip. Check his urine calcium levels to detect hypercalciuria.

Assess the I.V. site for burning, sloughing, or tissue necrosis—signs of infiltration into intramuscular or subcutaneous tissue—particularly when giving calcium chloride. If you see such signs, stop the infusion, infiltrate the area with 1% procaine and hyaluronidase to reduce vasospasm and dilute the calcium, and apply local heat.

After an I.V. injection, keep the patient supine for a short time in case of postural hypotension.

Calcium salts affect several laboratory tests. A plasma 11-hydroxycorticosteroid test using the Glenn-Nelson technique within 1 hour of calcium chloride administration will show increased levels. Serum amylase levels will rise with calcium chloride. Serum phosphate levels will decrease with large doses and prolonged use of calcium, and serum and urine magnesium tests may produce false-negative results when the Titan yellow method is used.

Chlorpheniramine maleate

(Chlor-Pro, Chlor-Trimeton, Phenetron)

Chlorpheniramine maleate treats allergic transfusion reactions and serves as an adjunct in the treatment of anaphylaxis. The drug works by competing with the H_1-receptors on effector cells to prevent—but not reverse—the histamine-mediated response. (See *How chlorpheniramine stops an allergic response*, page 31.)

When the drug is given I.V., peak levels are achieved at the end of the infusion. The duration of action lasts for 4 to 25 hours. The I.V. form has a serum half-life of 12 to 15 hours in adults and 10 to 13 hours in children. In patients with chronic renal failure, the half-life may increase to 330 hours. With oral administration, peak action occurs in 6 hours. The oral form has a half-life of 21 to 27 hours.

Chlorpheniramine is distributed rapidly and extensively throughout the body and central nervous system (CNS), with 69% to 72% of the drug binding to plasma proteins. The highest concentrations occur in the lungs, heart, kidneys, brain, spleen, and small intestine. The drug probably crosses the placenta. Metabolized in the liver, chlorpheniramine is almost completely excreted in urine, with 35% excreted within 48 hours, primarily as metabolites. The excretion rate falls as urine pH rises. Less than 1% of chlorpheniramine appears in feces or breast milk. (See *Chlorpheniramine: Indications and dosages*, page 30.)

DOSAGE FINDER

Chlorpheniramine: Indications and dosages

Treatment of allergic transfusion reactions

▶ For adults and children over age 12, give a single dose of 10 to 20 mg I.V., I.M., or S.C. Don't exceed 40 mg per day.

Adjunctive treatment of anaphylaxis

▶ For adults and children over age 12, wait until epinephrine and other measures have controlled acute symptoms. Then give a single dose of 10 to 20 mg I.V., I.M., or S.C. Or give 8 to 12 mg P.O. Don't exceed 24 mg per day.

▶ For children ages 6 to 12, give 2 mg I.V., I.M., or S.C. every 4 to 6 hours up to 12 mg per day.

Contraindications and cautions

Don't give chlorpheniramine to neonates, premature infants, or patients who have a hypersensitivity to chlorpheniramine or other antihistamines.

Give the drug cautiously to patients with narrow-angle glaucoma, stenotic peptic ulcer, pyloroduodenal obstruction, symptomatic prostatic hyperplasia, or bladder neck obstruction because chlorpheniramine may increase the severity of the symptoms. Also use it cautiously in patients with increased intraocular pressure, hyperthyroidism, cardiovascular disease, and bronchial asthma because the drug can produce an atropine-like effect. Because of the risk of increased toxicity, you should administer chlorpheniramine cautiously to patients with renal dysfunction. (See *Managing a chlorpheniramine overdose,* page 32.)

The risk of using chlorpheniramine during pregnancy hasn't been ruled out, so it's classified as a pregnancy risk category C drug.

Preparation

Chlorpheniramine comes in 1-ml ampules of either 10 mg/ml or 100 mg/ml. To prepare the drug for intermittent infusion, dilute the 10 mg/ml concentration in 50 to 100 ml of a compatible solution (most solutions are compatible). Use either concentration for I.M. or S.C. injection.

Oral chlorpheniramine comes in three forms—a liquid that contains 2 mg/ml, a 4-mg tablet, and a 2-mg chewable tablet.

You can refrigerate chlorpheniramine or store it at room temperature. Store oral forms of the drug in tight, light-resistant containers to prevent discoloration. Dispose of any drug that becomes discolored.

Incompatibilities

Chlorpheniramine is incompatible with calcium chloride, iodipamide meglumine, kanamycin sulfate, norepinephrine bitartrate, and phenobarbital sodium.

Administration

- *Direct injection:* Slowly inject the diluted drug into an I.V. line of a free-flowing, compatible solution.
- *Intermittent infusion:* Infuse the diluted drug slowly through an established I.V. line.
- *I.M. injection:* Inject the ordered dose deep into the muscle at any I.M. injection site.
- *S.C. injection:* Administer the ordered dose into any S.C. injection site.
- *Oral:* Give the drug with food, milk, or water to decrease stomach irritation.

Adverse reactions

- *Life-threatening:* anaphylaxis.

MECHANISM OF ACTION

How chlorpheniramine stops an allergic response

Although chlorpheniramine can't reverse symptoms of an allergic response, it can stop the progression of the response. Here's what happens.

Once sensitized to an antigen, a mast cell reacts to repeated antigen exposure by releasing chemical mediators. One of these mediators, histamine, binds to histamine-1 (H_1) receptors found on effector cells (the cells responsible for allergic symptoms). This initiates the allergic response that affects the respiratory, cardiovascular, GI, endocrine, and integumentary systems.

Chlorpheniramine competes with histamine for H_1 receptor sites on the effector cells. By attaching to these sites first, the drug prevents more histamine from binding to the effector cells.

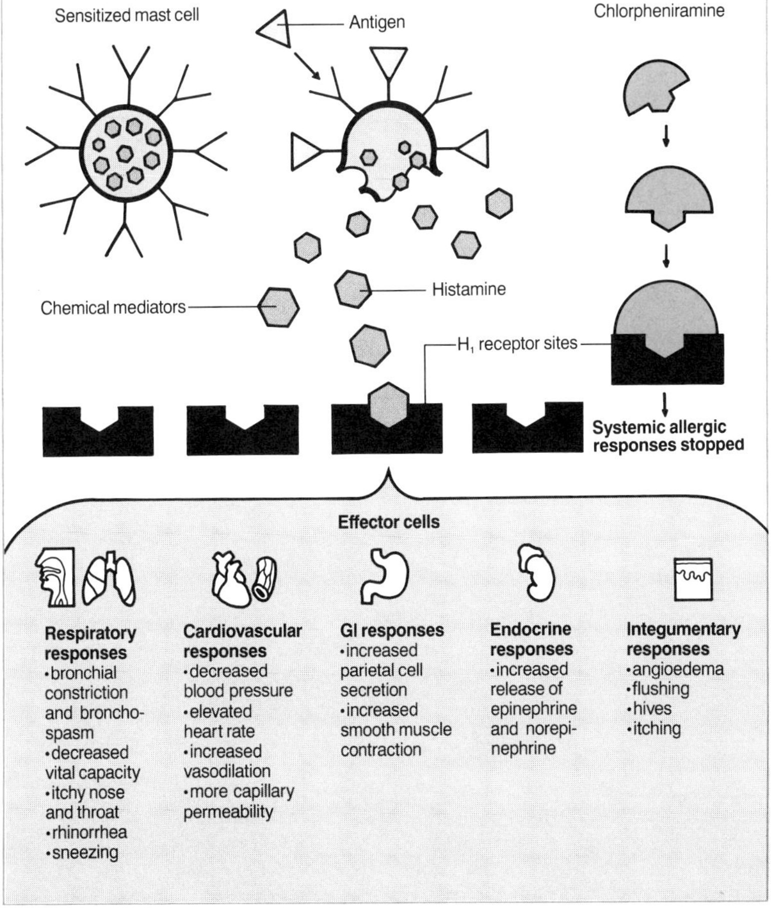

EMERGENCY INTERVENTION

Managing a chlorpheniramine overdose

An overdose of chlorpheniramine can cause a life-threatening reaction. Look for such signs and symptoms as ataxia, athetosis, dry mouth, excitation, fever, fixed and dilated pupils, a flushed face, hallucinations, incoordination, and tonic-clonic seizures. If the patient experiences such seizures, postictal depression can lead to coma, cardiorespiratory collapse, and death. A toxic reaction is most likely in young children and elderly patients.

If you note signs of chlorpheniramine toxicity, provide the following treatment as ordered:

- If the patient needs a vasopressor, use norepinephrine or phenylephrine—not epinephrine.
- Give physostigmine to help counteract central nervous system anticholinergic effects.
- If the seizures continue, treat them with I.V. diazepam.
- Bring down the fever with cold packs or sponges soaked in tepid water. Don't use alcohol sponges.

- *Other:* acute labyrinthitis; blurred vision; ***burning and stinging at injection site;*** chest tightness; chills; confusion; constipation; diaphoresis; diarrhea; diplopia; disturbed coordination; dizziness; ***drowsiness; dry mouth, nose, and throat;*** epigastric distress; euphoria; ***excitation;*** extrasystole; fatigue; headache; hypotension; hysteria; insomnia; irritability; nasal congestion; nausea; nervousness; neuritis; palpitations; paresthesia; photosensitivity; rash; restlessness; sedation; seizures; tachycardia; thickened bronchial secretions; tinnitus; tremor; urinary frequency and difficulty; urticaria; vertigo; vomiting; ***weak pulse after parenteral administration,*** wheezing.

Interactions

- *Alcohol and other CNS depressants:* deepened CNS depression.
- *Antimuscarinics:* potentiated effects.
- *Monoamine oxidase inhibitors:* prolonged and intensified anticholinergic effects.
- *Ototoxic drugs:* masked signs of ototoxicity.
- *Phenytoin:* increased phenytoin effects.

Special considerations

Keep in mind that Chlor-Pro contains benzyl alcohol.

During therapy, monitor the patient for hypotension and tachycardia.

Chlorpheniramine will alter the results of allergy skin tests so the patient should stop taking the drug 4 days before such a test.

Chlorpromazine hydrochloride

(Thorazine)

Chlorpromazine hydrochloride quiets severe hyperactive or excited states in psychotic patients by blocking postsynaptic dopaminergic receptors in the brain. It also controls vomiting—especially useful during surgery—primarily by inhibiting or blocking the dopamine receptors in the medullary chemoreceptor trigger zone and secondarily by blocking the vagus nerve in the GI tract. Chlorpromazine can also be used to control intractable hiccups and along with barbiturates to treat tetanus.

Chlorpromazine's onset and duration of action aren't known. The drug is widely distributed throughout most body fluids, concentrating in the brain, lungs, liver, kidneys, and spleen. Most of the drug—92% to 97%—binds to plasma proteins, and it readily crosses the placenta and the blood-brain barrier. In the liver, the drug undergoes hydroxylation, oxidation, demethylation, sulfoxide formation, and conjugation with gluconic acid—finally emerging primarily as inactive metabolites. Although excreted mainly in the urine, these metabolites and any unchanged chlorpromazine can also appear in feces and breast milk. (See *Chlorpromazine: Indications and dosages.*)

DOSAGE FINDER

Chlorpromazine: Indications and dosages

Treatment of severe psychosis

- For adults, give an I.M. injection of 25 mg. If necessary, give another 25- to 50-mg dose an hour later.
- For children between ages 5 and 12, give an I.M. injection of 0.55 mg/kg every 6 to 8 hours as needed, up to 75 mg a day. Increase the dosage in unmanageable cases.
- For children ages 6 months to 5 years, give an I.M injection of 0.55 mg/kg every 6 to 8 hours as needed. Don't exceed 40 mg a day.

Prevention of vomiting during surgery

- For adults, give an I.M. injection of 12.5 mg. If necessary, repeat the injection in 30 minutes. Or administer an I.V. infusion at a rate of 1 mg/minute up to a total dose of 25 mg.
- For children, administer 0.25 mg/kg I.M. If hypotension doesn't occur, repeat the dose in 30 minutes, as necessary. Or administer an I.V. infusion at a rate of 1 mg/2 minutes up to a total dose of 0.275 mg/kg.

Treatment of severe hiccups

- For adults, give an I.M. injection of 25 to 50 mg four times a day. If hiccups continue, start an I.V. infusion of 25 to 50 mg at 1 mg/minute.

Adjunctive treatment for tetanus

- For adults, administer an I.M. or I.V. injection of 25 to 50 mg.
- For children over age 6 months, administer 0.55 mg/kg I.M. or I.V. every 6 to 8 hours. Don't exceed 40 mg for children weighing less than 50 pounds (23 kg) or 75 mg for children between 50 pounds and 100 pounds (45 kg).

Contraindications and cautions

Don't give this drug to patients with a hypersensitivity to chlorpromazine or other phenothiazines, or to sulfites. Chlorpromazine is also contraindicated for patients with severe toxic central nervous system (CNS) depression, subcortical brain damage, bone marrow depression, or severe cardiovascular disorders because it can worsen these conditions. Avoid giving the drug to patients with such neurologic disorders as Reye's syndrome, meningitis, and encephalopathy because it can mask their symptoms.

Use the drug cautiously in patients with hypocalcemia to avoid dystonic reactions and in alcoholics and patients with respiratory disease because it can deepen CNS depression. Chlorpromazine also suppresses the cough reflex in respiratory patients. And because the drug can precipitate glaucoma, you should give it cautiously to patients who have or are susceptible to this condition.

Give chlorpromazine cautiously to patients with hepatic or renal disease because they metabolize and excrete the drug more slowly, increasing their risk of toxicity. (See *Managing a chlorpromazine overdose,* page 34.) Use the drug carefully in patients who've had a

EMERGENCY INTERVENTION

Managing a chlorpromazine overdose

An overdose of chlorpromazine can cause extrapyramidal reactions and hypotension. If you detect an overdose, give the patient an anticholinergic drug to control the extrapyramidal reactions and a vasopressor such as norepinephrine or phenylephrine to treat severe hypotension, as ordered. Don't give him epinephrine because it may lower his blood pressure.

severe reaction to insulin or electroconvulsive therapy.

The drug can also potentiate extrapyramidal effects in Parkinson's disease; aggravate peptic ulcer disease; exacerbate urine retention in some urinary disorders, including symptomatic prostatic hyperplasia; and lower the seizure threshold in seizure disorders. So you should give chlorpromazine carefully to a patient who has any of these conditions.

Because its safety during pregnancy hasn't been established, chlorpromazine is classified as a pregnancy risk category C drug. Give it carefully.

Preparation

Chlorpromazine is available in 1- and 2-ml ampules and 10-ml, multiple-dose vials containing 25 mg/ml. Store the drug below 104° F (40° C), preferably between 59° and 86° F (15° and 30° C). Protect it from light and freezing, and discard any solution that looks darker than light amber or has formed a precipitate.

To prepare the drug for direct injection, dilute it with 0.9% sodium chloride solution to a concentration of 1 mg/ml. To prepare it for infusion, dilute the ordered dose in 500 to 1,000 ml of 0.9% sodium chloride solution. To prepare the drug for an I.M. injection, dilute it with 0.9% sodium chloride solution or 2% procaine or both.

Incompatibilities

Chlorpromazine is incompatible with aminophylline, amphotericin B, ampicillin, atropine, chloramphenicol sodium succinate, chlorothiazide, cimetidine, dimenhydrinate, heparin, methicillin, methohexital, penicillin, pentobarbital, phenobarbital, thiopental, and solutions that have a pH between 4.0 and 5.0.

Administration

- *Direct injection:* Slowly inject the diluted drug into a patent I.V. line.
- *Continuous infusion:* Slowly infuse the ordered dose at the prescribed rate.
- *I.M. injection:* Slowly inject the ordered dose deep into the upper, outer quadrant of the buttock. Massage the site slowly after injection to prevent sterile abscess, and keep the patient supine for 30 minutes to prevent postural hypotension.

Adverse reactions

- *Life-threatening:* anaphylaxis, angioedema, bronchospasm, cardiac arrest, laryngeal edema, laryngospasm, neuroleptic malignant syndrome (altered blood pressure, altered mental status, hyperthermia, and tachycardia), severe hypotension.
- *Other:* anorexia, anxiety, ***blurred vision,*** cerebral edema, ***constipation,*** contact dermatitis, dizziness, drowsiness, ***dry mouth,*** dyspepsia, dystonia, electrocardiogram (ECG) changes, erythema, ***extrapyramidal effects,*** headache, hypotension, increased appetite, ***pain at I.M. injection site,*** paralytic ileus, ***photosensi-***

tivity, restlessness, ***sedation,*** seizures, sterile abscess at I.M. injection site, syncope, tachycardia, ***urine retention,*** urticaria.

Interactions

- *Alcohol, CNS depressants, and parenteral magnesium sulfate:* deepened CNS and respiratory depression.
- *Amantadine, antidyskinetics, antihistamines, and antimuscarinics (especially atropine and related compounds):* intensified antimuscarinic effects.
- *Amphetamines:* reduced stimulant effects.
- *Anticonvulsants, including barbiturates:* lowered seizure threshold requiring an anticonvulsant dosage adjustment.
- *Apomorphine:* deepened CNS depression and decreased emetic response to apomorphine.
- *Appetite suppressants:* antagonized anorectic effects.
- *Beta-adrenergic blockers:* elevated serum levels of both drugs.
- *Bone marrow depressants:* increased leukopenia or thrombocytopenia.
- *Bromocriptine:* inhibited effects because of increased serum prolactin levels.
- *Dopamine:* antagonized peripheral vasoconstriction with high dopamine doses.
- *Ephedrine and metaraminol:* reduced pressor response.
- *Epinephrine:* severe hypotension and tachycardia resulting from blocked alpha-adrenergic effects.
- *Guanadrel and guanethidine:* diminished hypotensive effects of these drugs.
- *Hypotension-producing drugs:* increased risk of severe hypotension.
- *Levodopa:* inhibited antiparkinson effects.
- *Lithium:* extrapyramidal symptoms and accelerated excretion of lithium.
- *Methoxamine and phenylephrine:* decreased pressor effects and reduced duration of action of these drugs.
- *Metrizamide:* lowered seizure threshold.
- *Monamine oxidase inhibitors and tricyclic antidepressants:* intensified sedative and antimuscarinic effects of chlorpromazine or of these drugs, and increased risk of neuroleptic malignant syndrome.
- *Other photosensitizing drugs:* additive photosensitivity.
- *Ototoxic drugs, especially antibiotics:* masked signs of ototoxicity.
- *Phenytoin:* increased risk of phenytoin toxicity.
- *Quinidine:* additive cardiac effects.
- *Riboflavin:* increased riboflavin requirements.
- *Systemic methoxsalen, trioxsalen, and tetracyclines:* potentiated intraocular photochemical damage.

Special considerations

To avoid dermatitis, make sure you don't touch the drug either during preparation or administration. Before administering the chlorpromazine, determine the patient's baseline blood pressure and heart rate.

Monitor the patient for tachycardia and hypotension during administration. Make sure he lies supine for 30 minutes after the injection, and tell him to change positions slowly. Monitor an elderly patient carefully because age increases a patient's vulnerability to hypotension and extrapyramidal symptoms. Typically, an elderly, debilitated, or emaciated patient will receive a lower dose of the drug.

Observe the patient for signs of acute dystonic reactions. Report such signs to the doctor, who may order I.V. diphenhydramine. Also monitor the patient for indications of neuroleptic malignant syndrome—a rare but frequently fatal reaction. Signs include elevated temperature, muscle rigidity, altered mental status, tachycardia, and arrhythmias. Over 60% of the patients who develop this syndrome are men.

Throughout chlorpromazine therapy, keep track of the patient's fluid intake and output to detect urine retention. Also monitor his ECG, which may show changes in the Q and T waves. And keep in mind that, because the drug suppresses vomiting, you may have difficulty recognizing conditions characterized by this sign.

After therapy, tell the patient to let you know if he experiences dizziness, nausea and vomiting, GI upset, pain, trembling in his hands and fingers, or controlled, repetitive movements of his mouth, tongue, or jaw. If he reports any of these signs or symptoms to you, notify the doctor.

If the patient received chlorpromazine during surgery, remember that he'll sleep longer postoperatively.

If the patient received the drug for severe psychosis, he should be switched to an oral form of the drug 24 to 48 hours after receiving an I.M. dose.

Chlorpromazine can alter the results of several laboratory tests. By increasing serum prolactin levels, it can blunt the response in the gonadorelin test. The metyrapone test may show a decreased secretion of corticotropin. Serum phenylalanine screening may show a false-positive result; urine pregnancy tests, a false-positive or false-negative result. Also, the white blood cell (WBC) count and WBC differential may decrease.

Cimetidine hydrochloride

(Tagamet)

A histamine-2 (H_2) receptor antagonist, cimetidine hydrochloride is used to treat active gastric and duodenal ulcers, stress ulcers, peptic esophagitis, and upper GI bleeding not caused by major vessel erosion. By competitively inhibiting histamine's action on the H_2 receptors of gastric parietal cells, the drug reduces gastric acid output and concentration. The result: Gastric pH rises to 5.0 or more. (See *How cimetidine reduces gastric acid,* page 38.)

After parenteral injection of cimetidine, the onset of action is immediate. Its duration of action lasts 4 to 5 hours, and the serum half-life is 2 to 3 hours.

Cimetidine is distributed throughout body tissues and across the placenta. About 15% to 20% binds to plasma proteins. The drug is metabolized in the liver to form sulfoxide and 5-hydroxymethyl derivatives. In 24 hours, between 80% and 90% of the drug is excreted in urine, primarily unchanged, with the remainder excreted in feces as two metabolites. It also appears in breast milk. (See *Cimetidine: Indications and dosages.*)

Contraindications and cautions

Don't give cimetidine to patients with a known hypersensitivity to the drug.

Give the drug cautiously to elderly patients and patients with renal or hepatic insufficiency because of an increased risk of toxicity. Also use the drug cautiously in patients under age 16; information on pediatric dosages is limited.

No evidence exists showing that cimetidine poses a risk to the fetus. Thus, it's classified as a pregnancy risk category B drug.

Preparation

Cimetidine is available in 2-ml, single-dose vials and disposable syringes containing 300 mg of the drug; in 8-ml, multidose vials containing 300 mg/2 ml; and in premixed polyvinylchloride (PVC) bags containing 300 mg/50 ml. Protect the drug from light.

For a direct injection, dilute the dose (including the single-dose form) with 20 ml of 0.9% sodium chloride solution. For an infusion, use the premixed PVC bags or dilute cimetidine with 50 to 100 ml of a compatible solution, such as amino acid solution, dextrose 5% in water, Ringer's injection, lactated Ringer's solution, invert sugar 5% in water, 0.9% sodium chloride solution, or dextrose 5% in 0.2%, 0.45%, or 0.9% sodium chloride solution.

Use a diluted solution within 48 hours. Check the expiration date on a commercially prepared solution. Store the solution at room temperature. Solutions may become cloudy if they're refrigerated.

Incompatibilities

Cimetidine is incompatible with aminophylline, amphotericin B, barbiturates, cefamandole nafate, cefazolin sodium, cephalothin sodium, chlorpromazine hydrochloride, pentobarbital sodium, and secobarbital sodium.

Administration

- *Direct injection:* Give the diluted drug over at least 2 minutes directly into a vein or through an I.V. line containing a free-flowing, compatible solution. Rapid injections may increase the risk of arrhythmias and hypotension.
- *Intermittent infusion:* Infuse 50 to 100 ml of diluted drug over 15 to 20 minutes, using an intermittent infusion device or an I.V. line containing a free-flowing, compatible solution.
- *I.M. injection:* Inject the ordered dose into any I.M. injection site. Keep in mind that an I.M. injection may be painful.

DOSAGE FINDER

Cimetidine: Indications and dosages

Treatment of active gastric and duodenal ulcers

▶ For adults, administer 300 mg I.M. or I.V. every 6 to 8 hours (every 12 hours if creatinine clearance is under 30 ml/minute). Don't exceed 2,400 mg daily. Adjust the dosage to maintain a gastric pH above 5.0.

▶ For children, give 5 to 10 mg/kg I.M. or I.V. every 6 to 8 hours.

Treatment of stress ulcers, peptic esophagitis, and upper GI bleeding not caused by major vessel erosion

▶ For adults, give 300 to 400 mg I.M. or I.V. four times daily.

Adverse reactions

- *Life-threatening:* arrhythmias, including sinus bradycardia, uniform and multiform premature ventricular contractions, ventricular fibrillation, and ventricular tachycardia; cardiac arrest; hypotension.
- *Other:* agitation, agranulocytosis, anxiety, aplastic anemia, arthralgias, atrial fibrillation, bradycardia, confusion, ***diarrhea,*** disorientation, dizziness, fever, hallucinations, headache, hepatotoxicity, maculopapular or acnelike rash, myalgias, nephrotoxicity, neutropenia, palpitations, premature atrial contractions, psychosis, somnolence, urticaria.

MECHANISM OF ACTION

How cimetidine reduces gastric acid

To stimulate gastric acid secretion, certain endogenous agents—primarily histamine, but also acetylcholine and gastrin—attach to receptors on the parietal cell surface. These agents activate the enzyme adenyl cyclase, which converts adenosine triphosphate (ATP) to the intracellular catalyst cyclic adenosine monophosphate (cAMP). This ultimately stimulates proton pump (H^+/K^+ ATPase) activity. Basically, the pump catalyzes the exchange of extracellular potassium (K^+) ions for intracellular hydrogen (H^+) ions. When the H^+ ions combine with extracellular chloride (Cl^-) ions, the result is HCl, or gastric acid.

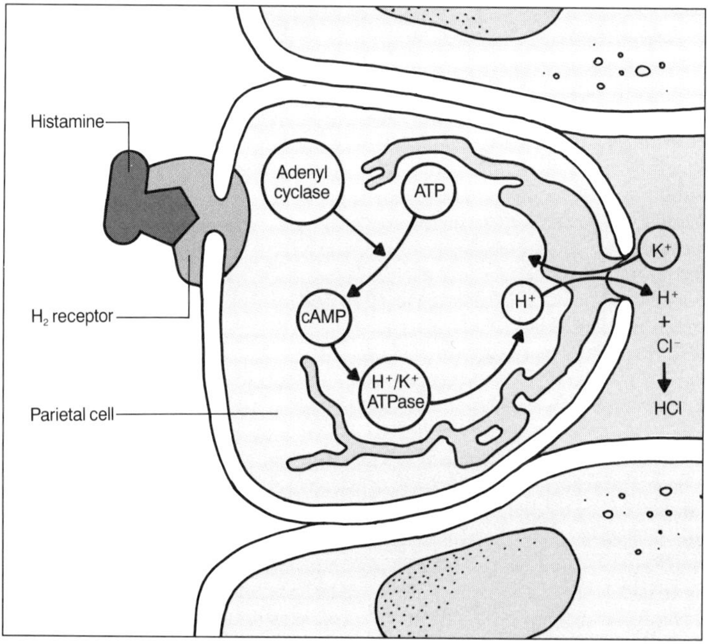

Cimetidine competitively binds to the H_2 receptor sites on the parietal cell surface, inhibiting the common pathway that histamine and the other agents must travel to stimulate proton pump activity and promote gastric acid secretion.

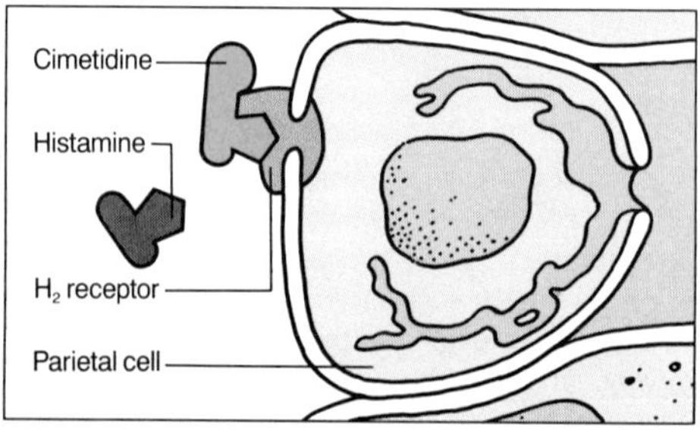

Interactions

- *Alprazolam, chlordiazepoxide, diazepam, flurazepam, triazolam, tricyclic antidepressants:* impaired metabolism.
- *Aminophylline, theophylline:* increased serum levels of these drugs.
- *Caffeine, ethanol:* increased central nervous system effects.
- *Calcium channel blockers, labetalol, lidocaine, metoprolol, propranolol, quinidine:* decreased metabolism.
- *Disulfiram, estrogen-containing oral contraceptives, isoniazid:* altered metabolism resulting from inhibition of hepatic microsomal enzymes.
- *Metronidazole, phenytoin, sulfonylureas, theophylline:* impaired metabolism.
- *Myelosuppressive drugs (alkylating agents, antimetabolites):* potentiated toxicity.
- *Procainamide:* reduced excretion.
- *Triamterene:* decreased metabolism and excretion.
- *Warfarin and similar anticoagulants:* elevated serum levels.

Special considerations

If a patient is receiving hemodialysis, administer the drug after a dialysis session and every 12 hours during the interdialysis period. A patient with renal or hepatic failure will require a dosage adjustment.

During therapy, watch the cardiac rhythm strip for arrhythmias. If administering cimetidine and coumarin together, closely monitor prothrombin time and adjust the coumarin dosage as necessary. Because cimetidine can cause transient healing of malignant gastric ulcers, closely monitor a patient with such ulcers. Remember that elderly patients may be more susceptible to cimetidine-induced confusion.

Cimetidine-induced, elevated gastric pH may permit candidal overgrowth in the stomach. The drug also may affect the bioavailability of many oral drugs.

Cimetidine affects several diagnostic tests. A patient receiving the drug may exhibit elevated serum alkaline phosphatase, creatinine, or prolactin levels, as well as elevated levels of alanine aminotransferase (ALT), formerly SGOT, or aspartate aminotransferase (AST), formerly SGPT. Parathyroid hormone concentrations may be depressed. The gastric acid stimulation test (using pentagastrin) may show depressed gastric acid levels. And a skin test for allergies may show false-negative results because of an inhibited cutaneous histamine response.

Dantrolene sodium

(Dantrium, Dantrium I.V.)

A hydantoin derivative, dantrolene sodium is given as an adjunct to treat malignant hyperthermia crisis and to relieve symptoms of neuroleptic malignant syndrome that are similar to those of malignant hyperthermia. Dantrolene works by interfering with calcium ion release from the sarcoplasmic reticulum. This reduces the myoplasmic concentration of calcium ions, thus helping to inactivate the catabolic processes associated with malignant hyperthermia crisis (see *How dantrolene reduces muscle rigidity*, page 41).

Peak plasma levels of dantrolene are reached almost immediately after administration. The drug's half-life is about 5 hours.

Dantrolene is distributed throughout the tissues, with substantial amounts reversibly bound to plasma proteins, especially albumin. The

DOSAGE FINDER

Dantrolene: Indications and dosage

Adjunctive treatment of malignant hyperthermia crisis or symptoms of neuroleptic malignant syndrome

▶ For adults and children, give 1 mg/kg I.V. initially. Repeat if needed up to a total dose of 10 mg/kg.

drug is metabolized in the liver to form 5-hydroxy derivatives and is excreted in the urine, mainly as metabolites. Dantrolene probably appears in breast milk. (See *Dantrolene: Indications and dosage*.)

Contraindications and cautions

Use dantrolene cautiously in patients with cardiac impairment because of the increased risk of pleural effusion or pericarditis.

A pregnancy risk category C drug, dantrolene should be used cautiously during pregnancy.

Preparation

Dantrolene is supplied in 20-mg vials. Reconstitute it with 60 ml of sterile water (without a bacteriostatic agent) to achieve a concentration of 0.333 mg/ml. The solution remains stable for 6 hours when stored between 59° and 86° F (15° to 30° C). Protect it from light.

Incompatibilities

Dantrolene is incompatible with dextrose 5% in water and 0.9% sodium chloride solution. Don't mix it and other drugs in a syringe.

Administration

- *Direct injection:* Rapidly inject the drug directly into a vein or through an I.V. line containing a free-flowing, compatible solution.

Adverse reactions

- *Life-threatening:* none reported.
- *Other:* chills, confusion, constipation, depression, ***diarrhea,*** dizziness, ***drowsiness,*** fatigue, fever, hallucinations, headache, light-headedness, ***muscle weakness,*** myalgia, nausea, nervousness, phlebitis, pleural effusion with pericarditis, pruritus, rash, seizures, sweating, tachycardia, thrombophlebitis, urinary difficulty (frequency, incontinence, or retention), visual disturbances.

Interactions

- *Calcium channel blockers:* ventricular fibrillation and cardiovascular collapse associated with severe hypokalemia.
- *Central nervous system (CNS) depressants:* excessive CNS depression.

Special considerations

When giving dantrolene, perform other interventions, as ordered. For instance, administer oxygen, treat metabolic acidosis, and use cooling measures. Give fluids to help maintain adequate urine output, and monitor serum electrolyte levels. Because of the solution's high pH, be sure to prevent extravasation.

A dantrolene overdose may cause respiratory depression, decreased level of consciousness, seizures, and cardiac arrhythmias. Keep a crash cart nearby for supportive treatment. Administer large amounts of fluids to prevent crystalluria.

After the initial therapy, the doctor may switch the patient to oral dantrolene to prevent the return of malignant hyperthermia crisis.

Dantrolene affects the results of certain tests. It elevates levels of blood urea nitrogen; serum alkaline phosphatase; lactate dehydrogenase; total bilirubin; aspartate aminotransferase (AST), formerly SGOT;

MECHANISM OF ACTION

How dantrolene reduces muscle rigidity

Dantrolene appears to decrease the number of calcium ions released from the sarcoplasmic reticulum. The lower the myoplasmic calcium level, the less energy produced when calcium prompts the muscle's actin and myosin filaments to interact. Less energy means a weaker muscle contraction.

By promoting muscle relaxation, dantrolene prevents or reduces the rigidity that contributes to the life-threatening body temperatures of malignant hyperthermia crisis and to similar symptoms of neuroleptic malignant syndrome.

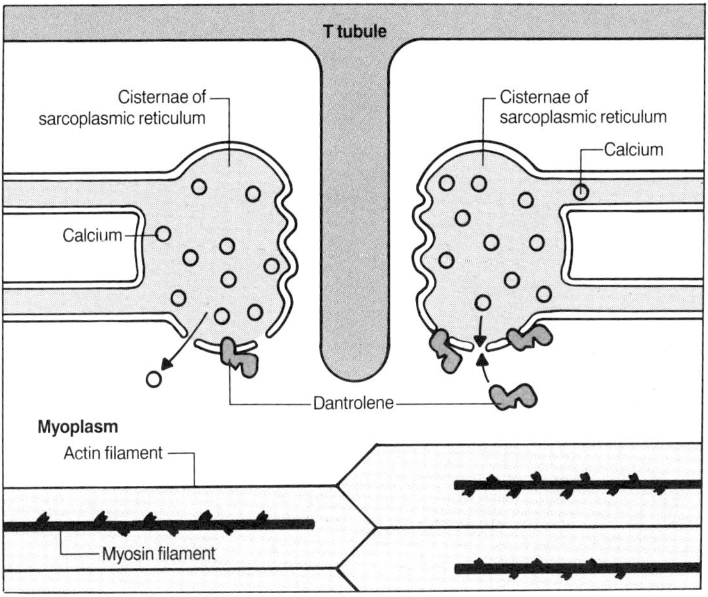

and alanine aminotransferase (ALT), formerly SGPT.

Dexamethasone sodium phosphate

(Decadron Phosphate)

A synthetic glucocorticoid, dexamethasone sodium phosphate is indicated as an adjunct in the treatment of shock and cerebral edema as well as for the treatment of inflammatory conditions and allergic reactions. The drug decreases inflammation by stabilizing leukocyte lysosomal membranes. It also suppresses the pituitary release of corticotropin, thus halting adrenocortical secretion of corticosteroids and stifling the immune response. The drug influences protein, fat, and carbohydrate metabolism.

DOSAGE FINDER

Dexamethasone: Indications and dosages

Adjunctive treatment of shock

▶ For adults, administer 1 to 6 mg/kg I.V. in a single dose, 40 mg I.V. every 2 to 6 hours, or 20 mg I.V. in a single dose followed by 3 mg/kg over 24 hours in a continuous infusion. The total daily dose shouldn't exceed 80 mg.

Adjunctive treatment of cerebral edema

▶ For adults, administer 10 mg I.V. or I.M. initially, with successive doses given I.M. Don't exceed 80 mg/day.

Treatment of inflammatory conditions or allergic reactions

▶ For adults, you'll usually give 0.5 to 9 mg I.V. or I.M. daily.

▶ For children, give 6 to 40 mcg/kg I.M. once or twice daily.

The onset of action is rapid, and the duration varies, depending on the dose, frequency of administration, and length of therapy. The half-life of the drug averages about 4 hours.

Dexamethasone is distributed throughout the muscles, liver, skin, intestines, and kidneys. It crosses the placenta and the blood-brain barrier. Metabolism occurs primarily in the liver and, to a lesser degree, in the kidneys and other tissues. The drug is then excreted in the urine as inactive metabolites, primarily glucuronides and sulfates, and as unconjugated products. Small amounts of unchanged drug are excreted in urine, and negligible amounts in bile. The drug also appears in breast milk. (See *Dexamethasone: Indications and dosages.*)

Contraindications and cautions

Don't give dexamethasone to patients with a sensitivity to sulfites or any other component of the drug.

Use the drug cautiously in patients with peptic ulcers; in those with diverticulitis or nonspecific ulcerative colitis who are at risk for perforation, abscess, or other pyogenic infections; in those with recent intestinal anastomoses because the drug may exacerbate complications or mask early signs; and in those with seizure disorders, diabetes mellitus, osteoporosis, or bacterial, viral, or fungal infections because dexamethasone can exacerbate these disorders. Also use the drug cautiously in patients with hypothyroidism or cirrhosis because of the risk of an exaggerated drug response; in those with cardiac disease, congestive heart failure (CHF), renal insufficiency, or hypertension because of the risk of fluid retention; and in those with thromboembolic disease because the drug increases blood coagulability and the risk of intravascular thrombosis.

Give dexamethasone carefully to patients with ocular herpes simplex because of the risk of corneal perforation; to those with a history of or a positive skin test for tuberculosis because the drug may reactivate the disease; to those with glaucoma because the drug can raise intraocular pressure; to those with hepatic impairment or hypo-albuminemia because of an increased risk of drug toxicity; and to those with hyperlipidemia because the drug can raise serum cholesterol or fatty-acid levels.

Dexamethasone is classified as a pregnancy risk category C drug.

Preparation

Dexamethasone is available in concentrations of 4, 10, 20, and 24 mg/

ml in vials and syringes of varying sizes. The 24-mg/ml concentration is for I.V. use only.

Usually clear, the solution may appear yellow at higher concentrations. Protect the drug from sunlight and freezing.

Dilute dexamethasone in dextrose 5% in water or 0.9% sodium chloride solution for intermittent or continuous infusion.

Incompatibilities

Dexamethasone is incompatible with amikacin, daunorubicin, doxorubicin, glycopyrrolate, metaraminol, and vancomycin.

Administration

- *Direct injection:* Give the prescribed dose of undiluted drug over at least 1 minute.
- *Intermittent infusion:* Administer the prescribed dose diluted in a compatible solution at the recommended rate.
- *Continuous infusion:* Administer the prescribed dose diluted in a large volume of compatible solution over 24 hours.
- *I.M. injection:* Inject the prescribed dose deep into the gluteal muscle.

Adverse reactions

- *Life-threatening:* anaphylaxis.
- *Other:* acne, cataracts, CHF, delayed wound healing, edema, ***euphoria, GI irritation,*** glaucoma, growth suppression in children, hyperglycemia, hypertension, ***hypokalemia,*** increased appetite, increased susceptibility to infection, ***insomnia,*** pancreatitis and pancreatic destruction (with high doses), peptic ulcer, psychotic behavior, weakness.

Interactions

- *Anticholinesterase drugs:* severe weakness in patients with myasthenia gravis.
- *Cardiac glycosides:* increased risk of arrhythmias.
- *Estrogen:* enhanced dexamethasone effects.
- *Hepatic enzyme inhibitors:* increased glucocorticoid metabolism.
- *Indomethacin and other ulcerogenic drugs:* increased risk of GI ulcers.
- *Insulin:* elevated serum levels, requiring dexamethasone dosage adjustment.
- *Iodine 131 (^{131}I):* reduced uptake.
- *Mexiletine:* accelerated metabolism.
- *Mitotane:* suppressed adrenocortical function, requiring higher doses of dexamethasone.
- *Potassium-depleting diuretics and other potassium-depleting drugs:* enhanced potassium loss.
- *Salicylates:* enhanced salicylate clearance, requiring dosage increase.
- *Toxoids and live or inactivated vaccines:* diminished response to vaccines.

Special considerations

During therapy, monitor the patient for signs of infection. Report any signs of GI bleeding.

Keep in mind that adverse reactions are uncommon with short-term therapy—even when massive doses are given. Long-term therapy may retard bone growth in infants and children and requires careful monitoring. Remember that most adverse reactions are dose- or duration-dependent. To reduce the risk of adverse reactions, titrate the drug to its lowest effective dose, as ordered.

Keep in mind that dexamethasone therapy can alter the findings of various laboratory tests. The values for the following tests may be decreased: plasma cortisol; corticotropin stimulation; basophil, eosinophil, lymphocyte, and monocyte counts;

iodine 123 uptake; protein-bound iodine; serum thyroxine; serum calcium and potassium; and urine 14-ketosteroids and 17-hydroxycorticosteroids. Also, the nitroblue tetrazolium test for systemic bacterial infection will produce false-negative results.

The results for these tests will be elevated: serum and urine glucose, polymorphonuclear leukocytes, serum cholesterol, serum fatty acids, serum sodium, and serum uric acid.

A platelet count may be increased or decreased, and gonadorelin test results may be altered because of the modified pituitary secretion of gonadatropins. When technetium 99m pertechnetate or technetium 99m medronate is used, radionuclide brain and skeletal imaging results will be altered. Also, reactions on skin tests will be suppressed.

Dextrose in water solutions, glucose solutions

Solutions containing dextrose (glucose) and water can provide calories and water to meet a patient's metabolic and hydration needs. These solutions are also ordered for hyperkalemia, conditions that require adequate calories but little water, cerebral edema, pregnancy-induced hypertension, renal disease, acute hypoglycemia, and acute symptomatic hypoglycemia. And you'll see these solutions prescribed as an adjunctive treatment for shock, as a sclerosing agent, and to promote diuresis.

The solutions vary in tonicity and concentration: Solutions of 2.5% are hypotonic; 5%, isotonic; and over 10%, hypertonic. (See *Dextrose in water solutions: Indications and dosages.*)

Contraindications and cautions

Hypertonic solutions are contraindicated for neurosurgical procedures, alcohol withdrawal syndrome with dehydration, and intracranial or intraspinal hemorrhage because hyperosmolar syndrome may result. These solutions are also contraindicated for patients with anuria because of the risk of circulatory overload.

All dextrose solutions are contraindicated for patients in diabetic coma because of the risk of exacerbation as well as for those with allergies to corn or corn products because the solutions are made from corn sugar.

Use any dextrose solution cautiously in patients with renal or cardiac disease or hypertension because of the risk of circulatory overload; in those with overt or subclinical diabetes mellitus because the solution may exacerbate hyperglycemia; in those with urinary tract obstruction because of excretion difficulties; and in those with carbohydrate intolerance because the solution may cause hyperosmolar syndrome.

Dextrose solutions are classified as pregnancy risk category C drugs.

Preparation

Dextrose solutions are available in 100-, 150-, 250-, 500-, and 1,000-ml bottles or polyvinylchloride bags in the following concentrations: 2.5%, 5%, 7.7%, 10%, 11.5%, 20%, 25%, 30%, 38%, 38.5%, 40%, 50%, 60%, and 70%. Because dextrose is an excellent medium for bacterial growth, store the solutions in a cool, dry place. Protect them from freezing and extreme heat. Don't administer cloudy solutions.

Incompatibilities

When mixed with ampicillin sodium, a dextrose solution must be used within 1 hour. These solutions are also incompatible with cisplatin, diazepam, erythromycin lactobionate, 10% and 25% fat emulsion solutions, phenytoin, procainamide, thiopental (solutions of 10% and above), and whole blood.

Administration

- *Direct injection:* Administer 50 ml of 50% solution at 3 ml/minute.
- *Continuous infusion:* Administer hypotonic and isotonic solutions through a peripheral line and hypertonic solutions through a central venous line. The rate depends on the concentration and the patient's age and condition. An hourly rate above 0.5 g/kg may cause glycosuria in healthy people. The maximum rate is 0.8 g/kg/hour.

Adverse reactions

- *Life-threatening:* none reported.
- *Other:* extravasation, fever (from contaminated solution), glycosuria or hyperglycemia (from prolonged infusion, hypertonic solution, or metabolic insufficiency), hyperosmolar syndrome (confusion, unconsciousness caused by rapid administration of hypertonic solution), hypervolemia, hypokalemia, hypovitaminosis, ***infusion site reaction (local pain, phlebitis, or sclerosed veins with prolonged infusion of hypertonic solution),*** metabolic acidosis or alkalosis, thrombosis, water intoxication (from prolonged infusion of hypotonic or isotonic solution).

Interactions

No interactions have been reported.

DOSAGE FINDER

Dextrose in water solutions: Indications and dosages

Provision of calories and water to meet metabolic and hydration needs
▶ For adults and children, administer a 2.5%, 5%, or 10% solution.

Treatment of hyperkalemia and conditions that require adequate calories but little water
▶ For adults and children, administer a 20% solution.

Promotion of diuresis
▶ For adults and children, administer a 20% to 50% solution.

Adjunctive treatment of shock
▶ For adults and children, administer a 40% to 70% solution.

Treatment of cerebral edema, pregnancy-induced hypertension, renal disease, and acute hypoglycemia and use as a sclerosing agent
▶ For adults and children, administer a 50% solution.

Treatment of acute symptomatic hypoglycemia
▶ For infants, administer a 10% to 25% solution.

Special considerations

Never infuse hypertonic solutions rapidly; doing so can cause hyperglycemia and fluid shift.

Monitor serum glucose levels, which may be elevated by the infusion of any of these solutions. Hypertonic solutions can also alter insulin requirements, and a prolonged infusion of nutrients can diminish insulin production and secretion. Assess the patient for signs and symptoms of hyperglycemia. If you note them, reduce the infusion rate and administer insulin, as indicated.

Monitor intake and output, and watch for signs of fluid overload (exacerbated hypertension, increased pulse pressure, shortness of breath), especially in elderly patients and patients with renal or cardiac disease. Expect osmotic diuresis with hypertonic solutions.

Monitor serum electrolyte and acid-base balance during prolonged administration. Give electrolyte supplements, as needed.

Check the infusion site for signs of extravasation—a complication that can cause tissue sloughing and necrosis. If you note such signs, intervene immediately.

To avoid rebound hypoglycemia, give dextrose 5% or 10% in water after discontinuing a hypertonic solution.

Diazepam

(Valium, Zetran)

This benzodiazepine acts as a central nervous system (CNS) depressant, producing effects that range from mild sedation to hypnosis and coma. Diazepam may be used to treat tetanus, status epilepticus, and recurrent seizures, and to provide short-term, symptomatic relief of anxiety. Also, the drug may be used as a skeletal muscle relaxant in patients who are allowed nothing by mouth, to treat psychoneurotic reactions and alcohol withdrawal syndrome, and as an amnesic agent in patients undergoing cardioversion or endoscopy.

As an anticonvulsant, diazepam suppresses the spread of impulses from irritable foci in the cortex, thalamus, and limbic structures. As a skeletal muscle relaxant, it apparently inhibits polysynaptic afferent pathways. Although the sites and mechanism of action aren't completely understood, the drug is thought to enhance or facilitate the action of the neurotransmitter gamma-aminobutyric acid, which depresses the CNS at the limbic and subcortical levels, producing an antianxiety effect. (See *How diazepam works,* page 48.)

The onset of action for diazepam is 1 to 5 minutes. The duration of action is 15 to 60 minutes, and the half-life ranges from 20 to 50 hours.

The drug is distributed widely throughout body tissues, with 80% to 99% binding to plasma proteins. Diazepam is metabolized in the liver to form the active metabolite desmethyldiazepam. Though it's excreted mainly in urine, small amounts of diazepam also are excreted in feces and pass into breast milk. (See *Diazepam: Indications and dosages.*)

Contraindications and cautions

Don't administer diazepam to patients with a known hypersensitivity to the drug. It's also contraindicated in those with acute narrow-angle glaucoma or untreated chronic open-angle glaucoma because of the drug's possible anticholinergic effects. Don't give the drug to patients in shock or in a coma because its hypotensive or hypnotic effects may be prolonged or worsened. And avoid giving diazepam to those with acute alcohol intoxication because the drug can deepen CNS depression.

Use diazepam with extreme caution in patients with limited pulmonary reserve because of the risk of apnea and cardiac arrest. Also give the drug cautiously to psychotic patients because of a possible paradoxical reaction; to depressed

DOSAGE FINDER

Diazepam: Indications and dosages

Short-term, symptomatic relief of anxiety and treatment of skeletal muscle spasm, psychoneurotic reactions, and alcohol withdrawal syndrome

▶ For adults and children over age 12, administer 2 to 10 mg (0.4 to 2 ml) I.V. or I.M. every 3 to 4 hours. The maximum dosage is 30 mg in 8 hours.

▶ For elderly patients or patients receiving another sedative, administer 2 to 5 mg every 3 to 4 hours.

As an amnesic agent before cardioversion

▶ For adults, administer 5 to 15 mg (1 to 3 ml) I.V., 5 to 10 minutes before the procedure.

As an amnesic agent before endoscopy

▶ For adults, give up to 20 mg I.V. immediately before the procedure or 5 to 10 mg I.M. about 30 minutes before the procedure.

Treatment of tetanus

▶ For adults and children age 5 and over, administer 5 to 10 mg I.V. or I.M. If necessary, repeat the dose in 3 to 4 hours. Larger doses may be required.

▶ For children ages 1 month to 5 years, administer 1 to 2 mg I.M. or I.V. every 3 to 4 hours.

Treatment of status epilepticus and recurrent seizures

▶ For adults, administer 5 to 10 mg by slow I.V. push at 2 to 5 mg/minute. If necessary, repeat the dose every 10 to 15 minutes. The maximum dose is 30 mg.

▶ For elderly or debilitated patients, give 2 to 5 mg I.M. or I.V. For recurrent seizures, the dose may be repeated in 20 to 30 minutes.

▶ For children age 5 and over, administer 0.5 to 1 mg I.V. every 2 to 5 minutes up to a total of 10 mg. This dosage may be repeated in 2 to 4 hours.

▶ For children ages 1 month to 5 years, administer 0.2 to 0.5 mg I.V. every 2 to 5 minutes up to a total of 5 mg. This dosage may be repeated in 2 to 4 hours.

patients because of the risk of deepened depression; to patients with myasthenia gravis or porphyria because of a possible exacerbation; to those with renal or hepatic impairment because of delayed drug elimination; and to those with hypoalbuminemia because of the greater risk of adverse drug effects. You should also use the drug cautiously in elderly and debilitated patients because they'll experience increased CNS effects. And you should give diazepam cautiously to patients who are prone to addiction.

Maternal use of the drug poses a risk to the fetus during the first trimester of pregnancy. For this reason, diazepam is classified as a pregnancy risk category D drug.

Preparation

Diazepam is available in a concentration of 5 mg/ml in 10-ml bottles, prefilled syringes, and 2-ml ampules. Never mix the drug with I.V. solutions. Protect diazepam from light, and don't store it in plastic syringes or administration sets because it interacts with plastic.

Incompatibilities

Diazepam is incompatible with all other drugs and I.V. solutions.

MECHANISM OF ACTION

How diazepam works

Diazepam's mechanism of action isn't fully understood. But the drug apparently acts as an agonist at benzodiazepine receptors, facilitating the action of gamma-aminobutyric acid (GABA), one of the major inhibitory neurotransmitters in the brain. Released from an inhibitory neuron, GABA opens the chloride channel of a supramolecular unit known as the benzodiazepine-GABA receptor-chloride ionophore complex. This mechanism controls the flow of chloride ions into and out of the neuron. As chloride ions flow into the neuron, the cell becomes hyperpolarized, which reduces neuronal activity.

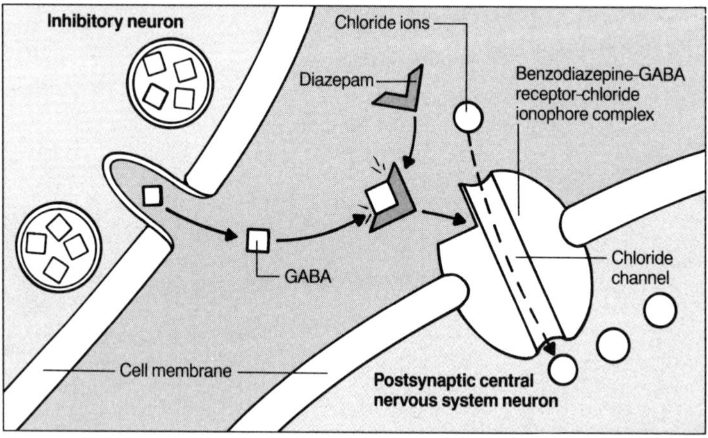

Administration

• *Direct injection:* Slowly administer the undiluted drug into a large vein or cannula at less than 5 mg/minute for adults or 0.25 mg/kg over 3 minutes for children. Check for extravasation. If you're injecting the drug into tubing, choose a site directly above the needle or cannula insertion site. Afterward, flush the tubing with 0.9% sodium chloride solution.

• *I.M. injection:* Inject the ordered dose deep into the deltoid muscle.

Adverse reactions

• *Life-threatening:* bradycardia, cardiovascular collapse, hypotension, respiratory depression.

• *Other:* **ataxia,** blurred or double vision, confusion, depression, desquamation, dizziness, ***drowsiness,*** dysarthria, fatigue, ***hangover,*** headache, ***lethargy,*** nausea, nightmares, nystagmus, ***pain and phlebitis at injection site,*** rash, slurred speech, syncope, tremor, urinary incontinence, urine retention, urticaria, vertigo, vomiting.

Interactions

• *Alcohol, barbiturates, general anesthetics, narcotics, phenothiazines:* intensified CNS depression.

• *Antihypertensives:* potentiated effects.

• *Cimetidine:* elevated diazepam levels resulting from diminished hepatic metabolism.
• *Isoniazid, rifampin:* increased serum diazepam levels.
• *Ketamine:* heightened risk of hypotension or respiratory depression.
• *Levodopa:* diminished therapeutic effects.
• *Magnesium sulfate:* potentiated CNS effects.
• *Monoamine oxidase inhibitors and other antidepressants:* deepened CNS depression.
• *Neuromuscular blocking drugs:* deepened respiratory depression.

Special considerations

Keep in mind that diazepam may contain benzyl alcohol.

Before administering diazepam, make sure you have emergency resuscitation equipment on hand. Next, obtain the patient's baseline respiratory rate and blood pressure measurement. Monitor these signs during administration and for 1 hour afterward. Notify the doctor if the respiratory rate falls below 12 breaths/minute. Keep in mind that hemodialysis won't remove the drug. (See *Managing a diazepam overdose.*)

If the patient is receiving a narcotic, reduce the dosage by at least one-third before giving diazepam. Stop giving diazepam if a paradoxical reaction occurs. Such a reaction may be marked by acute excitation, anxiety, hallucinations, increased muscle spasticity, insomnia, and violent behavior.

During and after administration, observe the I.V. injection site for signs of phlebitis. Remember, abrupt withdrawal after high doses or extended use can cause seizures and delirium. Keep the patient in bed for 3 hours after giving the drug.

EMERGENCY INTERVENTION

Managing a diazepam overdose

An overdose of diazepam may cause bradycardia, cardiovascular collapse, hypotension, and respiratory depression. If you suspect an overdose, take the following actions:
• Check the patency of the airway and administer supplemental oxygen, if necessary. If the patient can't maintain a patent airway, assist the doctor with intubation.
• Monitor the patient's vital signs and cardiac rhythm.
• If his respiratory rate falls below 8 breaths/minute, arouse him and encourage him to breathe at a rate of 10 to 12 breaths/minute. If he can't, use a hand-held respirator to maintain that rate.
• Administer a vasopressor—such as dopamine, metaraminol, or norepinephrine—for severe hypotension, as ordered.

Diazepam may alter certain diagnostic test results. For example, an electroencephalogram will show minor changes in wave patterns, usually low-voltage fast activity, during and after therapy. Liver function tests and serum bilirubin levels also will be affected.

Diazoxide

(Hyperstat)

Rapid I.V. infusion of diazoxide produces an emergency blood pressure reduction in patients with malignant hypertension or hypertensive crisis. The drug acts directly on arterial smooth muscle, causing vasodilation. It also reduces peripheral re-

DOSAGE FINDER

Diazoxide: Indications and dosages

Treatment of malignant hypertension or hypertensive crisis

▶ For adults, give 1 to 3 mg/kg I.V. up to a total of 150 mg. Repeat every 5 to 15 minutes as needed. Administer maintenance doses every 4 to 24 hours as needed up to 1.2 g/day.

▶ For children, give 1 to 3 mg/kg I.V. every 5 to 15 minutes as needed. Administer maintenance doses every 4 to 24 hours as needed.

sistance by inhibiting alpha-adrenergic receptors. Diazoxide isn't effective in reducing blood pressure when the hypertension is caused by monoamine oxidase inhibitors or pheochromocytoma.

The onset of action for the drug is 1 minute; its duration of action varies from 30 minutes to 72 hours, with an average of 3 to 12 hours. The half-life of the drug is 21 to 45 hours—longer in patients with renal impairment and possibly shorter in children.

The highest concentrations of diazoxide are found in the kidneys, liver, and adrenal glands. About 90% binds to plasma proteins. Diazoxide crosses the placenta and the blood-brain barrier. Metabolism occurs in the liver by oxidation and conjugation. The drug is excreted in urine by glomerular filtration; about 50% is excreted unchanged. Whether the drug appears in breast milk is unknown. (See *Diazoxide: Indications and dosages.*)

Contraindications and cautions

Don't administer diazoxide to a patient with a known hypersensitivity to this drug or other thiazide diuretics or sulfonamide-type agents. The drug is also contraindicated for a patient with hypertension associated with aortic coarctation or an arteriovenous shunt. In these cases, therapy should focus on the underlying cause.

Use diazoxide cautiously in a woman who's in labor because the drug can stop uterine contractions. Also administer it carefully to patients with impaired cerebral or cardiac function because it can cause transient cerebral or myocardial ischemia, to patients with uremia because hypotensive effects may be potentiated, and to diabetic patients because the drug can aggravate hyperglycemia, requiring insulin or oral hyperglycemic dosage adjustment. Also give the drug carefully to any patient who could be harmed by transient fluid and sodium retention, rapid blood pressure reduction, tachycardia, decreased perfusion, or renal impairment.

A pregnancy risk category C drug, diazoxide should be given cautiously to pregnant women.

Preparation

Diazoxide is available in 20-ml ampules of 300 mg. Store the drug between 59° and 86° F (15° and 30° C). Protect it from freezing temperatures, heat, and light.

Incompatibilities

No incompatibilities have been reported.

Administration

• *Direct injection:* Rapidly administer the undiluted drug directly into a peripheral vein or peripheral I.V. line over 10 to 30 seconds. A slower injection rate may reduce or shorten the antihypertensive effect because of extensive drug binding to plasma proteins.

Adverse reactions

• *Life-threatening:* anaphylaxis, congestive heart failure (CHF), excessive hypotension (with overdose).
• *Other:* abdominal discomfort, altered taste, angina, anorexia, anxiety, arrhythmias, back pain, burning, chest pain, confusion, constipation, diabetic ketoacidosis (with renal impairment), diarrhea, dizziness, drowsiness, dry mouth, edema, excessive salivation, facial flushing or redness, generalized or localized warmth, ***headache, hyperglycemia,*** ileus, light-headedness, ***nausea,*** orthostatic hypotension, pain at injection site, paralysis, paresthesia, pruritus, retention of nitrogenous wastes, seizures, severe muscle cramps, ***sodium and water retention,*** sweating, tachycardia, tinnitus, unconsciousness, urine retention, ***vomiting,*** weakness, weight gain.

Interactions

• *Allopurinol, colchicine, probenecid, sulfinpyrazone:* possible decreased effectiveness resulting from elevated serum uric acid levels.
• *Anticoagulants (coumarin or indanedione derivatives):* possible enhanced effect.
• *Antihypertensives:* intensified hypotensive effect if given within 6 hours of diazoxide.
• *Anti-inflammatory analgesics, nonsteroidal anti-inflammatory drugs (especially indomethacin):* antagonized hypotensive effects of diazoxide.
• *Beta blockers:* increased risk of hypotension; prevention of diazoxide-induced tachycardia.
• *Insulin, oral antidiabetic drugs:* reversed hyperglycemic effects of diazoxide.
• *Phenytoin:* subtherapeutic levels or toxicity and risk of hyperglycemia, resulting from altered metabolism or plasma protein binding.
• *Thiazide and loop diuretics:* possible increased antihypertensive, hyperglycemic, and hyperuricemic effects of diazoxide.

Special considerations

Diazoxide is commonly administered along with a diuretic—particularly a loop diuretic such as furosemide or ethacrynic acid—to achieve the maximum antihypertensive effect and to prevent CHF from sodium and water retention. In such a case, administer 40 to 80 mg of the diuretic about 30 to 60 minutes before administering diazoxide.

Keep the patient supine during therapy and for 15 to 30 minutes afterward. If you note significant hypotension, have him remain supine for at least 1 hour. If he received a diuretic along with diazoxide, keep him supine for 8 to 10 hours.

Record the patient's blood pressure during and after diazoxide administration. Continue to monitor his pressure closely until he's stable, then hourly. Also monitor his intake and output for evidence of fluid retention.

Monitor a diabetic patient for signs of severe hyperglycemia or hyperosmolar nonketotic syndrome. Administer insulin as necessary (see *Managing a diazoxide overdose,* page 52).

If extravasation occurs, apply cold packs to the area or, as ordered, infiltrate the area with 0.9% sodium chloride solution and then apply warm compresses. Relieve pain by infiltrating a local anesthetic, as ordered.

Diazoxide therapy can alter many laboratory test results. For example, blood urea nitrogen, serum alkaline phosphatase, free fatty acids, glucose, sodium, uric acid, and aspartate aminotransferase (AST),

EMERGENCY INTERVENTION

Managing a diazoxide overdose

A diazoxide overdose may cause severe hypotension and possibly hyperglycemia. If you note these signs, take the following actions, as ordered:

- For hypotension, administer a vasopressor such as metaraminol or norepinephrine.
- For hyperglycemia, administer insulin.
- Because of diazoxide's prolonged half-life, closely monitor the patient's blood glucose level for at least 7 days to ensure stabilization.

formerly SGOT, values may be elevated. Creatinine clearance, hematocrit, hemoglobin, immunoglobulin G, and urine bicarbonate, chloride, and potassium values may be decreased. An insulin response to glucagon will show a false-negative result.

Digoxin

(Lanoxin)

A cardiac glycoside, digoxin is indicated for the emergency treatment of congestive heart failure (CHF), atrial flutter and fibrillation, and atrial tachycardias – including paroxysmal atrial tachycardia. The drug has two important actions: It enhances myocardial contractility and helps control atrial arrhythmias (see *How digoxin increases myocardial contractility*, page 54).

Following I.V. administration of digoxin, the onset of action occurs in 5 to 30 minutes. The peak effect is achieved in 1 to 5 hours, and the half-life ranges from 34 to 44 hours in patients with normal renal function.

Digoxin is distributed throughout the body tissues. High concentrations appear in the skeletal muscle, liver, heart, brain, and kidneys. About 20% to 30% binds to plasma proteins. The drug doesn't accumulate in adipose tissue. It does cross the placenta. Metabolized in the liver and the biliary tract at varying rates, digoxin is excreted in urine by glomerular filtration and active renal tubular secretion. About 50% to 70% of the drug is excreted unchanged. Small amounts of the drug and metabolites are also excreted in bile, and the drug appears in breast milk. (See *Digoxin: Indications and dosages.*)

Contraindications and cautions

Digoxin is contraindicated for patients with a known hypersensitivity to the drug. It's also contraindicated for patients with digitalis-induced toxicity because of the risk of increased toxicity, and for those with ventricular tachycardia or fibrillation (unless it's caused by CHF) because of the risk of exacerbating the arrhythmia.

Administer digoxin with extreme caution to patients with idiopathic hypertrophic subaortic stenosis because of the risk of increased left ventricular outflow obstruction and to those with heightened carotid sinus sensitivity because of the increased vagal tone. Administer it cautiously to all patients at increased risk for digoxin-induced arrhythmias, including elderly patients; to patients who've received any digitalis preparation within the past 3 weeks; and to patients with acute myocardial infarction, incomplete atrioventricular (AV) block, sick sinus syndrome, acute myocarditis, chronic constric-

DOSAGE FINDER

Digoxin: Indications and dosages

Treatment of congestive heart failure, atrial flutter and fibrillation, and atrial tachycardias, including paroxysmal atrial tachycardia

▶ For adults and children over age 10, administer a loading dose of 0.5 to 1 mg I.V. or I.M. (or 0.008 to 0.012 mg/kg) and a maintenance dose of 0.125 to 0.5 mg daily. The usual maintenance dose is 0.25 mg.

▶ For children ages 5 to 10, administer a loading dose of 0.015 to 0.03 mg/kg I.V. and a daily maintenance dose that's 25% to 35% of the loading dose.

▶ For children ages 2 to 5, administer a loading dose of 0.025 to 0.035 mg/kg I.V. and a daily maintenance dose that's 25% to 35% of the loading dose.

▶ For children ages 1 month to 2 years, administer a loading dose of 0.03 to 0.05 mg/kg I.V. and a daily maintenance dose that's 25% to 35% of the loading dose.

▶ For full-term neonates under age 1 month, administer a loading dose of 0.02 to 0.03 mg/kg I.V. and a daily maintenance dose that's 25% to 35% of the loading dose.

▶ For premature infants, administer a loading dose of 0.015 to 0.025 mg/kg I.V. and a daily maintenance dose that's 20% to 30% of the loading dose.

tive pericarditis, renal insufficiency, severe pulmonary disease, hypoxia, hypothyroidism, myxedema, or Wolff-Parkinson-White syndrome with atrial fibrillation.

Also use digoxin cautiously in patients at increased risk for toxicity, such as those with acute glomerulonephritis, CHF, hypokalemia, hypomagnesemia, or hypercalcemia.

Risks associated with using digoxin during pregnancy haven't been ruled out; thus it's classified as a pregnancy risk category C drug.

Preparation

Digoxin is available in 1- and 2-ml ampules (0.25 mg/ml) for adults and in 1-ml ampules (0.1 mg/ml) for children. Store the drug at room temperature.

Dilute digoxin with 10 ml of dextrose 5% in water, 0.9% sodium chloride solution, or sterile water. Or give digoxin undiluted. Administer diluted digoxin immediately to avoid precipitation. This problem occurs more commonly with dilution ratios of less than one part digoxin to four parts diluent.

Incompatibilities

Digoxin is incompatible with dobutamine. The manufacturer, however, recommends not mixing digoxin with any other drug or administering it in the same I.V. line with any other drug.

Administration

• *Direct injection:* Administer the drug over at least 5 minutes. If you're using an existing line, inject the drug as close to the I.V. site as possible.

• *I.M. injection:* Administer the ordered dose deep into any I.M. injection site. Then massage the site to help reduce pain. Because absorption after I.M. administration is slow and erratic, this route is recommended only when I.V. injection isn't possible. Administer no more than 2 ml at any one site.

MECHANISM OF ACTION

How digoxin increases myocardial contractility

Digoxin works by directly increasing the force and velocity of myocardial contractions. It does this by inhibiting sodium/potassium adenosine triphosphatase (Na+/K+ ATPase) enzyme activity. This increases intracellular sodium (Na^+) ions and impairs the sodium/calcium exchange pump, causing an increase in intracellular calcium (Ca^{++}) ions. The result of this ion activity is an increase in myocardial fiber activity.

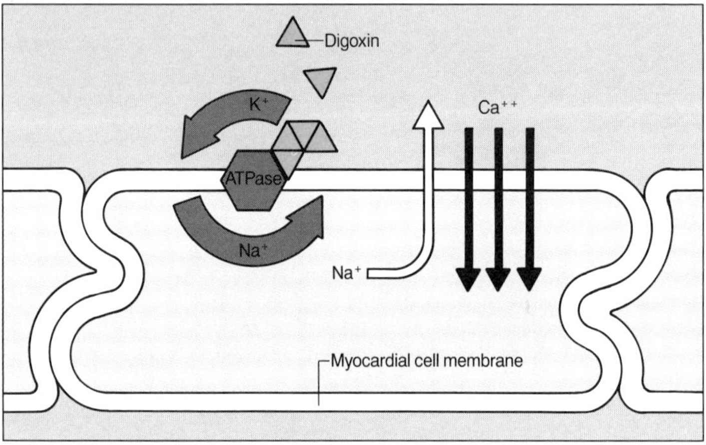

Digoxin also indirectly controls atrial rhythm by enhancing parasympathetic (vagal) tone and decreasing sympathetic tone. This increases the rate of depolarization of the sinoatrial (SA) node; it also slows the conduction rate and prolongs the refractory period of the atrioventricular (AV) node.

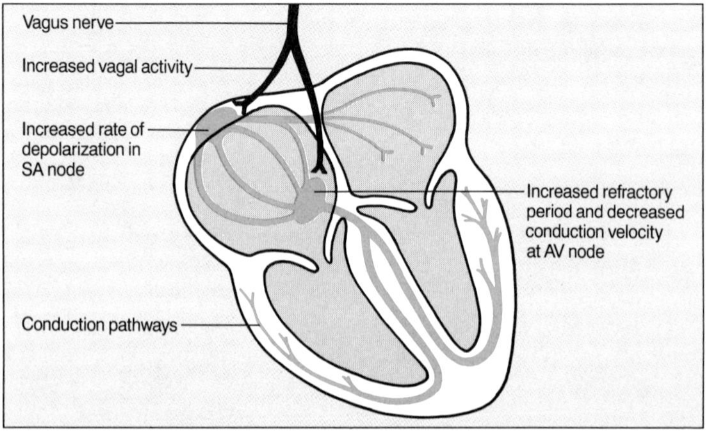

Adverse reactions

- *Life-threatening:* anaphylaxis, AV block, profound sinus bradycardia, ventricular tachycardia.
- *Other:* ***agitation, anorexia, atrial and junctional tachycardia, blurred vision,*** diarrhea, diplopia, dizziness, ***fatigue, generalized weakness,*** gynecomastia, hallucinations, headache, hypotension, light flashes, malaise, nausea, paresthesia, photophobia, premature ventricular contractions, rash, stupor, urticaria, vertigo, vomiting, ***yellow-green halos around visual images.***

Interactions

- *Amiodarone, captopril, diltiazem, nifedipine, quinidine, verapamil:* increased digoxin levels.
- *Amphotericin B, carbenicillin, corticosteroids, diuretics, ticarcillin:* possible digitalis toxicity associated with hypokalemia.
- *Bretylium tosylate:* aggravated arrhythmias associated with digitalis toxicity.
- *Calcium salts:* severe arrhythmias caused by effects on cardiac contractility and excitability.
- *Edrophonium:* possible excessively slowed heart rate.
- *Heparin:* partially counteracted anticoagulant effect.
- *Pancuronium, rauwolfia alkaloids, succinylcholine, sympathomimetics:* possible heightened risk of arrhythmias.

Special considerations

Divide the loading dose. Begin by giving 50% of it. Then, 4 to 8 hours later, give 25%, and 4 to 8 hours after that, give the other 25%. The loading dose may be omitted in patients with CHF and reduced in patients with renal failure.

Keep in mind that digoxin has a low therapeutic index, requiring an individualized dosage based on the

EMERGENCY INTERVENTION

Managing a digoxin overdose

A potentially life-threatening condition, digoxin toxicity requires early detection and prompt intervention. Monitor the patient for signs and symptoms, particularly anorexia, arrhythmias, diarrhea, nausea and vomiting, and a pulse rate under 60 beats/minute. In children, the most common sign of toxicity is an arrhythmia. If you note these signs and symptoms, take the following actions:

- Discontinue the digoxin.
- Monitor the patient's cardiac rhythm strip continuously and maintain his serum potassium level between 3.5 and 5 mEq/liter.
- Treat bradycardia with 0.5 to 1 mg of I.V. atropine, as ordered.
- Treat ventricular arrhythmias with phenytoin (the drug of choice) or with lidocaine, procainamide, or propranolol, as ordered.
- If symptomatic bradycardia or atrioventricular block occurs, the doctor may use temporary transvenous pacing.
- For a life-threatening overdose, you may administer digoxin immune Fab, as ordered, to bind with the digoxin and reduce its toxicity.

patient's ideal body weight and his response to the drug. Therapeutic blood levels of digoxin range from 0.5 to 2 ng/ml in adults.

Before administering each dose of digoxin, check the patient's apical pulse for a full minute. Report any significant changes, such as a pulse rate below 60 beats/minute or above 100 beats/minute, or irregular beats. A pulse rate below 60 beats/minute in an adult may indicate toxicity. (See *Managing a digoxin overdose.*)

Report any blood pressure

changes. And monitor the patient's cardiac rhythm strip for arrhythmias. If they develop, notify the doctor immediately.

Be aware that elderly patients occasionally experience hallucinations, delusions, and severe anxiety from digoxin toxicity. If such symptoms occur, notify the doctor immediately. Protect the patient by raising the bed rails and checking on him often. Try to reorient and reassure him. Use restraints if ordered.

Diphenhydramine hydrochloride

(Benadryl)

Indicated for allergic reactions, diphenhydramine hydrochloride competes with histamine for histamine-1 (H_1)-receptor sites on effector cells to prevent, but not reverse, the actions of histamine. The drug's anticholinergic properties are probably responsible for its antiemetic and sedative effects.

The onset of action for diphenhydramine is 15 to 20 minutes; the duration of action, 4 to 6 hours. The drug's half-life averages 5 hours.

The distribution of diphenhydramine isn't fully understood. The highest concentrations appear in the lungs, spleen, and brain; lower concentrations, in the heart, muscles, and liver. The drug crosses the placenta. About 82% of the drug binds to plasma proteins.

Diphenhydramine is metabolized in the liver, where it apparently undergoes first-pass biotransformation to form dephenylmethoxyacetic acid and N-demethyl and N,N-didemethyl derivatives. Most of the drug is excreted in urine as metabolites within 24 hours. Small amounts appear in breast milk. (See *Diphenhydramine: Indication and dosages.*)

Contraindications and cautions

Diphenhydramine is contraindicated for patients with a hypersensitivity to diphenhydramine or other antihistamines as well as for neonates and premature infants because of the increased risk of antimuscarinic effects (such as central nervous system [CNS] excitation) and seizures.

Administer the drug cautiously to patients with lower respiratory tract symptoms, including asthma, because the drug thickens and dries secretions, making expectoration difficult. Also use diphenhydramine cautiously in patients with narrow-angle glaucoma, stenosing peptic ulcer, pyloroduodenal obstruction, symptomatic prostatic hyperplasia, bladder neck obstruction, cardiovascular disease, or hypertension because the drug can worsen their symptoms.

Risks associated with using diphenhydramine during pregnancy haven't been ruled out, so it's classified as a pregnancy risk category C drug.

Preparation

Diphenhydramine is available in 10- and 50-mg/ml vials. Store the drug between 59° and 86° F (15° to 30° C). Protect it from light and freezing.

Further dilution isn't required for direct injection. For infusion, dilute the drug with any compatible solution.

Incompatibilities

Diphenhydramine is incompatible with the following drugs: amobarbital sodium, amphotericin B, cephalothin sodium, hydrocortisone sodium succinate, iodides, iodipamide meglumate, pentobarbital sodium, phenytoin sodium, secobarbital sodium, and thiopental sodium.

Administration

• *Direct injection:* Administer the drug over 3 to 5 minutes directly into a vein or into an I.V. line containing a free-flowing, compatible solution.
• *Intermittent infusion:* Administer the diluted drug slowly.
• *Continuous infusion:* Administer the appropriate dose slowly.
• *I.M. injection:* Inject the ordered dose deep into a large muscle. Alternate injection sites to prevent irritation.

Adverse reactions

• *Life-threatening:* agranulocytosis, anaphylaxis, hemolytic anemia, thrombocytopenia.
• *Other:* acute labyrinthitis, anorexia, blurred vision, chest tightness, chills, clumsiness, confusion, constipation, diaphoresis, diarrhea, diplopia, dizziness, ***drowsiness, dry mouth, dry nose, dry throat,*** epigastric distress, euphoria, excitation, extrasystole, fatigue, headache, hypotension, hysteria, insomnia, irritability, nasal congestion, ***nausea,*** neuritis, nightmares, palpitations, paresthesia, photosensitivity, rash, restlessness, sedation, seizures, tachycardia, thickened bronchial secretions, tinnitus, tremor, urinary difficulty, urine retention, urticaria, vertigo, vomiting, wheezing.

Interactions

• *Alcohol, hypnotics, sedatives, tranquilizers, other CNS depressants:* deepened CNS depression.
• *Antimuscarinics:* possible potentiated effects.
• *Apomorphine:* decreased emetic effects.
• *Monoamine oxidase inhibitors:* prolonged and intensified anticholinergic effects.
• *Ototoxic drugs (such as cisplatin, vancomycin):* masked signs of ototoxicity.

DOSAGE FINDER

Diphenhydramine: Indication and dosages

Treatment of allergic reactions
▶ For adults, administer 10 to 50 mg I.V. or I.M., up to 100 mg per dose, every 4 to 6 hours. Or you can infuse the total daily dose over 24 hours. The maximum daily dosage is 400 mg.
▶ For children, administer 1.25 mg/kg I.M. every 6 hours. The maximum daily dosage is 300 mg.

Special considerations

Have the patient lie down for an infusion. During the infusion, monitor his vital signs and level of consciousness. Also observe him for signs of an overdose (see *Managing a diphenhydramine overdose*).

EMERGENCY INTERVENTION

Managing a diphenhydramine overdose

Signs of a diphenhydramine overdose can vary from central nervous system (CNS) depression in an elderly patient to CNS stimulation in a child. Other indications of toxicity may include dry mouth; fixed, dilated pupils; flushing; GI symptoms; and hypotension.

If you note such signs, treat the patient symptomatically with oxygen and I.V. fluids. Administer a vasopressor for hypotension, as ordered. Avoid giving epinephrine because it can potentiate hypotension. Also avoid analeptic agents because of the risk of seizures.

Keep in mind that diphenhydramine can cause false-negative results in skin tests using allergen extracts.

Dobutamine hydrochloride

(Dobutrex)

Dobutamine hydrochloride, a direct-acting inotropic agent, is used for short-term treatment of cardiac decompensation caused by depressed contractility from either heart disease or cardiac surgery. The drug works by stimulating $beta_1$ receptors in the heart to increase myocardial contractility and stroke volume, thus increasing cardiac output. Preload decreases because of the reduced ventricular filling pressure, and afterload decreases because of the reduced systemic vascular resistance. Dobutamine also produces mild chronotropic, hypertensive, arrhythmogenic, and vasodilatory effects.

The drug's onset of action is 1 to 2 minutes; it may take up to 10 minutes with a slow infusion. The duration of action lasts a few minutes, and the half-life is about 2 minutes.

Distributed in plasma, dobutamine is metabolized in the liver and other tissues to form the inactive compound 3/0-methyldobutamine. The drug also undergoes conjugation with glucuronic acid. Whether the drug crosses the placenta is unknown.

Dobutamine is excreted primarily in urine as metabolites; however, small amounts of it can also appear in feces. It's not known if dobutamine is excreted in breast milk. (See *Dobutamine: Indication and dosage.*)

Contraindications and cautions

Dobutamine is contraindicated for patients with a hypersensitivity to the drug or to sulfites and for patients with idiopathic hypertrophic subaortic stenosis because the drug may exacerbate symptoms.

Administer dobutamine cautiously to patients with atrial fibrillation because the drug facilitates atrioventricular conduction and rapid ventricular response, to hypertensive patients because of the risk of an exaggerated pressor response, to patients who've sustained a myocardial infarction because high doses may intensify oxygen demand and increase ischemia, and to those with premature ventricular contractions (PVCs) because the drug may worsen the arrhythmia.

The risk of using this drug during pregnancy hasn't been ruled out. Thus, it's classified as a pregnancy risk category C drug.

Preparation

Dobutamine is supplied in 250-mg/20-ml vials. Before reconstituting the drug, store it at room temperature. Reconstitute it with 10 ml of sterile water or dextrose 5% in water (D_5W) to a concentration of 25 mg/ml. The reconstituted solution remains potent for 6 hours at room temperature and up to 48 hours if refrigerated.

Before administration, further dilute dobutamine with at least 50 ml of D_5W, dextrose 5% in 0.45% sodium chloride solution, 0.9% sodium chloride solution, or ⅙ M sodium lactate. For a desired concentration of 250 mcg/ml, mix 250 mg of dobutamine in a 1,000-ml solution; for 500 mcg/ml, mix 250 mg in a 500-ml solution; for 1 mg/ml, mix

250 mg in a 250-ml solution. The maximum concentration for infusion is 5 mg/ml. Use the diluted solution within 24 hours. It may turn pink from slight drug oxidation, but this won't significantly affect its potency. Avoid freezing the drug because crystals may form in the solution.

Incompatibilities

Dobutamine is incompatible with alkaline solutions, aminophylline, bretylium tosylate, bumetanide, calcium chloride, calcium gluconate, cefamandole nafate, cefazolin sodium, diazepam, digoxin, ethacrynate sodium, furosemide, heparin sodium, hydrocortisone sodium succinate, magnesium sulfate, cephalothin sodium, penicillin G sodium, phenytoin sodium, potassium chloride, potassium phosphate, regular insulin, sodium bicarbonate, and verapamil hydrochloride.

Administration

- *Continuous infusion:* To ensure delivery of the appropriate dosage, infuse dobutamine through a central I.V. line using an infusion pump. (See *Drip rates for dobutamine infusions,* pages 60 and 61.)

Adverse reactions

- *Life-threatening:* PVCs.
- *Other:* angina, dyspnea, headache, increased blood pressure, ***increased heart rate,*** mild leg cramps, nausea, ***palpitations,*** paresthesia, vomiting.

Interactions

- *Anesthetics (cyclopropane and halothane):* increased risk of ventricular arrhythmias.
- *Beta-adrenergic blockers:* antagonized beta$_1$ effects of dobutamine.
- *Guanadrel, guanethidine:* elevated blood pressure and arrhythmias, resulting from diminished hypotensive effects of these drugs and from potentiated pressor effects of dobutamine.
- *Insulin:* increased insulin requirements in diabetic patients.
- *Monoamine oxidase inhibitors, tricyclic antidepressants:* enhanced pressor effects of dobutamine.
- *Nitroprusside:* additive effects, including higher cardiac output and lower pulmonary wedge pressure.
- *Rauwolfia alkaloids:* prolonged effect of dobutamine because these alkaloids prevent dobutamine uptake into storage granules.

DOSAGE FINDER

Dobutamine: Indication and dosage

Short-term treatment of cardiac decompensation caused by depressed contractility from either heart disease or cardiac surgery

▶ For adults and children, administer 2.5 to 15 mcg/kg/minute, with the exact dosage titrated individually.

Special considerations

Before administering dobutamine to a hypovolemic patient, give him a volume expander. Also, administer digitalis to a patient who exhibits a rapid ventricular response to atrial fibrillation.

During administration, monitor the patient's blood pressure, heart rate, and cardiac rhythm strip continuously. Also monitor his cardiac output and pulmonary wedge pressure. If you detect tachycardia or a markedly altered blood pressure, suspect an overdose and reduce the infusion rate or discontinue therapy until the patient's vital signs stabilize. Because dobutamine has such a short half-life, you don't need to take other measures.

Drip rates for dobutamine infusions

A doctor's order for dobutamine may be in micrograms per minute or micrograms per kilograms per minute. Using this chart, you can convert either to the drip rate you need for a standard concentration of 250 mg in a 500-ml solution.

For an order in micrograms per minute, use the first column of the chart on this page. Find the number closest to the ordered number of micrograms per minute. Then look to the right to find the correct drip rate. For example, for an order of 200 mcg/minute, you'd scan down the first column to the line for 208.333 mcg/minute. Looking to the right, you'd find the corresponding drip rate is 25 microdrops/minute.

PRESCRIBED DOSAGE (mcg/minute)	DRIP RATE (microdrops/ minute)	PATIENT'S WEIGHT kg 35 / lb 77	kg 40 / lb 88	kg 45 / lb 99	kg 50 / lb 110	kg 55 / lb 121	kg 60 / lb 132	kg 65 / lb 143
		PRESCRIBED DOSAGE (mcg/kg/minute)						
41.667	5	1.190	1.042	0.926	0.833	0.758	0.694	0.641
83.333	10	2.381	2.083	1.851	1.667	1.515	1.389	1.282
125.000	15	3.571	3.125	2.778	2.500	2.273	2.083	1.923
166.667	20	4.762	4.167	3.704	3.333	3.030	2.778	2.564
208.333	25	5.952	5.208	4.630	4.167	3.788	3.472	3.205
250.000	30	7.143	6.250	5.556	5.000	4.545	4.167	3.846
291.667	35	8.333	7.292	6.481	5.833	5.303	4.861	4.487
333.333	40	9.524	8.333	7.407	6.667	6.061	5.556	5.128
375.000	45	10.714	9.375	8.333	7.500	6.818	6.250	5.769
416.667	50	11.905	10.417	9.259	8.333	7.576	6.944	6.410
458.333	55	13.095	11.458	10.185	9.167	8.333	7.639	7.051
500.000	60	14.286	12.500	11.111	10.000	9.091	8.333	7.692
541.667	65	15.476	13.542	12.037	10.833	9.848	9.028	8.333
583.333	70	16.667	14.583	12.963	11.667	10.606	9.722	8.974
625.000	75	17.857	15.625	13.889	12.500	11.364	10.417	9.615
666.667	80	19.048	16.667	14.815	13.333	12.121	11.111	10.256
708.333	85	20.238	17.708	15.741	14.167	12.879	11.806	10.897
750.000	90	21.429	18.750	16.667	15.000	13.636	12.500	11.538
791.667	95	22.619	19.792	17.593	15.833	14.394	13.194	12.179
833.333	100	23.810	20.833	18.519	16.667	15.152	13.889	12.821

Dopamine hydrochloride

(Dopastat, Intropin, Revimine)

Because dopamine hydrochloride increases cardiac output, blood pressure, and urine flow, it's used as an adjunct in treating shock persisting after fluid volume replacement and shock in which oliguria doesn't respond to other vasopressors. The drug is also used for acute exacerbation of chronic refractory congestive heart failure, occlusive vascular disease, and severe illness.

The onset of action is 5 minutes; the duration, less than 10 minutes; and the half-life, about 2 minutes.

Dopamine is distributed throughout the body but doesn't cross the blood-brain barrier. Whether it crosses the placenta is unknown. The drug is metabolized in the liver, kidneys, and plasma by monoamine

For an order in micrograms per kilograms per minute, first find the number closest to the patient's weight (in kilograms or pounds). Follow that column down until you find the number closest to the prescribed dosage. Follow that line across to the drip rate column to find the appropriate rate. For example, if a doctor ordered 4 mcg/kg/minute for a 200-lb patient, you'd locate the column for 198 lb. Then you'd follow that column down to the line for 4.167 mcg/kg/minute. Finally, you'd follow this line across to the left and learn that you need a drip rate of 45 microdrops/minute.

DRIP RATE (microdrops/ minute)	PATIENT'S WEIGHT								
kg	70	75	80	85	90	95	100	105	110
lb	154	165	176	187	198	209	220	231	242
	PRESCRIBED DOSAGE (mcg/kg/minute)								
5	0.595	0556	0.521	0.490	0.463	0.439	0.417	0.397	0.370
10	1.190	1.111	1.042	0.980	0.926	0.877	0.833	0.794	0.758
15	1.786	1.667	1.563	1.471	1.389	1.316	1.250	1.190	1.136
20	2.381	2.222	2.083	1.961	1.852	1.754	1.667	1.587	1.515
25	2.976	2.278	2.604	2.451	2.315	2.193	2.083	1.984	1.894
30	3.571	3.333	3.125	2.941	2.778	2.632	2.500	2.381	2.273
35	4.167	3.889	3.646	3.431	3.241	3.070	2.917	2.778	2.652
40	4.762	4.444	4.167	3.922	3.704	3.509	3.333	3.175	3.030
45	5.357	5.000	4.688	4.412	4.167	3.947	3.750	3.571	3.409
50	5.952	5.556	5.208	4.902	4.630	4.386	4.167	3.968	3.788
55	6.548	6.111	5.729	5.392	5.093	4.825	4.583	4.365	4.167
60	7.143	6.667	6.250	5.882	5.556	5.263	5.000	4.762	4.545
65	7.738	7.222	6.771	6.373	6.019	5.702	5.417	5.159	4.924
70	8.333	7.778	7.292	6.863	6.481	6.140	5.833	5.556	5.303
75	8.929	8.333	7.813	7.353	6.944	6.579	6.250	5.952	5.682
80	9.524	8.889	8.333	7.843	7.407	7.018	6.667	6.349	6.061
85	10.119	9.444	8.854	8.333	7.870	7.456	7.083	6.746	6.439
90	10.714	10.000	9.375	8.824	8.333	7.895	7.500	7.143	6.818
95	11.310	10.556	9.896	9.314	8.796	8.333	7.917	7.540	7.197
100	11.905	11.111	10.417	9.804	9.259	8.772	8.333	7.937	7.576

oxidase (MAO) and catechol-o-methyltransferase to form inactive compounds. About 25% of the drug forms norepinephrine in adrenergic nerve terminals. Dopamine is excreted primarily in urine, with about 80% removed in 24 hours as metabolites; a small amount is excreted unchanged. (See *Dopamine: Indications and dosages,* page 62.)

Contraindications and cautions

Because dopamine contains sulfite, it's contraindicated for patients with a hypersensitivity to sulfites. The drug also shouldn't be given to patients with pheochromocytoma because of the risk of severe hypertension.

Use dopamine cautiously in patients with tachyarrhythmias or ventricular arrhythmias because it may worsen these conditions. Also use the drug cautiously in patients with occlusive diseases (such as Raynaud's disease and arterial em-

DOSAGE FINDER

Dopamine: Indications and dosages

Adjunctive treatment for shock that persists after adequate fluid volume replacement or shock in which oliguria doesn't respond to other vasopressors

▶ For adults and children, infuse 1 to 5 mcg/kg/minute initially. Increase the dosage by 1 to 4 mcg/kg/minute at 10- to 30-minute intervals until the desired response is achieved. The maintenance dosage is usually less than 20 mcg/kg/minute.

Treatment of acute exacerbation of chronic refractory congestive heart failure

▶ For adults and children, infuse 0.5 to 2 mcg/kg/minute until the desired response is achieved.

Treatment of occlusive vascular disease

▶ For adults, infuse 1 mcg/kg/minute. Increase the dosage by 5 to 10 mcg/kg/minute until the desired response is achieved. The maximum dosage is 50 mcg/kg/minute.

Treatment of severe illness

▶ For adults, administer 5 mcg/kg/minute initially. Increase the dosage by 5 to 10 mcg/kg/minute until the desired response is achieved. The maximum dosage is 50 mcg/kg/minute.

bolism) because it may impair circulation.

Because the risks associated with using dopamine during pregnancy haven't been ruled out, it's classified a pregnancy risk category C drug.

Preparation

Dopamine is available in 5-ml vials, single-dose vials, and prefilled syringes of 200 mg (40 mg/ml), 400 mg (80 mg/ml), and 800 mg (160 mg/ml). Because the injectable solution is light-sensitive, it comes in protective containers. Dopamine also comes premixed with dextrose 5% in water (D_5W) in concentrations of 0.8, 1.6, and 3.2 mg/ml in 250- and 500-ml glass or polyvinylchloride containers. Don't use solutions that appear darker than light yellow or have any other discoloration. Protect all forms of the drug from light.

Dilute dopamine concentrate to 200 mg/50 ml or 200 mg/500 ml, using 0.9% sodium chloride solution, D_5W, dextrose 5% in 0.9% sodium chloride solution, lactated Ringer's solution, dextrose 5% in lactated Ringer's solution, or ⅙ M sodium lactate. Dilution with 250 ml yields an 800-mcg/ml solution. The diluted solution is stable for 24 hours.

Incompatibilities

Dopamine is incompatible with amphotericin B, cephalothin, gentamicin, iron salts, oxidizing agents, and sodium bicarbonate and other alkaline solutions. Dopamine is also incompatible with ampicillin sodium and penicillin G potassium, though it can be infused through a Y site with either of these drugs.

Because of the risk of incompatibility, don't mix additives with a dopamine and dextrose solution.

Administration

• *Continuous infusion:* To prevent an inadvertent bolus of dopamine, use an infusion control device. Administer the diluted concentration through a long I.V. catheter into a large vein—one in the antecubital fossa, for instance. Avoid using a hand or ankle vein because of the risk of extravasation. (See *Drip rates for dopamine infusions,* pages 64 and 65.)

Adverse reactions

- *Life-threatening:* conduction abnormalities, ***hypotension,*** ventricular arrhythmias (with high doses).
- *Other:* allergic reactions (in preparations containing sulfites), angina, anxiety, azotemia, dyspnea, ectopic heartbeats, gangrene in extremities (with high doses in occlusive vascular disease), headache, hypertension, nausea, piloerection, tachycardia, vomiting, widened QRS complex.

Interactions

- *Alpha-adrenergic blockers (such as phenoxybenzamine):* decreased peripheral vasoconstriction (with high doses).
- *Anesthetics (chloroform, cyclopropane, halothane, trichloroethylene):* increased risk of severe arrhythmias or hypertension.
- *Antihypertensives:* reduced antihypertensive effect if dopamine dosage is sufficient to produce alpha-adrenergic effects.
- *Beta-adrenergic blockers, sympathomimetics:* decreased cardiac effects.
- *Cardiac glycosides, levodopa:* increased risk of arrhythmias.
- *Diatrizoate, iothalamate, ioxaglate:* if given after dopamine, increased neurologic effects during aortography.
- *Diuretics:* enhanced diuresis.
- *Doxapram, oxytocin:* increased vasopressor effects.
- *Ergonovine, methylergonovine, methysergide:* increased vasopressor effects and possible enhanced vasoconstriction.
- *Ergotamine:* increased vasopressor effects and possible peripheral vascular ischemia and gangrene.
- *Guanadrel, guanethidine, mazindol, mecamylamine, methyldopa, methylphenidate, trimethaphan:* increased vasopressor effects.
- *MAO inhibitors (such as phenelzine):* prolonged and intensified effects of dopamine.
- *Maprotiline, tricyclic antidepressants:* possible potentiation of dopamine's cardiovascular effects.
- *Nitrates:* reduced antianginal effects.
- *Phenytoin:* possible hypotension and bradycardia.
- *Thyroid hormones:* possible heightened effects of hormones or of dopamine.

Special considerations

Before starting dopamine therapy, correct hypovolemia.

Before and during therapy, monitor the patient's heart rate, blood pressure, urine flow, peripheral perfusion, central venous pressure or pulmonary capillary wedge pressure, and cardiac output.

If you detect severe hypertension—a sign of dopamine overdose—immediately reduce the infusion rate or temporarily discontinue the infusion until the blood pressure decreases. If this doesn't lower the patient's blood pressure, you may administer a short-acting alpha-adrenergic blocker, such as phentolamine, as ordered. Additional measures aren't usually necessary because of dopamine's short duration of action.

Closely observe the infusion site for extravasation, which can lead to gangrene. If extravasation occurs, use a small-gauge needle to infiltrate the area with 10 to 15 ml of 0.9% sodium chloride solution containing 5 to 10 mg of phentolamine.

Keep in mind that high doses of dopamine can increase renal vasoconstriction and peripheral resistance. Also, when discontinuing therapy, reduce the infusion rate gradually to help prevent severe hypotension.

Drip rates for dopamine infusions

A doctor's order for dopamine may be in micrograms per minute or micrograms per kilograms per minute. Using this chart, you can convert either to the drip rate you need for a standard dopamine concentration of 200 mg in a 500-ml solution.

For an order in micrograms per minute, use the first column of the chart on this page. Find the number closest to the ordered number of micrograms per minute. Then look to the right to find the correct drip rate. For example, for an order of 350 mcg/minute, you'd scan down the first column to the line for 366.667 mcg/minute. Looking to the right, you'd find the corresponding drip rate is 55 microdrops/minute.

PRESCRIBED DOSAGE (mcg/minute)	DRIP RATE (microdrops/ minute)	PATIENT'S WEIGHT							
		kg	35	40	45	50	55	60	65
		lb	77	88	99	110	121	132	143
		PRESCRIBED DOSAGE (mcg/kg/minute)							
33.333	5		0.952	0.833	0.741	0.667	0.606	0.556	0.513
66.667	10		1.905	1.667	1.481	1.333	1.212	1.111	1.026
100.000	15		2.857	2.500	2.222	2.000	1.818	1.667	1.538
133.333	20		3.810	3.333	2.963	2.667	2.424	2.222	2.051
166.667	25		4.762	4.167	3.704	3.333	3.030	2.778	2.564
200.000	30		5.714	5.000	4.444	4.000	3.636	3.333	3.077
233.333	35		6.667	5.833	5.185	4.667	4.242	3.889	3.590
266.667	40		7.619	6.667	5.926	5.333	4.848	4.444	4.103
300.000	45		8.571	7.500	6.667	6.000	5.455	5.000	4.615
333.333	50		9.524	8.333	7.407	6.667	6.061	5.556	5.128
366.667	55		10.476	9.167	8.148	7.333	6.667	6.111	5.641
400.000	60		11.429	10.000	8.889	8.000	7.273	6.667	6.154
433.333	65		12.381	10.833	9.630	8.667	7.879	7.222	6.667
466.667	70		13.333	11.667	10.370	9.333	8.485	7.778	7.179
500.000	75		14.286	12.500	11.111	10.000	9.091	8.333	7.692
533.333	80		15.238	13.333	11.852	10.667	9.697	8.889	8.205
566.667	85		16.190	14.167	12.593	11.333	10.303	9.444	8.718
600.000	90		17.143	15.000	13.333	12.000	10.909	10.000	9.231
633.333	95		18.095	15.833	14.074	12.667	11.515	10.556	9.744
666.667	100		19.048	16.667	14.815	13.333	12.121	11.111	10.256

Ephedrine sulfate

Ephedrine sulfate is used to treat bronchospasm and hypotension and to temporarily support the ventricular rate in bradycardia, atrioventricular block, carotid sinus syndrome, or Stokes-Adams syndrome. It exerts direct and indirect sympathomimetic effects, stimulating alpha- and beta-adrenergic receptors (see *How ephedrine works,* page 67).

Peak levels are achieved almost immediately when given I.V.; the effects last about 1 hour. The half-life ranges from 3 to 6 hours.

Ephedrine is rapidly and completely absorbed after oral, S.C., or I.M. administration. The exact distribution of the drug isn't understood, but ephedrine seems to cross the placenta. The drug is metabolized slowly in the liver. Small quan-

For an order in micrograms per kilograms per minute, first find the number closest to the patient's weight (in kilograms or pounds). Follow that column down until you find the number closest to the prescribed dosage. Follow that line across to the drip rate column to find the appropriate rate. For example, if a doctor ordered 6 mcg/kg/minute for a 150-lb patient, you'd locate the column for 154 lb. Then you'd follow that column down to the line for 6.190 mcg/kg/minute. Finally, you'd follow this line across to the left and learn that you need a drip rate of 65 microdrops/minute.

DRIP RATE (microdrops/minute)	PATIENT'S WEIGHT									
	kg	70	75	80	85	90	95	100	105	110
	lb	154	165	176	187	198	209	220	231	242
	PRESCRIBED DOSAGE (mcg/kg/minute)									
5		0.476	0.444	0.417	0.392	0.370	0.351	0.333	0.317	0.303
10		0.952	0.889	0.833	0.784	0.741	0.702	0.667	0.635	0.606
15		1.429	1.333	1.250	1.176	1.111	1.053	1.000	0.952	0.909
20		1.905	1.778	1.667	1.569	1.481	1.404	1.333	1.270	1.212
25		2.381	2.222	2.083	1.961	1.852	1.754	1.667	1.587	1.515
30		2.857	2.667	2.500	2.353	2.222	2.105	2.000	1.905	1.818
35		3.333	3.111	2.917	2.745	2.593	2.456	2.333	2.222	2.121
40		3.810	3.556	3.333	3.137	2.963	2.807	2.667	2.540	2.424
45		4.286	4.000	3.750	3.529	3.333	3.158	3.000	2.857	2.727
50		4.762	4.444	4.167	3.922	3.704	3.509	3.333	3.175	3.030
55		5.238	4.889	4.583	4.314	4.074	3.860	3.667	3.492	3.333
60		5.714	5.333	5.000	4.706	4.444	4.211	4.000	3.810	3.636
65		6.190	5.778	5.417	5.098	4.815	4.561	4.333	4.127	3.939
70		6.667	6.222	5.833	5.490	5.185	4.912	4.667	4.444	4.242
75		7.143	6.667	6.250	5.882	5.556	5.263	5.000	4.762	4.545
80		7.619	7.111	6.667	6.275	5.926	5.614	5.333	5.079	4.848
85		8.095	7.556	7.083	6.667	6.296	5.965	5.667	5.397	5.152
90		8.571	8.000	7.500	7.059	6.667	6.316	6.000	5.714	5.455
95		9.048	8.444	7.917	7.451	7.037	6.667	6.333	6.032	5.758
100		9.524	8.889	8.333	7.843	7.407	7.018	6.667	6.349	6.061

tities are metabolized by oxidative deamination, demethylation, aromatic hydroxylation, and conjugation. Within 48 hours, ephedrine is excreted in urine, mostly as the unchanged drug and its metabolites. The rate of excretion depends on urine pH. The drug also appears in breast milk. (See *Ephedrine: Indications and dosages,* page 66.)

Contraindications and cautions

Don't give ephedrine to patients with a known hypersensitivity to the drug. It's also contraindicated for patients with narrow-angle glaucoma because of the risk of increased intraocular pressure, for patients with psychoneurosis because the drug may aggravate central nervous system (CNS) effects, and for patients with cardiac disease because the drug increases oxygen consumption and stimulates the heart.

Administer ephedrine with ex-

DOSAGE FINDER

Ephedrine: Indications and dosages

Treatment of bronchospasm
▶ For adults, administer 25 to 50 mg P.O. every 3 to 4 hours or 12.5 to 25 mg I.V., I.M., or S.C. Subsequent doses will be based on the patient's response. The maximum parenteral dosage is 150 mg every 24 hours.
▶ For children, administer 3 mg/kg I.V., S.C., or P.O. every 4 to 6 hours.

Treatment of hypotension and temporary support of ventricular rate in bradycardia, atrioventricular block, carotid sinus syndrome, or Stokes-Adams syndrome
▶ For adults, administer 5 to 25 mg I.V. Repeat the dose in 5 to 10 minutes, if needed. The maximum daily dosage is 150 mg. As an alternative, administer 25 to 50 mg I.M. or S.C. Repeat the dose, if necessary. The maximum daily dosage is 150 mg.
▶ For children, administer 3 mg/kg I.V. or S.C. every 4 to 6 hours.

treme caution to patients with hypertension or hyperthyroidism because of the increased risk of adverse reactions. Use the drug cautiously in elderly patients with prostatic hyperplasia because of the risk of urine retention, in diabetic patients because the drug raises serum glucose levels, and in patients with cardiovascular disease or pheochromocytoma because of ephedrine's pressor effects.

Risks associated with using ephedrine during pregnancy haven't been ruled out. Thus, it's classified as a pregnancy risk category C drug.

Preparation
Ephedrine is available in 1-ml vials with concentrations of 25 and 50 mg/ml. Store the drug between 59° and 86° F (15° and 30° C). Because the drug gradually decomposes and darkens with exposure to light, store it in light-resistant containers. Discard any unused, cloudy, or precipitated solutions. Ephedrine is compatible with most common I.V. solutions.

Incompatibilities
Ephedrine is incompatible with fructose, hydrocortisone sodium succinate, meperidine, pentobarbital sodium, secobarbital sodium, thiopental, and Ionosol B, D/CM, D, and G solutions.

Administration
- *Direct injection:* Slowly inject the ordered dose directly into a vein or an I.V. line containing a free-flowing, compatible solution.
- *I.M. injection:* Inject the ordered dose into any appropriate I.M. injection site.
- *S.C. injection:* Inject the ordered dose into any appropriate S.C. injection site.
- *Oral:* Give the last oral dose at least 2 hours before bedtime to prevent insomnia.

Adverse reactions
- *Life-threatening:* anaphylaxis, extrasystole, potentially fatal arrhythmias (including ventricular fibrillation).
- *Other:* acute urine retention, agitation, anginal pain (in coronary insufficiency or ischemic heart disease), anorexia, anxiety, breathing difficulty, confusion, delirium, dizziness, dry nose and throat, euphoria, fear, fever, hallucinations, headache, hyperactive reflexes, ***insomnia,*** irritability, light-headedness, mild epigastric distress, nausea, ***nervousness,*** painful urination, pallor, ***palpitations,*** precordial pain, rest-

MECHANISM OF ACTION

How ephedrine works

Ephedrine works by triggering the release of norepinephrine from adrenergic nerve cell terminals and by stimulating alpha- and beta-adrenergic receptors on the postsynaptic sites of these nerve cells.

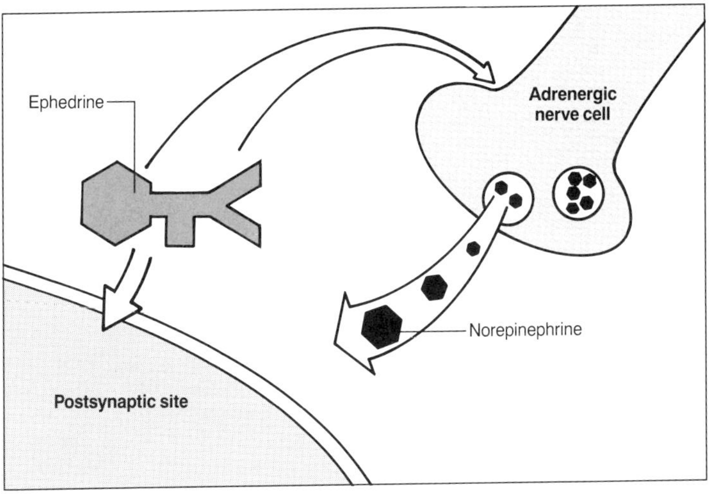

The key effects of alpha- and beta-adrenergic stimulation include:

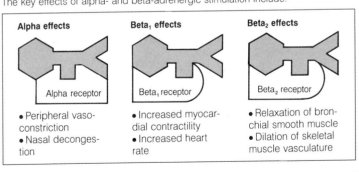

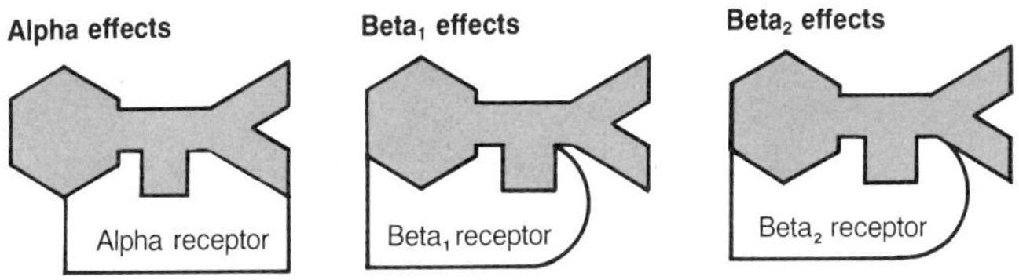

Alpha effects
- Peripheral vasoconstriction
- Nasal decongestion

Beta$_1$ effects
- Increased myocardial contractility
- Increased heart rate

Beta$_2$ effects
- Relaxation of bronchial smooth muscle
- Dilation of skeletal muscle vasculature

lessness, seizures, tachycardia, talkativeness, tremor, vomiting.

Interactions

- *Alpha-adrenergic blockers:* possible decreased pressor response to ephedrine.
- *Antihypertensives:* possible reduced effects.
- *Atropine:* enhanced pressor response to ephedrine.
- *Beta-adrenergic blockers:* possible reduced ephedrine effects, heightened risk of hypertension, and ex-

EMERGENCY INTERVENTION

Managing an ephedrine overdose

If you detect signs of impending cardiovascular collapse, suspect an ephedrine overdose and take these steps:
- Maintain a patent airway and ensure adequate perfusion.
- Monitor the patient's vital signs carefully.
- As ordered, administer a beta blocker by slow I.V. infusion to correct arrhythmias.
- Give phentolamine mesylate or nitroprusside for hypertension.
- Administer diazepam or paraldehyde for seizures.
- Give I.V. fluids and vasopressors for hypotension.
- Apply cold compresses and administer I.V. dexamethasone for fever, as necessary.

cessive bradycardia with heart block.
- *Cardiac glycosides:* sensitization of myocardium to sympathomimetic effects.
- *CNS stimulants (such as amphetamines):* possible excessive CNS stimulation.
- *Corticosteroids:* possible increased metabolic clearance.
- *Diatrizoate, iothalamate, ioxaglate:* enhanced CNS effects, such as paraplegia, if given after ephedrine.
- *Doxapram, guanadrel, guanethidine:* possible increased pressor effects.
- *Ergot alkaloids:* possible enhanced vasodilation, peripheral vascular ischemia, and potentiated pressor effects, causing severe hypertension.
- *Furosemide and other diuretics:* possible reduced arterial responsiveness to ephedrine.
- *General anesthetics (cyclopropane, halogenated hydrocarbons):* possible increased cardiac irritability.
- *Levodopa:* increased risk of arrhythmias.
- *Mazindol, methylphenidate:* possible enhanced CNS stimulation and potentiated pressor effects.
- *Mecamylamine, methyldopa, trimethaphan:* possible diminished hypotensive effects of these drugs and enhanced pressor effects of ephedrine.
- *Monoamine oxidase inhibitors:* potentiated pressor effects of ephedrine.
- *Nitrates:* possible reduced effects.
- *Rauwolfia alkaloids:* possible diminished hypotensive effects of these drugs and decreased pressor effects of ephedrine.
- *Sympathomimetics:* possible additive effects and increased risk of toxicity.
- *Thyroid hormones:* possible heightened thyroid hormone or ephedrine effects and enhanced risk of coronary insufficiency in coronary artery disease.
- *Urine alkalizers (such as carbonic anhydrase inhibitors, sodium bicarbonate):* prolonged ephedrine effects.
- *Xanthines:* possible increased incidence of adverse reactions.

Special considerations

Before administering ephedrine, correct hypovolemia as indicated. Also keep in mind that hypoxia, hypercapnia, and acidosis may reduce the effectiveness of ephedrine.

Before, during, and after ephedrine therapy, monitor the patient's blood pressure and cardiac status, watching for signs of overdose. Intervene promptly if you detect early signs of cardiovascular collapse. (See *Managing an ephedrine overdose.*)

Epinephrine hydrochloride

(Adrenalin)

A sympathomimetic, epinephrine hydrochloride stimulates alpha- and beta-adrenergic receptors, producing relaxation of bronchial smooth muscle, cardiac stimulation, and dilation of the skeletal muscle vasculature. The drug's primary emergency indications include bronchospasm, hypersensitivity reactions, anaphylactic shock, and cardiac arrest.

Epinephrine takes effect immediately, although the duration of action is brief. Distributed widely and rapidly, epinephrine crosses the placenta but not the blood-brain barrier and is metabolized in sympathetic nerve endings, the liver, and other tissues to inactive metabolites. The drug is excreted in urine—about 40% as metabolites, mostly as sulfate conjugates. Small amounts are excreted unchanged. Epinephrine appears in breast milk. (See *Epinephrine: Indications and dosages,* page 70.)

Contraindications and cautions

Epinephrine is contraindicated for patients with shock (other than anaphylactic shock) because of the increased myocardial oxygen demand. Other contraindications include organic brain damage, cerebral arteriosclerosis, organic heart disease, cardiac dilation, coronary insufficiency, and most arrhythmias because the drug may worsen these conditions. Epinephrine also is contraindicated for patients with narrow-angle glaucoma because it may increase intraocular pressure.

Give the drug cautiously to patients with hyperthyroidism—especially elderly patients—because of the heightened risk of adverse reactions. Because epinephrine also causes hyperglycemia, patients with diabetes mellitus who take the drug may require an increased insulin dosage or a hypoglycemic drug. Epinephrine may also exacerbate cardiovascular disorders, such as angina pectoris, tachycardia, congestive heart failure, coronary artery disease (CAD), and hypertension.

Epinephrine increases the risk of hypersensitivity in patients sensitive to sulfites or sympathomimetic amines. In patients with psychoneurosis, the drug may cause symptoms to worsen. And in patients with Parkinson's disease, epinephrine may temporarily increase rigidity or tremor.

A pregnancy risk category C drug, epinephrine should be given cautiously to pregnant patients.

Preparation

Epinephrine is available in 1- and 30-ml vials in concentrations of 0.1 mg/ml (1:10,000), 0.5 mg/ml (1:2,000), and 1 mg/ml (1:1,000). It also comes in prefilled syringes containing 1 to 2 ml of 1 mg/ml concentration, 10 ml of 0.1 mg/ml, and 5 ml of 0.01 mg/ml.

Protect the drug from light, and keep vials in the carton until you're ready to use them. Discard solutions that have turned brown or contain a precipitate.

To obtain a solution of 4 mcg/ml for infusion, add 1 mg of the drug to 250 ml of dextrose 5% in water (D_5W) or 0.9% sodium chloride solution. For direct I.V. or intracardiac injection, dilute 0.5 ml of a 1:1,000 solution in 10 ml of 0.9% sodium chloride solution. Epinephrine is

DOSAGE FINDER

Epinephrine: Indications and dosages

Treatment of bronchospasm

▶ For adults, give 0.1 to 0.25 mg (1 to 2.5 ml of a 1:10,000 dilution) I.V. slowly over 5 to 10 minutes. As ordered, follow this with an infusion of 1 to 4 mcg/minute.

For S.C. administration, give 200 to 500 mcg every 20 minutes to 4 hours up to a maximum of 1 mg.

For oral inhalation, give two to three inhalations of a 2.25% solution. Then, if necessary, give two to three inhalations four to six times a day.

With a nebulizer, give 5 ml of a 0.1% solution for a period of 15 minutes every 3 to 4 hours.

▶ For children, give 0.1 mg (10 ml of a 1:100,000 dilution) I.V. slowly over 5 to 10 minutes. As ordered, follow this with an infusion of 0.1 mcg/kg/minute; this may be increased as necessary to a maximum of 1.5 mcg/kg/minute.

For S.C. administration, give 10 mcg/kg up to a maximum of 500 mcg at 15-minute intervals for two doses, then every 4 hours as needed.

Inhalation dosages for children age 4 and over are the same as those for an adult; for children under age 4, the dosage must be individualized.

Treatment of a hypersensitivity reaction

▶ For adults, give 200 to 500 mcg I.M. or S.C. As needed, repeat the dose every 15 minutes. If necessary, the dose may be increased to a maximum of 1 mg.

▶ For children, give 10 mcg/kg I.M. or S.C. up to a maximum of 300 mcg. If necessary, the dose may be repeated every 5 minutes.

Treatment of anaphylactic shock

▶ For adults, give 0.1 to 0.25 mg (1 to 2.5 ml of a 1:10,000 dilution) I.V. slowly over 5 to 10 minutes. If needed, follow this with an infusion of 1 to 4 mcg/minute.

Or give 500 mcg I.M. or S.C. initially; repeat this dose every 5 minutes, if necessary. If needed, follow the I.M. or S.C. dose with an I.V. infusion at an initial rate of 1 mcg/minute; the rate may be increased to 4 mcg/minute.

▶ For children, give 0.1 mg (10 ml of a 1:100,000 dilution) I.V. slowly over 5 to 10 minutes.

If needed, follow this with an infusion of 0.1 mcg/kg/minute; this dosage may be increased as necessary to a maximum of 1.5 mcg/kg/minute. Or give 10 mcg/kg up to a maximum of 300 mcg; repeat this dose every 5 minutes, if necessary.

Treatment of cardiac arrest

▶ For adults, 0.1 to 1 mg (1 to 10 ml of 1:10,000 dilution) may be given by the I.V., intracardiac, or endotracheal route. The dose may be repeated every 5 minutes as necessary. Then, if needed, an I.V. infusion of 1 mcg/minute may be given; this dosage may be increased as necessary to 4 mcg/minute.

▶ For children, 0.01 mg/kg (0.1 ml/kg of a 1:10,000 dilution) may be given by the I.V., intracardiac, or endotracheal route. The dose may be repeated every 5 minutes as necessary. Then, if needed, an I.V. infusion of 0.1 mcg/kg/minute may be administered; this may be increased as necessary by 0.1 mcg/kg/minute to a maximum of 1 mcg/kg/minute.

▶ For neonates, 0.01 to 0.03 mg/kg (0.1 to 0.3 ml/kg of a 1:10,000 dilution) may be given by the I.V., intracardiac, or endotracheal route. The dose may be repeated every 5 minutes as necessary.

compatible with most other I.V. solutions.

To avoid settling, use a suspension immediately after drawing it into the syringe.

Assemble a metered-dose inhaler according to the package instructions for patient use. For use in a nebulizer, add the ordered amount to the medication cup.

Incompatibilities

Epinephrine is rapidly destroyed by alkalies or oxidizing agents, including halogens, nitrates, nitrites, permanganates, sodium bicarbonate, and salts of easily reducible metals (such as iron, copper, and zinc). The drug is incompatible with aminophylline, cephapirin, hyaluronidase, mephentermine sulfate, warfarin, Ionosol D-CM, Ionosol PSL, and Ionosol T in D_5W.

Administration

- *Direct injection:* Slowly inject the drug directly into the vein or into an I.V. line containing a free-flowing, compatible solution.
- *Intermittent infusion:* Piggyback an appropriately diluted concentration into a compatible I.V. solution, infusing it at 1 to 4 mcg/minute. (See *Drip rates for epinephrine infusions,* pages 72 and 73.)
- *I.M. injection:* Immediately after drawing the drug into the syringe, inject it into any I.M. site, except the buttocks.
- *S.C. injection:* Immediately after drawing the drug into a tuberculin syringe with a 26G, ½" needle, inject it into the subcutaneous tissue.
- *Endotracheal administration:* Stop chest compressions and deliver several breaths with a manual resuscitation bag. Using a syringe with a long catheter inserted deep into the endotracheal tube, instill the ordered dose of a 1:10,000 solution. Then deliver several more breaths to distribute the drug into the lungs.
- *Intracardiac administration:* After the doctor injects the drug directly into the right ventricle, deliver cardiac compressions to ensure that the drug enters the coronary circulation.
- *Inhalation:* While the patient presses down the cartridge on the metered-dose inhaler, have him inhale the drug and hold his breath for 2 to 3 seconds. Or add the drug solution to a nebulizer, place the mouthpiece over the patient's mouth, turn on the gas source, and have the patient inhale slowly and hold his breath for 2 to 3 seconds, then exhale. Repeat the inhalation procedure until all the medication is delivered.

Adverse reactions

- *Life-threatening:* anaphylaxis, cerebral hemorrhage, ventricular arrhythmias.
- *Other:* agitation, anxiety, blurred vision, bradycardia, breathing difficulty, chest pain, chills, disorientation, dizziness, excitability, fever, hallucinations, ***headache, hyperglycemia,*** hypertension, impaired memory, insomnia, light-headedness, mood changes, muscle cramps, nausea, ***nervousness, pallor, palpitations,*** restlessness, sweating, ***tachycardia,*** tremor, vomiting, weakness.

Interactions

- *Alpha-adrenergic blockers:* reversed epinephrine effects.
- *Antihistamines, tricyclic antidepressants:* potentiated epinephrine effects.
- *Beta-adrenergic blockers:* antagonized cardiac and bronchodilatory effects of epinephrine.
- *Cardiac glycosides:* anginal pain (in coronary insufficiency).
- *Diatrizoate, iothalamate, ioxaglate:*

Drip rates for epinephrine infusions

A doctor's order for epinephrine may be in micrograms per minute or micrograms per kilograms per minute. Using this chart, you can convert either to the drip rate you need for a standard concentration of 1 mg in 250 ml of solution.

For an order in micrograms per minute, use the first column of the chart. Find the number that's closest to the number of micrograms per minute in the order. Then look to the right to find the appropriate drip rate. For example, if a doctor ordered 2 mcg/minute, you'd scan down the first column and find the line for 2.0 mcg/minute. Looking to the right, you'd find that the corresponding drip rate is 30 microdrops/minute.

PRESCRIBED DOSAGE (mcg/minute)	DRIP RATE (microdrops/minute)	PATIENT'S WEIGHT kg 35 / lb 77	kg 40 / lb 88	kg 45 / lb 99	kg 50 / lb 110	kg 55 / lb 121	kg 60 / lb 132	kg 65 / lb 143
		PRESCRIBED DOSAGE (mcg/kg/minute)						
0.333	5	0.010	0.008	0.007	0.007	0.006	0.006	0.005
0.667	10	0.019	0.017	0.015	0.013	0.012	0.011	0.010
1.000	15	0.029	0.025	0.022	0.020	0.018	0.017	0.015
1.333	20	0.038	0.033	0.030	0.027	0.024	0.022	0.021
1.667	25	0.048	0.042	0.037	0.033	0.030	0.028	0.026
2.000	30	0.057	0.050	0.044	0.040	0.036	0.033	0.031
2.333	35	0.067	0.058	0.052	0.047	0.042	0.039	0.036
2.667	40	0.076	0.067	0.059	0.053	0.048	0.044	0.041
3.000	45	0.086	0.075	0.067	0.060	0.055	0.050	0.046
3.333	50	0.095	0.083	0.074	0.067	0.061	0.056	0.051
3.667	55	0.105	0.092	0.081	0.073	0.067	0.061	0.056
4.000	60	0.114	0.100	0.089	0.080	0.073	0.067	0.062
4.333	65	0.124	0.108	0.096	0.087	0.079	0.072	0.067
4.667	70	0.133	0.117	0.104	0.093	0.085	0.078	0.072
5.000	75	0.143	0.125	0.111	0.100	0.091	0.083	0.077
5.333	80	0.152	0.133	0.119	0.107	0.097	0.089	0.082
5.667	85	0.162	0.142	0.126	0.113	0.103	0.094	0.087
6.000	90	0.171	0.150	0.133	0.120	0.109	0.100	0.092
6.333	95	0.181	0.158	0.141	0.127	0.115	0.106	0.097
6.667	100	0.190	0.167	0.148	0.133	0.121	0.111	0.103

possible increased central nervous system (CNS) effects, such as paraplegia, if given after epinephrine.
- *Doxapram, guanadrel, guanethidine:* possible increased pressor effects.
- *Ergot alkaloids:* possible enhanced vasoconstriction, peripheral ischemia, and pressor effects, resulting in severe hypertension.
- *General anesthetics (cyclopropane, halogenated hydrocarbons):* increased risk of ventricular arrhythmias.
- *Levodopa:* possible heightened risk of arrhythmias.
- *Mazindol, methylphenidate:* possible increased CNS stimulation and pressor effects of epinephrine.
- *Mecamylamine, methyldopa, trimethaphan:* possible decreased antihypertensive effects and heightened pressor effects of epinephrine.
- *Other CNS stimulants and xan-*

For an order in micrograms per kilograms per minute, first find the number closest to the patient's weight (in kilograms or pounds). Follow that column down until you find the number closest to the prescribed dosage. Follow that line to the drip rate column to find the appropriate rate. For example, if a doctor ordered 0.03 mcg/kg/minute for a 180-lb patient, you'd locate the column for 176 lb. Then you'd follow that column down to the line for 0.029 mcg/kg/minute. Finally, you'd follow this line to the left and learn that you need a drip rate of 35 microdrops/minute.

DRIP RATE (microdrops/ minute)	PATIENT'S WEIGHT									
	kg	70	75	80	85	90	95	100	105	110
	lb	154	165	176	187	198	209	220	231	242
	PRESCRIBED DOSAGE (mcg/kg/minute)									
5		0.005	0.004	0.004	0.004	0.004	0.004	0.003	0.003	0.003
10		0.010	0.009	0.008	0.008	0.007	0.007	0.007	0.006	0.006
15		0.014	0.013	0.013	0.012	0.011	0.011	0.010	0.010	0.009
20		0.019	0.018	0.017	0.016	0.015	0.014	0.013	0.013	0.012
25		0.024	0.022	0.021	0.020	0.019	0.018	0.017	0.016	0.015
30		0.029	0.027	0.025	0.024	0.022	0.021	0.020	0.019	0.018
35		0.033	0.031	0.029	0.027	0.026	0.025	0.023	0.022	0.021
40		0.038	0.036	0.033	0.031	0.030	0.028	0.027	0.025	0.024
45		0.043	0.040	0.038	0.035	0.033	0.032	0.030	0.029	0.027
50		0.048	0.044	0.042	0.039	0.037	0.035	0.033	0.032	0.030
55		0.052	0.049	0.046	0.043	0.041	0.039	0.037	0.035	0.033
60		0.057	0.053	0.050	0.047	0.044	0.042	0.040	0.038	0.036
65		0.062	0.058	0.054	0.051	0.048	0.046	0.043	0.041	0.039
70		0.067	0.062	0.058	0.055	0.052	0.049	0.047	0.044	0.042
75		0.071	0.067	0.063	0.059	0.056	0.053	0.050	0.048	0.045
80		0.076	0.071	0.067	0.063	0.059	0.056	0.053	0.051	0.048
85		0.081	0.076	0.071	0.067	0.063	0.060	0.057	0.054	0.052
90		0.086	0.080	0.075	0.071	0.067	0.063	0.060	0.057	0.055
95		0.090	0.084	0.079	0.075	0.070	0.067	0.063	0.060	0.058
100		0.095	0.089	0.083	0.078	0.074	0.070	0.067	0.063	0.061

thines: additive CNS effects.
- *Sympathomimetics:* additive effects and heightened risk of epinephrine or sympathomimetic toxicity.
- *Thyroid hormones:* possible increased thyroid hormone or epinephrine effects and enhanced risk of coronary insufficiency (in CAD).

Special considerations

Because of the many concentrations available, read the label carefully before administering the drug. Using the wrong concentration can result in an overdose. (See *Managing an epinephrine overdose,* page 74.)

Take the patient's baseline vital signs, then monitor vital signs during drug administration. Epinephrine may widen the pulse pressure. Observe the patient for this adverse effect, and modify the dosage, as ordered.

EMERGENCY INTERVENTION

Managing an epinephrine overdose

An epinephrine overdose may cause severe metabolic acidosis (from elevated lactic acid levels), renal shutdown, and circulatory collapse. To manage a patient's epinephrine overdose, follow these guidelines, as ordered:

- To help counteract marked hypotension, administer a rapid-acting vasodilator—such as a nitrite or sodium nitroprusside—or an alpha-adrenergic blocker. For a patient with prolonged hypotension, you may need to give another pressor agent, such as norepinephrine.
- To help treat epinephrine-induced pulmonary edema, give a rapid-acting alpha-adrenergic blocker, such as phentolamine, or administer intermittent positive-pressure ventilation.
- For arrhythmias, give a beta-adrenergic blocker, such as propranolol. For an asthmatic patient, you may need to give a more cardioselective beta-adrenergic agent, such as atenolol or metoprolol.

Monitor arterial blood gas levels, and keep in mind that epinephrine is less effective in an acidic environment. Also, monitor blood glucose levels in diabetic patients because epinephrine can alter the patient's insulin requirements. Epinephrine also increases blood lactic acid levels and causes electrocardiogram alterations, including decreased T-wave amplitude.

Avoid intra-arterial injection of epinephrine, which can cause marked vasoconstriction and result in gangrene. Also, repeated injections at the same site may cause necrosis because of vascular constriction.

Ergonovine maleate

(Ergotrate)

An ergot alkaloid, ergonovine maleate directly stimulates uterine and vascular smooth muscle, causing uterine contraction and vasoconstriction. The drug is used primarily to treat emergency postpartum or postabortion hemorrhage caused by uterine atony or subinvolution. Ergonovine also is given as an adjunct to coronary arteriography to diagnose coronary artery spasm in patients with variant angina and no coronary obstruction.

This drug takes effect in less than 1 minute. The duration of action lasts up to 45 minutes, although rhythmic uterine contractions may persist for 3 hours.

Distributed rapidly into plasma, extracellular fluid, and tissues, ergonovine is thought to be metabolized in the liver and is excreted primarily in feces. Elimination of the drug may be prolonged in neonates. Ergonovine appears in breast milk but not in sufficient quantities to affect infants who are breast-feeding. (See *Ergonovine: Indications and dosages.*)

Contraindications and cautions

Ergonovine is contraindicated before placental expulsion because placental captivation may occur. It's also contraindicated for inducing labor because of the risks of uterine tetany or rupture, cervical and perineal lacerations, amniotic fluid embolism, and fetal trauma. The drug shouldn't be given to a patient at risk for a spontaneous abortion or a patient with hypersensitive or idiosyncratic reactions to ergonovine or methylergonovine. Other conditions that contraindicate ergonovine use include hypertension, heart disease, atrioventricular shunts, mitral valve stenosis, and obliterative vascular disease.

Give ergonovine cautiously to patients with sepsis or hepatic or renal impairment because the drug may accumulate. Also give it cautiously to patients with hypocalcemia, which may alter the response to ergonovine.

Preparation

Ergonovine is supplied in 1-ml ampules containing 0.2 mg/ml. It should be stored below 46° F (8° C) in light-resistant containers. Avoid freezing it. Dilute the drug with 5 ml of 0.9% sodium chloride solution before an I.V. infusion. Ergonovine solution should be clear and colorless. Discard a solution that has become discolored or formed a precipitate.

Incompatibilities

Although ergonovine has no known incompatibilities, the drug shouldn't be mixed with any I.V. infusions.

Administration

- *Direct injection:* Slowly inject the diluted drug directly into the vein over a period of at least 1 minute. If the injection is too rapid, severe cardiovascular effects can occur.
- *I.M. injection:* Inject the ordered dose into any I.M. site.

Adverse reactions

- *Life-threatening:* anaphylaxis or hypersensitivity reaction, severe arrhythmias, and cerebrovascular accident (in eclampsia).
- *Other:* arm, back, chest, or leg pain; confusion; diaphoresis; dizziness; dyspnea; ergotism; gangrene of fingers and toes; headache; hypertension; nausea; palpitations; seizures; tinnitus; vomiting.

DOSAGE FINDER

Ergonovine: Indications and dosages

Emergency treatment of postpartum or postabortion hemorrhage caused by uterine atony or subinvolution

▶ For adults, administer 0.2 mg I.V. or I.M. in a single dose. Repeat the dose every 2 to 4 hours as necessary up to five doses.

Adjunct to coronary arteriography in diagnosis of coronary artery spasm in patients with variant angina and no coronary obstruction

▶ For adults, administer 0.05 to 0.2 mg I.V. in a single dose. Repeat the dose every 5 minutes until chest pain occurs or a total dose of 0.4 mg has been given.

Interactions

- *Other ergot alkaloids, vasoconstrictors, vasopressors:* enhanced vasoconstriction, requiring dosage adjustment of either drug.
- *Regional anesthetics, vasoconstrictors:* heightened risk of hypertension and headache.
- *Tobacco:* increased vasoconstriction with heavy smoking.

Special considerations

Because of the risk of severe adverse effects, the I.V. route is recommended only when uterine bleeding is excessive. Review the patient's history for factors that may alter the drug's effectiveness. A hypocalcemic patient, for instance, may not respond to ergonovine until she receives I.V. calcium.

After giving the drug, closely monitor the patient's blood pressure and pulse. If ergonovine-induced hypertension develops, expect to administer I.V. hydralazine or chlorpromazine. Also, closely monitor the patient's uterine contractions and muscle tone. If appropriate, give analgesics.

If an overdose develops, monitor the patient's vital signs, arterial blood gas levels, electrolyte levels, and cardiac rhythm strip. As ordered, give nitroglycerin for myocardial ischemia, diazepam for seizures, nitroprusside or phentolamine for peripheral ischemia, and chlorpromazine for severe hypotension.

Use of this drug may decrease serum prolactin levels.

Esmolol hydrochloride

(Brevibloc)

An ultra-short-acting beta blocker, esmolol hydrochloride is indicated for the rapid, short-term control of atrial fibrillation or flutter. This drug blocks the agonist effect of sympathetic neurotransmitters by competing for beta$_1$-receptor sites, chiefly in the cardiac muscle. Because it primarily blocks beta$_1$ receptors, esmolol is considered to be cardioselective. However, at high doses, the drug does begin to block beta$_2$ receptors as well.

The drug takes effect in 2 minutes and lasts 10 to 20 minutes, with a plasma half-life of about 9 minutes. Because of this rapid action, the drug is easy to titrate. (See *How esmolol regulates heart rate.*)

Esmolol is distributed rapidly into plasma, with 55% bound to plasma proteins. The drug probably crosses the placenta. Metabolized by rapid hydrolysis by red blood cell esterases, esmolol is excreted in the urine in 24 hours. Any renal dysfunction will prolong elimination. (See *Esmolol: Indication and dosages.*)

DOSAGE FINDER

Esmolol: Indication and dosages

Rapid, short-term control of atrial fibrillation or flutter

▶ For adults, give a loading dose of 500 mcg/kg/minute infused over 1 minute, followed by a 4-minute maintenance infusion of 50 mcg/kg/minute. If the patient's response isn't adequate within 5 minutes, repeat the loading dose and increase the maintenance infusion to 100 mcg/kg/minute over 4 minutes. Repeat this regimen until the desired heart rate or blood pressure is achieved. Usually, the maintenance dose shouldn't exceed 200 mcg/kg/minute. Esmolol can be given for up to 48 hours. Depending on the patient's response, titration intervals may be increased to 10 minutes.

Contraindications and cautions

Esmolol is contraindicated for patients with a known hypersensitivity to the drug. It's also contraindicated for patients with sinus bradycardia or second- or third-degree heart block because of the chronotropic effects of beta blockade, and for patients with cardiogenic shock or overt heart failure because beta blockade further depresses myocardial contractility.

Give esmolol cautiously to patients with bronchospastic disease because of the risk of exacerbating it. In patients with diabetes mellitus and hypoglycemia, esmolol may mask tachycardia during hypoglycemic episodes.

Also use caution when giving esmolol to elderly patients and to patients with renal impairment

MECHANISM OF ACTION

How esmolol regulates heart rate

Esmolol regulates heart rate by blocking $beta_1$-adrenergic receptor sites. Because the drug has a rapid onset of action and short half-life, the esmolol plasma level responds quickly to any change in the infusion rate. So regulating the degree of blockade, and thus the heart rate, is fairly easy. As the graph shows, beta blockade rises in direct proportion to the esmolol plasma level, and the heart rate drops as the blockade increases.

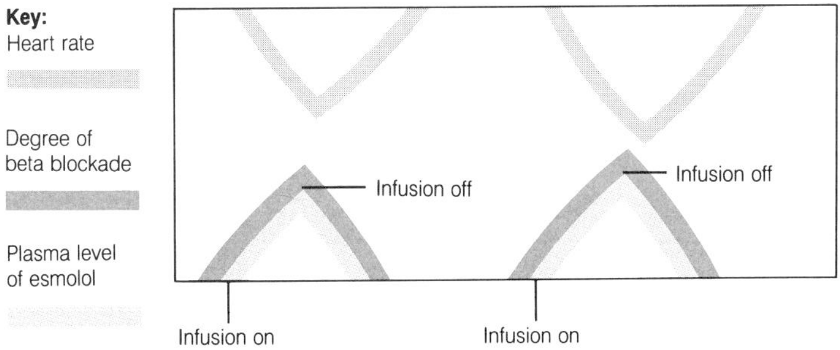

because of the increased risk of toxicity. Base the dosage on the patient's clinical response.

Don't give esmolol to pediatric patients; its safety in children hasn't been established.

Because esmolol is a pregnancy risk category C drug, use it cautiously in pregnant patients.

Preparation

Esmolol is available in 10-ml ampules containing 250 mg/ml. Freezing doesn't affect the drug; however, you shouldn't expose it to high temperatures.

Before infusion, reconstitute two ampules with 20 ml of diluent to yield a concentration of 10 mg/ml. Concentrations of 20 mg/ml or higher are associated with venous irritation and thrombophlebitis.

Compatible solutions include dextrose 5% in water, dextrose 5% in lactated Ringer's, lactated Ringer's, dextrose 5% in 0.45% sodium chloride, and 0.45% or 0.9% sodium chloride. Diluted solution will remain stable for 24 hours at room temperature.

Incompatibilities

Esmolol is incompatible with furosemide and sodium bicarbonate.

Administration

- *Continuous infusion:* Using an I.V. catheter and an infusion pump, give a loading dose over 1 minute and a maintenance dose over 4 minutes. If a reaction occurs at the infusion site, stop the infusion and restart it at another site. Avoid using a winged infusion needle.

Adverse reactions

- *Life-threatening:* none reported.
- *Other:* agitation, anxiety, bradycardia, bronchospasm, chest pain, cold hands and feet, confusion,

EMERGENCY INTERVENTION

Managing an esmolol overdose

Because of esmolol's short duration of action, signs of an overdose may disappear quickly once you decrease the infusion rate or discontinue the drug and thus may not require treatment. But if severe signs—bradycardia, premature ventricular contractions (PVCs), cardiac failure, hypotension, and bronchospasm—occur, also take these steps, as ordered:
- Give atropine or another anticholinergic for severe bradycardia; lidocaine or phenytoin for PVCs; a diuretic or a cardiac glycoside for cardiac failure; I.V. fluids or a vasopressor, such as epinephrine, dobutamine, or dopamine, for hypotension; and a $beta_2$ agonist or a theophylline derivative for bronchospasm.
- Closely monitor the patient's blood pressure and heart rate and rhythm. Assess him frequently for signs of neurologic deficit.

depression, dizziness, drowsiness, dyspnea, fatigue, headache, ***hypotension, nausea,*** seizures, sweating, thrombophlebitis, venous irritation, vomiting.

Interactions
- *Antihypertensives:* potentiated effects of both drugs.
- *Cardiac glycosides:* increased serum digoxin concentrations.
- *Catecholamine-depleting drugs, such as reserpine:* possible enhanced effects of both drugs.
- *Insulin:* masked symptoms of hypoglycemia (except sweating and dizziness).
- *Monoamine oxidase inhibitors:* significant hypertension may occur if taken within 14 days of each other.
- *Morphine:* esmolol levels increased by about 50%.
- *Nondepolarizing neuromuscular blockers:* possible prolonged action.
- *Phenytoin:* possible additive cardiac depression.
- *Sympathomimetics:* possible inhibited esmolol and sympathomimetic effects.
- *Xanthines (especially aminophylline and theophylline):* impaired esmolol and xanthine effects.

Special considerations
Monitor the patient's cardiac rhythm strip and blood pressure during the infusion. As many as 50% of patients treated with esmolol develop hypotension. Hypotension can usually be reversed within 30 minutes by decreasing the dose or, if necessary, by stopping the infusion.

Be alert for bradycardia, premature ventricular contractions, and other signs of esmolol overdose. Be prepared to intervene appropriately. (See *Managing an esmolol overdose.*)

Esmolol is recommended only for short-term use (no longer than 48 hours). After the heart rate stabilizes, substitute a longer-acting antiarrhythmic, as ordered. After starting the new drug, gradually reduce the esmolol infusion over 1 hour.

Ethacrynate sodium
(Edecrin)

A loop diuretic, ethacrynate sodium is used to treat edema associated with congestive heart failure. The drug works by inhibiting the reabsorption of electrolytes, including sodium and chloride, in the proximal tubule and ascending limb of the loop of Henle, while increasing potassium excretion in the distal tubule. Ethacrynate also may directly affect electrolyte transport at the proximal tubule.

The onset of action occurs within 5 minutes. The duration of action lasts about 2 hours.

The drug is dispersed rapidly but probably accumulates only in the liver, where it's metabolized. Highly protein-bound, the drug doesn't cross the blood-brain barrier. About 30% to 65% of ethacrynate is secreted by the proximal renal tubules and excreted in urine. As urine pH rises, urinary excretion increases. About 35% to 40% of the drug is excreted in bile. (See *Ethacrynate: Indication and dosages.*)

DOSAGE FINDER

Ethacrynate: Indication and dosages

Treatment of edema associated with congestive heart failure

▶ For adults, give 50 mg or 0.5 to 1 mg/kg I.V. The maximum dose is 100 mg. The dose may be repeated hourly, if necessary.

▶ For children, give 1 mg/kg I.V.

Contraindications and cautions

Ethacrynate is contraindicated for patients who are hypersensitive to ethacrynate or thimerosal (a preservative). The drug is also contraindicated for patients who have an electrolyte imbalance, hypotension, dehydration with low serum sodium concentrations, or metabolic alkalosis with hypokalemia. Ethacrynate would worsen these conditions. Avoid giving ethacrynate to patients with anuria, azotemia, or oliguria because of the heightened risk of toxicity.

Give the drug cautiously to patients with diabetes mellitus because ethacrynate may impair glucose tolerance. Also use caution when giving the drug to patients with hepatic impairment because dehydration and electrolyte imbalance may result, precipitating hepatic coma. Use caution, too, if a patient has an acute myocardial infarction because diuresis may trigger shock.

Because ethacrynate may raise serum uric acid levels, give it cautiously to patients with hyperuricemia or gout. And because the drug may exacerbate pancreatitis or lupus erythematosus, give it cautiously to patients with a history of these disorders.

Classified as a pregnancy risk category B drug, ethacrynate should be given cautiously to pregnant patients.

Preparation

Ethacrynate comes in 50-mg vials. For a direct injection, reconstitute a vial with 50 ml of 0.9% sodium chloride solution or dextrose 5% in water (D_5W) to a concentration of 1 mg/ml. Don't use a cloudy solution.

For an intermittent infusion, reconstitute the drug in the same manner or use 10 ml of 0.9% sodium chloride solution, then further dilute the drug with 40 ml of a compatible solution. Such solutions include dextran 75 6% in 0.9% sodium chloride, D_5W, dextrose 5% in 0.9% sodium chloride, Normosol R, Ringer's injection, lactated Ringer's, and 0.9% sodium chloride. Store the reconstituted solution at room temperature and discard any unused solution after 24 hours.

Incompatibilities

Ethacrynate is incompatible with

hydralazine, Normosol M, procainamide, reserpine, tolazoline, triflupromazine, whole blood and its derivatives, and any solution or drug with a pH below 5.0.

Administration

• *Direct injection:* Administer the drug directly into the vein over several minutes. To reduce the risk of thrombophlebitis, use different I.V. sites for subsequent doses.
• *Intermittent infusion:* Administer the drug slowly over 20 to 30 minutes through I.V. tubing carrying a free-flowing, compatible solution.

Adverse reactions

• *Life-threatening:* acute necrotizing pancreatitis, agranulocytosis, hepatic coma, profound diuresis.
• *Other:* carbohydrate intolerance, chills, ***dehydration,*** dermatitis, diarrhea (severe, profuse, watery), fever, ***fluid and electrolyte depletion,*** GI bleeding, hematuria, local irritation, metabolic alkalosis, orthostatic hypotension, ototoxicity, pain, rash, thrombophlebitis, tinnitus, transient deafness (with rapid I.V. injection), vertigo.

Interactions

• *Alcohol, antihypertensive drugs:* enhanced hypotensive and diuretic effects.
• *Aminoglycosides, amphotericin B, other ototoxic and nephrotoxic drugs:* increased risk of ototoxicity and nephrotoxicity and intensified electrolyte imbalance.
• *Amiodarone, cardiac glycosides:* increased risk of arrhythmias associated with hypokalemia.
• *Anticoagulants, thrombolytics:* enhanced anticoagulant effects and risk of GI bleeding.
• *Antidiabetic agents, insulin:* interference with hypoglycemic effects.
• *Antigout drugs:* possible elevated serum uric acid levels.
• *Antihistamines, antivertigo agents, phenothiazines, thioxanthenes, trimethobenzamide:* masked signs of ototoxicity.
• *Corticosteroids:* possible decreased natriuresis and diuresis and intensified electrolyte imbalance.
• *Dopamine:* increased diuresis.
• *Lithium:* heightened risk of lithium toxicity because of reduced clearance.
• *Neuromuscular blocking drugs:* prolonged blockade resulting from hypokalemia.
• *Nonsteroidal anti-inflammatory drugs, probenecid:* antagonized natriuresis and diuresis and heightened risk of renal failure.
• *Sodium bicarbonate:* enhanced risk of hypochloremic alkalosis.
• *Sympathomimetics:* reduced antihypertensive effects of ethacrynate.

Special considerations

Monitor the patient's blood pressure, blood urea nitrogen (BUN) and electrolyte levels, intake and output, and weight. Note any signs of an ethacrynate overdose, including excessive diuresis with dehydration and electrolyte depletion. Correct a fluid and electrolyte imbalance and treat the patient's symptoms. Severe, watery diarrhea may necessitate discontinuing the drug.

In patients with renal edema and hypoproteinemia, give salt-poor albumin to enhance the response to ethacrynate. In patients at high risk for metabolic alkalosis, give ammonium chloride or arginine chloride.

Ethacrynate affects several diagnostic tests. Expect BUN, serum uric acid, and urine uric acid levels to be elevated. Serum and urine glucose levels also will increase, whereas serum calcium, chloride, magnesium, potassium, and sodium levels will be diminished.

Furosemide

(Lasix, Lasix Special)

A loop diuretic, furosemide is given to treat edema associated with congestive heart failure, pulmonary edema, and hypertensive crisis. The drug inhibits reabsorption of electrolytes, including sodium and chloride, in the ascending limb of the loop of Henle. Furosemide also increases potassium excretion in the distal tubule and directly affects electrolyte transport at the proximal tubule. Plus, the drug may cause renal vasodilation and a transient rise in the glomerular filtration rate. (See *How furosemide reduces edema*, page 82.)

The onset of action occurs within 5 minutes, and the duration of action lasts about 2 hours. The drug's half-life varies, although it's usually about 1 to 1½ hours for a patient with normal renal function.

Furosemide's distribution isn't fully understood. But about 95% of the drug is bound to plasma proteins, and the drug crosses the placenta. A small amount of furosemide is metabolized in the liver. The drug is then excreted in urine by glomerular filtration and secretion from the proximal tubule; 80% to 88% of the drug and its metabolites is excreted in urine in 24 hours (mostly in the first 4 hours). About 12% is eliminated in bile, some as unchanged drug. The drug also passes into breast milk. (See *Furosemide: Indications and dosages*.)

DOSAGE FINDER

Furosemide: Indications and dosages

Treatment of edema associated with congestive heart failure and pulmonary edema

▶ For adults, initially give 40 mg I.V. or I.M. After 1 hour, increase the dose to 80 mg, if needed.

▶ For infants and children, initially administer 1 mg/kg I.V. or I.M. Increase the dose by 1 mg/kg every 2 hours, if needed. Don't exceed a dose of 6 mg/kg.

Treatment of hypertensive crisis in patients who have normal renal function

▶ For adults, give 40 to 80 mg I.V.

Treatment of hypertensive crisis in patients with pulmonary edema or renal failure

▶ For adults, give 100 to 200 mg I.V.

Contraindications and cautions

Furosemide is contraindicated for patients with anuria, hypersensitivity to furosemide or sulfonamides, and worsening azotemia or oliguria.

Give the drug cautiously to patients with diabetes mellitus because it may impair glucose tolerance, and to patients with hepatic impairment because dehydration and electrolyte imbalance may precipitate hepatic coma. Also use caution when giving the drug to a patient with an acute myocardial infarction because diuresis may precipitate shock.

Because furosemide may raise serum uric acid levels, give it cautiously to patients with hyperuricemia or a history of gout. Because the drug also may exacerbate pancreatitis or lupus erythematosus, use caution when giving it to patients with a history of these disorders.

Classified as a pregnancy risk category C drug, furosemide should be given cautiously to pregnant patients.

MECHANISM OF ACTION

How furosemide reduces edema

Furosemide, a loop diuretic, treats edema associated with congestive heart failure (CHF). The upper portion of this flowchart shows the three paths leading from inadequate cardiac output and tissue ischemia to increased intracellular fluid. The lower portion shows how furosemide reduces renal salt and water retention.

Furosemide acts on the ascending limb of the loop of Henle, inhibiting sodium and water reabsorption, thereby promoting the excretion of sodium, water, chloride, and potassium. The drug also temporarily increases glomerular filtration by renal and peripheral vasodilation and reduces extracellular fluid and venous pressure. This creates the hydrostatic pressure that forces fluid into the interstitium.

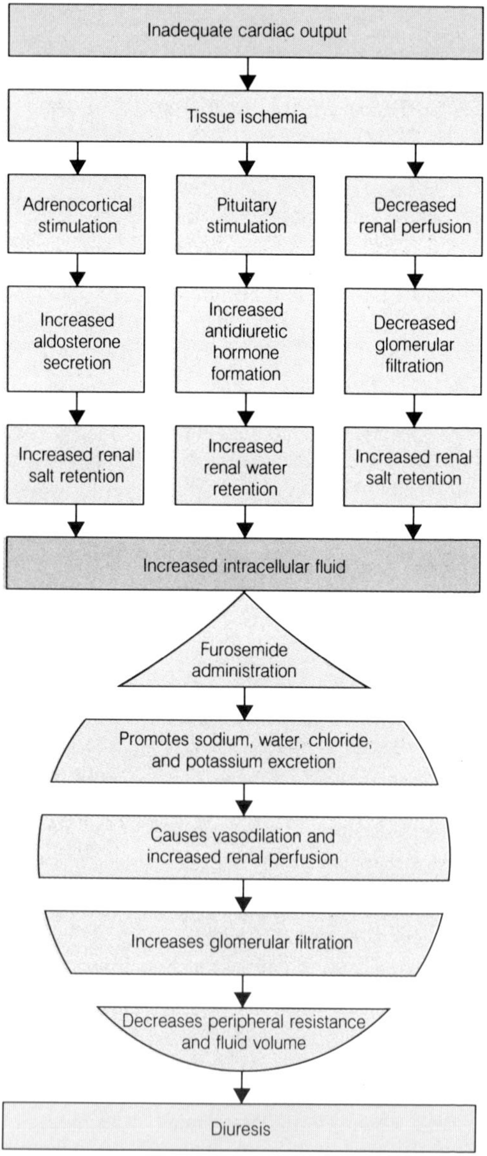

Preparation

Furosemide is available in 2-ml, 4-ml, and 10-ml ampules with a 10 mg/ml concentration. Store the drug at room temperature, and protect it from light. Use it within 42 days of the date of manufacture.

For an infusion, dilute the drug in one of the following solutions: dextrose 5% in water, lactated Ringer's, dextrose 5% in lactated Ringer's, dextrose 5% in Ringer's injection, or 0.9% sodium chloride. Filter the infusion solution to remove any glass particles. Discard any solution that's discolored or contains a precipitate.

Incompatibilities

Furosemide is incompatible with bleomycin, dobutamine, esmolol, fructose 10% and water, gentamicin, highly acidic solutions, invert sugar 10% and Electrolyte #2, metoclopramide, and netilmicin.

Administration

- *Direct injection:* Over a period of 1 to 2 minutes, inject furosemide directly into the vein or into I.V. tubing with a free-flowing, compatible solution.
- *Intermittent infusion:* Administer the diluted drug at the appropriate rate, which shouldn't exceed 4 mg/minute.
- *I.M. injection (not preferred):* Inject the ordered dose into any I.M. injection site.

Adverse reactions

- *Life-threatening:* agranulocytosis, cardiac arrest.
- *Other:* abdominal pain (in children), allergic interstitial nephritis, anemia, bladder spasm, blurred vision, dizziness, ***electrolyte depletion,*** erythema multiforme, exfoliative dermatitis, headache, hypovolemia, increased perspiration, leukopenia, light-headedness, metabolic alkalosis, muscle spasm, necrotizing angiitis, neutropenia, orthostatic hypotension, ototoxicity, paresthesia, photosensitivity, pruritus, purpura, rash, restlessness, thrombocytopenia, urinary frequency, urticaria, vertigo, weakness, xanthopsia.

Interactions

- *Alcohol, antihypertensive drugs:* possible enhanced hypotensive and diuretic effects.
- *Aminoglycosides, amphotericin B, other nephrotoxic or ototoxic drugs:* increased risk of nephrotoxicity and ototoxicity and intensified electrolyte imbalance.
- *Amiodarone, cardiac glycosides:* enhanced risk of arrhythmias associated with hypokalemia.
- *Anticoagulants, thrombolytics:* possible increased anticoagulant effects and risk of GI bleeding.
- *Antidiabetic agents, insulin:* possible interference with hypoglycemic effects.
- *Antigout agents:* possible elevated serum uric acid levels.
- *Antihistamines, antivertigo agents, phenothiazines, thioxanthenes, trimethobenzamide:* possible masked signs of ototoxicity.
- *Chloral hydrate:* possible diaphoresis, hot flashes, and variable blood pressure.
- *Clofibrate:* possible enhanced effects of both drugs.
- *Corticosteroids:* possible increased natriuresis and diuresis and intensified electrolyte imbalance.
- *Dopamine:* possible enhanced diuresis.
- *Lithium:* heightened risk of lithium toxicity because of reduced clearance.
- *Neuromuscular blockers:* possible enhanced blockade because of furosemide-induced hypokalemia.
- *Nonsteroidal anti-inflammatory drugs, probenecid:* antagonism of

DOSAGE FINDER

Glucagon: Indication and dosages

Treatment of severe hypoglycemia in diabetic patients

▶ For adults, give 0.5 to 1 unit (0.5 to 1 mg) I.V., I.M., or S.C. Larger doses may be necessary. If the patient doesn't awaken within 20 minutes, repeat the dose. If necessary, the dose can be repeated again.

▶ For children, give 0.025 unit/kg I.V., I.M., or S.C. The maximum dose is 1 unit. If the patient doesn't awaken within 20 minutes, repeat the dose. If necessary, the dose can be repeated again.

natriuresis and diuresis and increased risk of renal failure.
- *Sympathomimetics:* possible reduced antihypertensive effects of furosemide.

Special considerations

Give furosemide slowly because a rapid injection or infusion can cause ototoxicity.

During therapy, monitor the patient's blood urea nitrogen (BUN), serum uric acid, glucose, and electrolyte levels, as well as the results of his liver and kidney function tests. Also monitor his weight, intake and output, and vital signs. Be alert for signs of potassium depletion, such as muscle weakness and cramps.

Note any signs of a furosemide overdose, including excessive diuresis with dehydration and electrolyte depletion. Correct a fluid and electrolyte imbalance, as ordered, and treat the patient's symptoms.

Furosemide affects several diagnostic tests. BUN, serum glucose, and uric acid levels will be elevated. Urine glucose and uric acid levels also will be increased, whereas serum calcium, chloride, magnesium, potassium, and sodium levels will be decreased.

Glucagon

Indicated for severe hypoglycemia in diabetic patients, glucagon promotes hepatic glycogenolysis and gluconeogenesis, raising serum glucose levels. To produce this antihypoglycemic effect, glucagon requires hepatic stores of glycogen. (See *How glucagon raises glucose levels.*)

The drug's onset of action occurs in 5 to 30 minutes. The duration of action lasts 1 to 2 hours. The drug's half-life is short—about 3 to 10 minutes.

Glucagon is distributed to most tissues and plasma. Whether the drug crosses the placenta isn't known. Metabolism occurs primarily in the liver but also in the kidneys, tissues, and plasma through enzymatic proteolysis. The drug is excreted by the kidneys, mostly as metabolites. Whether glucagon passes into breast milk isn't known. (See *Glucagon: Indication and dosages.*)

Contraindications and cautions

Glucagon is contraindicated for patients with a known hypersensitivity to the drug. It's also contraindicated for treating hypoglycemia in premature infants and infants with intrauterine growth retardation.

Give the drug cautiously to patients who are allergic to beef or porcine proteins because they also may be allergic to glucagon. Use glucagon cautiously in patients with a history of insulinoma because severe hypoglycemia may occur. Also

MECHANISM OF ACTION

How glucagon raises glucose levels

When adequate stores of glycogen are present, glucagon can raise glucose levels in patients with severe hypoglycemia associated with diabetes mellitus. This illustration shows glucagon stimulating the reaction that produces the enzyme active phosphorylase; the enzyme then initiates hepatic glycogenolysis, which breaks down the glycogen so it can enter the blood.

Here's what happens: Initially, glucagon stimulates the formation of adenylate cyclase in the liver cell. The adenylate cyclase then converts adenosine triphosphate (ATP) to cyclic adenosine monophosphate (cAMP). This product initiates a series of reactions that result in an active phosphorylated glucose molecule.

In this phosphorylated form, the large glucose molecule can't pass through the cell membrane. Through glycogenolysis, the liver removes the phosphate group and allows the glucose to enter the bloodstream. This increases the glucose available to other tissues for short-term energy needs.

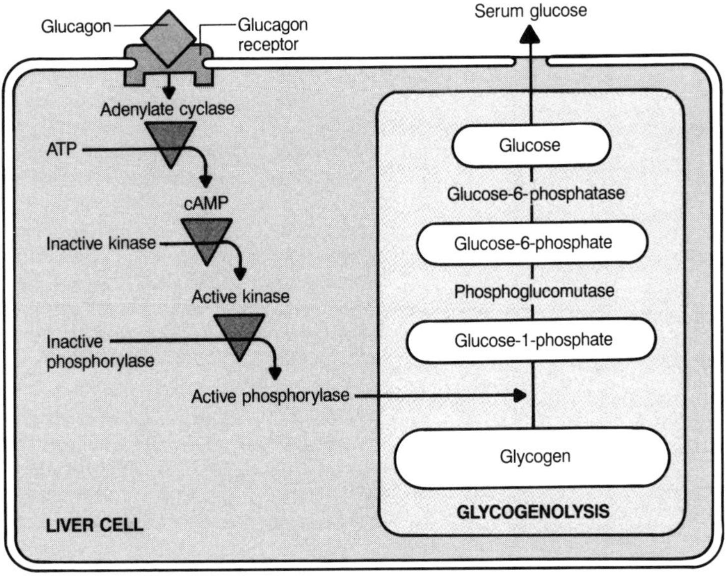

give it cautiously to patients with pheochromocytoma because of the risk of a marked increase in blood pressure.

Classified as a pregnancy risk category B drug, glucagon should be given cautiously to pregnant patients.

Preparation

The drug is available as a powder in 1- and 10-unit vials and should be stored at room temperature. The powder contains lactose. Reconstitute glucagon with the provided diluent — a clear, sterile fluid that contains 0.2% phenol as a preservative and 1.6% glycerin.

Don't reconstitute the drug until you need it, although the reconstituted solution will remain stable for up to 3 months when stored at 36° to 46° F (2.2° to 7.8° C).

Incompatibilities
Glucagon is incompatible with sodium chloride solution and other solutions with a pH between 3.0 and 9.5 because a precipitate may form.

Administration
• *Direct injection:* Inject the drug over a period of 2 to 5 minutes directly into the vein or into I.V. tubing with a free-flowing, compatible solution. Interrupt the primary infusion during glucagon injection if you're using the same I.V. line.
• *I.M. injection:* Inject the ordered dose into any I.M. injection site.
• *S.C. injection:* Inject the ordered dose into any S.C. injection site.

Adverse reactions
• *Life-threatening:* none reported.
• *Other:* dizziness, dyspnea, lightheadedness, nausea, rash, tachycardia, vomiting.

Interactions
• *Anticoagulants (such as coumarin or indanedione derivatives):* possible potentiated anticoagulant effects.
• *Epinephrine:* enhanced and prolonged hyperglycemic effect.

Special considerations
Because glucagon's half-life is so short, treatment of an overdose is symptomatic. Monitor the patient's serum electrolytes, especially potassium, and serum glucose. If necessary, replace potassium and any fluids lost through vomiting.

Also monitor the patient's blood pressure because rapid glucagon administration can reduce it. If the patient is taking coumarin as well as glucagon, monitor his prothrombin time.

If a hypoglycemic patient doesn't respond to glucagon, give him I.V. dextrose, as ordered. Glucagon may fail to relieve coma because of markedly depleted hepatic stores of glycogen or irreversible brain damage caused by prolonged hypoglycemia.

To prevent secondary hypoglycemia, provide oral supplemental glucose when the patient is sufficiently alert and oriented. After hypoglycemia has resolved, give him foods containing carbohydrates and proteins. Keep in mind that glucagon also may cause hyperglycemia.

Teach the hypoglycemic patient's family members how to give glucagon in an emergency. Instruct them to use a standard insulin syringe, employing a 90-degree approach (rather than the usual S.C. one) to deliver a deeper injection and achieve a faster response.

Glycopyrrolate
(Robinul)

This drug inhibits the muscarinic effects of acetylcholine on autonomic effectors innervated by postganglionic cholinergic nerves. Because glycopyrrolate produces such inhibition in cardiac muscle and the sinoatrial and atrioventricular nodes, it's given to control arrhythmias during surgery. And because the drug decreases GI motility and tone and reduces gastric secretions, it's used as an adjunctive treatment for peptic ulcers. The drug also is used to block the adverse muscarinic effects of neostigmine and pyridostigmine.

Glycopyrrolate's onset of action

occurs in about 1 minute. The vagal effects last 2 to 3 hours, salivary inhibition lasts up to 7 hours, and other anticholinergic effects last 8 to 12 hours. The drug's half-life is less than 5 minutes.

Distribution is rapid and widespread, with high levels found in the stomach and intestines. The drug crosses the placenta and appears in cerebrospinal fluid in low concentrations. Metabolized in small amounts to form several metabolites, glycopyrrolate is excreted primarily unchanged in feces and urine. Whether or not the drug appears in breast milk isn't known. (See *Glycopyrrolate: Indications and dosages.*)

DOSAGE FINDER

Glycopyrrolate: Indications and dosages

Control of arrhythmias during surgery
▶ For adults, give 0.1 mg I.V. Repeat the dose every 2 to 3 minutes, as needed.
▶ For children, give 0.0044 mg/kg I.V. (up to a maximum of 0.1 mg). Repeat this every 2 to 3 minutes, as needed.

Adjunctive treatment of peptic ulcers
▶ For adults and children age 12 and over, give 0.1 to 0.2 mg I.V. or I.M. every 6 to 8 hours. The daily maximum is four doses.

Blockade of adverse muscarinic effects of neostigmine or pyridostigmine
▶ For adults and children, give 0.2 mg I.V. for each 1 mg of neostigmine or 5 mg of pyridostigmine, using the same syringe.

Contraindications and cautions

Glycopyrrolate is contraindicated for patients with a known hypersensitivity to the drug. And because the drug blocks vagal inhibition of the sinoatrial node, avoid giving it to patients with tachycardia stemming from cardiac insufficiency, thyrotoxicosis, or acute hemorrhage and to patients with an unstable cardiovascular status. Similarly, patients with tachyarrhythmias, congestive heart failure, or coronary artery disease shouldn't receive glycopyrrolate.

Because the drug diminishes intestinal motility and heightens the risk of obstruction, it's contraindicated for patients with severe ulcerative colitis, toxic megacolon, obstructive GI disease, cardiospasm, paralytic ileus, and intestinal atony. Glycopyrrolate also shouldn't be given to patients with angle-closure glaucoma because it may raise intraocular pressure, or to patients with obstructive uropathy or prostatic hyperplasia because it may worsen urine retention. Also avoid giving the drug to patients with myasthenia gravis because it may exacerbate muscle weakness.

Give glycopyrrolate cautiously to febrile patients and to those exposed to high temperatures because of the risk of hyperthermia. Administer the drug carefully to children—especially those under age 2—because of the increased risk of adverse reactions. Also use caution when giving glycopyrrolate to children with brain damage because the drug may exacerbate central nervous system effects, and to children with spastic paralysis because they may have an increased drug response.

For patients with Down's syndrome, give glycopyrrolate carefully because of the risk of tachycardia. For elderly patients, give the drug cautiously because it may cause paradoxical excitement, agitation, increased drowsiness, or acute glaucoma.

Also use caution when giving glycopyrrolate to patients with the following conditions: hyperthyroidism because tachycardia may worsen; hypertension because of possible aggravation; hepatic or renal impairment because of the heightened risk of adverse reactions; and chronic pulmonary disease because the drug may promote mucus plug formation.

Because of glycopyrrolate's effects on the GI system, give the drug cautiously to patients with esophageal reflux or hiatal hernia, gastric ulcer, known or suspected GI infection, and mild or moderate ulcerative colitis. Glycopyrrolate promotes gastric retention and aggravates reflux, leading to delayed gastric emptying and possibly antral stasis. It also diminishes GI motility, prolonging retention of infection-causing organisms or toxins and possibly producing paralytic ileus or toxic megacolon. Give the drug carefully to patients with diarrhea because this sign may be an early indicator of intestinal obstruction.

For patients with autonomic or partial obstructive uropathy, give glycopyrrolate carefully because it may aggravate or precipitate urine retention. Also give the drug carefully to patients with xerostomia because salivary flow may be further curtailed.

Finally, because glycopyrrolate is classified as a pregnancy risk category B drug, give it cautiously to pregnant patients.

Preparation

Glycopyrrolate is available as a clear, colorless sterile solution in 1-ml, 2-ml, 5-ml, and 20-ml vials with a concentration of 0.2 mg/ml. Store the drug at room temperature.

With a pH of 2.0 to 3.0, glycopyrrolate is most stable in acidic solutions and unstable in solutions with a pH above 6.0. It may be mixed in a syringe and administered with dextrose 5% in water (D_5W) or dextrose 10% in water, 0.9% sodium chloride solution, meperidine, morphine sulfate, fentanyl with droperidol, hydroxyzine, neostigmine, or pyridostigmine.

For an infusion, mix the drug with D_5W, dextrose 5% in 0.45% sodium chloride, 0.9% sodium chloride, or lactated Ringer's solution. A concentration of 0.8 mg/liter in one of these solutions will remain stable at room temperature for 48 hours.

Incompatibilities

Glycopyrrolate is incompatible with drugs having an alkaline pH. Other incompatibilities include chloramphenicol sodium succinate, dexamethasone sodium phosphate, diazepam, dimenhydrinate, methohexital sodium, methylprednisolone sodium succinate, pentazocine lactate, pentobarbital sodium, secobarbital sodium, sodium bicarbonate, and thiopental sodium.

Administration

- *Direct injection:* Inject the drug into a vein or an I.V. line containing a free-flowing, compatible solution.
- *Intermittent infusion:* Infuse glycopyrrolate at the ordered rate.
- *I.M. injection:* Inject the ordered dose into any I.M. injection site.

Adverse reactions

- *Life-threatening:* anaphylaxis, respiratory paralysis.
- *Other:* anhidrosis, bloated sensation, ***blurred vision,*** breathing difficulty, confusion, ***constipation,*** cycloplegia, decreased lactation, ***dilated pupils,*** dizziness, drowsiness, ***dry mouth,*** dysphagia, dysuria, excitement, fever, flushing, headache, hypertension, hypotension, increased ocular tension, insomnia,

loss of taste, marked photophobia, memory loss (especially in elderly patients), mydriasis, nausea, palpitations, rash, tachycardia, thirst, ***urinary hesitancy, urine retention,*** urticaria, vomiting, weakness, xerostomia.

Interactions

- *Alphaprodine, amantadine, antidyskinetics, antihistamines, phenothiazines, quinidine, tricyclic antidepressants, other antimuscarinics:* additive anticholinergic effects.
- *Antimyasthenics:* reduced intestinal motility.
- *Antipsychotics, benzodiazepines, disopyramide, glutethimide, monoamine oxidase inhibitors:* increased anticholinergic effects.
- *Cyclopropane anesthetics:* ventricular arrhythmias.
- *Guanadrel, guanethidine, reserpine:* antagonized inhibitory action of glycopyrrolate on gastric acid.
- *Ketoconazole:* impaired absorption because of increased gastric pH.
- *Metoclopramide:* antagonized effect on GI motility.
- *Opioid analgesics:* heightened risk of severe constipation and additive anticholinergic effects.
- *Potassium chloride (Slow K, wax-matrix preparations):* increased severity of GI mucosal lesions.
- *Urinary alkalizers (such as antacids, carbonic anhydrase inhibitors):* delayed excretion of glycopyrrolate.

Special considerations

Keep in mind that glycopyrrolate may contain benzyl alcohol.

Remember that elderly and debilitated patients usually require lower doses of glycopyrrolate.

Monitor the patient's intake, output, vital signs, and bowel habits. Watch for signs of an overdose and intervene appropriately (see *Managing a glycopyrrolate overdose*).

EMERGENCY INTERVENTION

Managing a glycopyrrolate overdose

The signs of a glycopyrrolate overdose include excitement or delirium, lowered blood pressure, and respiratory distress. If you note such signs, provide the following symptomatic and supportive treatment, as ordered:
- To reverse anticholinergic symptoms in an adult, give 0.5 to 2 mg of physostigmine I.V. at a rate of no more than 1 mg/minute. The total dose shouldn't exceed 5 mg. Or give 0.5 mg to 2 mg of neostigmine I.V. or I.M. every 2 to 3 hours as needed.
- To control excitement or delirium, administer a short-acting barbiturate, such as thiopental.
- To help restore blood pressure, administer norepinephrine by I.V. infusion.
- If the patient develops severe respiratory depression, you may need to initiate mechanical ventilation.
- To help ensure adequate hydration, give I.V. fluids.

If the patient receives glycopyrrolate within 24 hours of a gastric acid secretion test, the results will reflect the antagonized effects of pentagastrin. And in patients with hyperuricemia or gout, serum uric acid levels will be decreased.

Haloperidol, Haloperidol lactate

(Haldol)

Indicated for acute psychosis, haloperidol apparently achieves its antipsychotic effect by producing a strong postsynaptic blockade of do-

DOSAGE FINDER

Haloperidol: Indication and dosage

Treatment of acute psychosis

▶ For adults, give 2 to 5 mg I.M. initially. Repeat the dose at 1-hour intervals if necessary, or at 4- to 8-hour intervals if symptoms are controlled.

pamine receptors in the central nervous system (CNS). This action inhibits dopamine-mediated effects.

Haloperidol also produces both alpha and ganglionic blockade and counteracts histamine- and serotonin-mediated activity. Plus, the drug produces weak peripheral anticholinergic effects and antiemetic effects.

About 70% of an I.M. dose is absorbed in 30 minutes. Peak plasma levels occur in 30 to 45 minutes.

Haloperidol is widely distributed in the body, with high concentrations appearing in adipose tissue. Between 91% and 99% of the drug is protein-bound. Haloperidol is metabolized extensively by the liver. About 40% of a dose is excreted in urine within 5 days. About 15% is excreted in feces via the biliary tract. (See *Haloperidol: Indication and dosage.*)

Contraindications and cautions

Haloperidol is contraindicated for patients with a hypersensitivity to the drug, phenothiazines, or related compounds. The drug is also contraindicated for those with jaundice because haloperidol may impair liver function. Because the drug may cause agranulocytosis, it shouldn't be given to patients with blood dyscrasias and bone marrow depression.

Haloperidol also is contraindicated for patients in a coma or with brain damage or CNS depression because the drug would increase CNS depression, and for patients with Parkinson's disease because the drug would aggravate symptoms. Because of the drug's hypotensive and arrhythmogenic effects, it shouldn't be given to patients with circulatory collapse or cerebrovascular disease.

Haloperidol isn't recommended for children under age 3 because they're especially prone to the extrapyramidal adverse reactions of the drug.

Give haloperidol cautiously to patients with cardiac conditions, such as arrhythmias, congestive heart failure, angina pectoris, valvular disease, or heart block. Also use caution when giving the drug to patients with encephalitis, Reye's syndrome, a head injury, respiratory disease, seizure disorder, glaucoma, prostatic hyperplasia, urine retention, hepatic or renal dysfunction, pheochromocytoma, or hypocalcemia.

Haloperidol is classified as a pregnancy risk category C drug and should be given carefully to pregnant patients.

Preparation

Haloperidol is available in 1-ml ampules and disposable syringes and 10-ml multiple-dose vials in a concentration of 5 mg/ml. Store the drug between 59° and 86° F (15° and 30° C). Protect it from light and freezing. A slight yellowing that commonly occurs doesn't affect the drug's potency. Discard any markedly discolored haloperidol solutions.

Incompatibility

Haloperidol is incompatible with heparin.

Administration

- *I.M. injection:* Inject the ordered dose deep into the gluteal region using a 21G needle. Don't inject more than 3 ml at any one I.M. site.

Adverse reactions

- *Life-threatening:* agranulocytosis, arrhythmias, asystole, extrapyramidal symptoms (akathisia, dystonia, torticollis), hypersensitivity, jaundice, neuroleptic malignant syndrome, orthostatic hypotension.
- *Other:* anorexia, ***blurred vision,*** constipation, contact dermatitis from concentrate, diarrhea, dizziness, drowsiness, ***dry mouth,*** exacerbation of psychotic symptoms, ***extrapyramidal effects,*** gynecomastia, headache, hypermenorrhea, hyperprolactinemia, increased anginal pain, increased appetite or weight gain, increased intraocular pressure, insomnia, muscle necrosis at injection site, mydriasis, nausea, photosensitivity, sedation, tinnitus, urine retention, vomiting.

Interactions

- *Antiarrhythmic agents, including disopyramide and procainamide:* increased incidence of arrhythmias and conduction defects.
- *Atropine or other anticholinergic drugs, including antidepressants, antihistamines, antiparkinsonian agents, meperidine, monoamine oxidase inhibitors, and phenothiazines:* oversedation, paralytic ileus, visual changes, and severe constipation.
- *Beta blockers:* inhibition of haloperidol metabolism, increasing plasma levels and toxicity.
- *Bromocriptine:* antagonized therapeutic effect of bromocriptine on prolactin secretion.
- *Clonidine, guanabenz, guanadrel, guanethidine, methyldopa, and reserpine:* inhibited blood pressure response.
- *CNS depressants, including alcohol, analgesics, barbiturates, general and spinal anesthetics, narcotics, parenteral magnesium sulfate, and tranquilizers:* additive effects, such as oversedation, respiratory depression, and hypotension.
- *Dopamine:* reduced vasoconstrictive effect of high-dose dopamine.
- *Heavy smoking:* increased metabolism.
- *Levodopa:* decreased effectiveness and increased toxicity of levodopa (by dopamine blockade).
- *Lithium:* severe neurologic toxicity with an encephalitis-like syndrome and decreased therapeutic response to haloperidol.
- *Metrizamide:* increased risk of seizures.
- *Nitrates:* hypotension.
- *Phenobarbital:* pharmacokinetic alterations and subsequent decreased therapeutic response to haloperidol.
- *Phenytoin:* inhibited phenytoin metabolism and increased toxicity.
- *Propylthiouracil:* increased risk of agranulocytosis.
- *Sympathomimetics, including appetite suppressants, ephedrine (often found in nasal sprays), epinephrine, phenylephrine, and phenylpropanolamine:* decreased stimulatory and pressor effects.

Special considerations

Keep in mind that elderly patients usually require lower initial doses and more gradual dosage titration.

Don't withdraw the drug abruptly unless you must, or the patient may experience adverse reactions. But if you detect signs of an overdose, stop the drug and intervene appropriately. (See *Managing a haloperidol overdose,* page 92.) Also discontinue the drug immediately if any life-threatening adverse effects develop; if severe extrapyramidal symptoms occur after the dosage

EMERGENCY INTERVENTION

Managing a haloperidol overdose

You'll recognize a haloperidol overdose by the exaggerated adverse drug effects it produces. The most obvious finding is central nervous system depression, characterized by a deep sleep or possibly a coma. The patient also may exhibit hypotension or hypertension, extrapyramidal symptoms, agitation, seizures, arrhythmias, hypothermia or hyperthermia, and autonomic nervous system dysfunction. The patient's electrocardiogram may show a prolonged Q-T interval and torsades de pointes.

If your patient experiences an overdose, take the following actions, as ordered:

- Provide symptomatic and supportive treatment, focusing your efforts on maintaining his airway, vital signs, and fluid and electrolyte balance.
- Regulate the patient's body temperature as needed.
- Treat hypotension with I.V. fluids. Don't give epinephrine because it may cause paradoxical hypotension.
- Treat seizures with parenteral diazepam or barbiturates.
- Treat arrhythmias with parenteral phenytoin (1 mg/kg with the rate titrated to the patient's blood pressure).
- Treat extrapyramidal reactions with barbiturates, benztropine, or parenteral diphenhydramine.

has been lowered; and 48 hours before and 24 hours after myelography using metrizamide because of the risk of seizures.

Watch for signs of neuroleptic malignant syndrome, a rare but often fatal complication. Signs and symptoms include difficult or unusually rapid breathing, rapid or irregular pulse, high fever, a change in blood pressure, increased sweating, loss of bladder control, severe muscle stiffness, seizures, unusual tiredness or weakness, and unusually pale skin. The development of this syndrome isn't necessarily related to the length of drug use.

Keep in mind that haloperidol has the weakest sedative effect of all the antipsychotic drugs.

Haloperidol causes quinidine-like effects on an electrocardiogram.

Heparin calcium
(Calcilean)

Heparin sodium
(Hepalean)

The emergency indications for this anticoagulant include treating venous thrombosis, pulmonary embolism, and disseminated intravascular coagulation (DIC). Heparin works by potentiating the effects of antithrombin, thus inhibiting the conversion of fibrinogen to fibrin. The drug also inhibits the action of Factors IX, X, XI, and XII; inactivates fibrin-stabilizing factor; and prevents the formation of a stable fibrin clot. (See *How heparin alters the clotting mechanism,* page 94.) Heparin doesn't have a fibrinolytic action, so it can't dissolve existing clots. But it can be used along with thrombolytic therapy to prevent the formation of new thrombi.

The serum half-life averages 1 to 6 hours. Peak plasma levels remain steady with a continuous infusion.

Distributed in plasma with extensive protein binding, heparin doesn't cross the placenta. Apparently, the drug is partly metabolized in the liver but is mainly removed from circulation by the reticuloendothelial system. Heparin is excreted

DOSAGE FINDER

Heparin: Indications and dosages

The exact heparin dosage depends on the patient's weight, disease, hepatorenal function, and activated partial thromboplastin time (APTT). The following dosages are guidelines:

Treatment of venous thrombosis or pulmonary embolism

▶ For adults, first give 5,000 units as an I.V. bolus. Then give a continuous infusion of 20,000 to 40,000 units in 1,000 ml of 0.9% sodium chloride solution over 24 hours. Or give 10,000 units as an I.V. bolus, then give an intermittent infusion of 5,000 to 10,000 units every 4 to 6 hours. Or give 5,000 units as an I.V. bolus, then give 10,000 to 20,000 units S.C., followed by 8,000 to 10,000 units every 8 hours or 15,000 to 20,000 units every 12 hours or a dosage based on the coagulation tests.

▶ For children, first give 50 units/kg I.V. Then give 100 units/kg I.V. every 4 hours or a continuous infusion of 20,000 units/m² over 24 hours. Or give 100 units/kg initially, then give 50 to 100 units/kg every 4 hours.

Treatment of disseminated intravascular coagulation

▶ For adults, give 50 to 100 units/kg I.V. every 4 hours. Discontinue the drug after 4 to 8 hours if no improvement occurs.

▶ For children, give 25 to 50 units/kg I.V. every 4 hours. Discontinue the drug after 4 to 8 hours if no improvement occurs.

in urine both as unchanged drug and as metabolites. The drug doesn't appear in breast milk. (See *Heparin: Indications and dosages.*)

Contraindications and cautions

Heparin is contraindicated for patients with heparin hypersensitivity—except in life-threatening situations. The drug also is contraindicated for patients with uncontrollable bleeding (except when caused by DIC), for patients with severe thrombocytopenia because of possible exacerbation, and for patients with severe, uncontrolled hypertension because of the increased risk of cerebral hemorrhage.

Avoid using heparin if coagulation tests can't be performed regularly.

In neonates, avoid using commercially available heparin sodium injections and heparin lock flush solutions that contain benzyl alcohol. This preservative has caused death in premature infants.

Give heparin with extreme caution to patients with hemorrhage that can be controlled surgically or mechanically and to those at risk for hemorrhage because of surgery or GI conditions, such as ulcerative colitis. Also give the drug carefully to women over age 60 because the risk of hemorrhage is highest in this age-group, and to diabetic patients undergoing medical or dental procedures because of the risk of bleeding.

Give heparin cautiously to patients with a history of allergies because of a possible hypersensitivity reaction and to patients with mild hepatic disease because of the risk of toxicity. Because of possible hyperkalemia, give heparin cautiously to patients with hypoaldosteronism. Also give the drug cautiously to pa-

MECHANISM OF ACTION

How heparin alters the clotting mechanism

Normally, damage to the endothelium of a blood vessel sets in motion a chain of biochemical reactions, called the coagulation cascade, resulting in a clot. Heparin prevents clots from forming by accelerating the activity of antithrombin III, a circulating plasma protein that neutralizes the activity of thrombin and other proteins involved in the coagulation cascade. Heparin does this by acting on Factors II (prothrombin), V, IX, and X.

As illustrated, the coagulation cascade consists of intrinsic and extrinsic pathways. Activation of the intrinsic pathway begins when Factor XII comes in contact with collagen; activation of the extrinsic pathway, when tissue factor (or thromboplastin) acts on Factor VII. Both pathways ultimately activate Factor X. Coagulation then proceeds along a common pathway and ends with the formation of an insoluble fibrin clot at the injury site.

Normally, clot formation activates the body's fibrinolytic system to keep the clot from enlarging and to dissolve further clots as they form. But if the fibrinolytic system fails to work correctly, anticoagulant drugs, such as heparin, may be needed to reverse or head off the clotting mechanism.

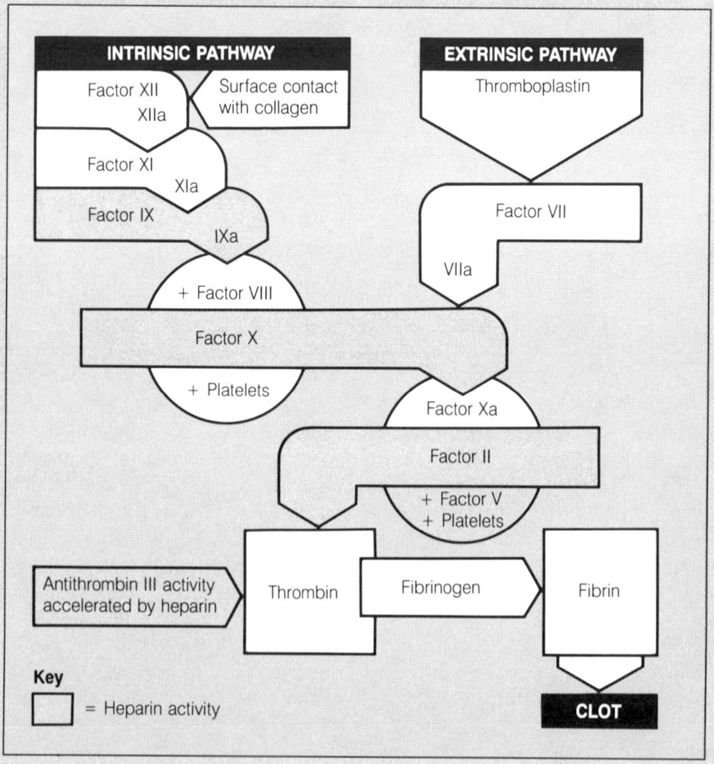

tients with renal insufficiency because of decreased renal clearance.

Classified as a pregnancy risk category C drug, heparin should be given cautiously to pregnant women—especially during the last trimester because of possible maternal hemorrhage. Give it cautiously postpartum for the same reason.

Preparation

Heparin is available in 0.5- and 1-ml ampules, vials, and prefilled syringes as well as in 1-ml, 2-ml, 5-ml, 10-ml, and 30-ml multidose vials, with concentrations ranging from 1,000 to 40,000 units/ml. Heparin flush concentrations range from 10 to 100 units/ml.

For an infusion, dilute the drug with 0.9% sodium chloride or another compatible solution, such as dextrose and Ringer's combination, dextrose 2.5% in water, dextrose 5% in water, fructose 10%, Ringer's injection, or lactated Ringer's, to achieve the prescribed concentration and volume. When diluting heparin, invert the container at least six times to ensure adequate mixing and prevent pooling of the heparin.

Store commercially available heparin preparations at room temperature. Avoid exposure to excessive heat. Don't freeze heparin solutions.

Before administration, inspect the heparin for particles and marked discoloration. Discard the solution if you find either. Slight discoloration doesn't affect the drug's potency.

Incompatibilities

Never mix another drug with heparin in a syringe. Never piggyback other drugs into an infusion line while a heparin infusion is running. Many antibiotics and other drugs inactivate heparin.

Heparin is incompatible with the following drugs: amikacin, ampicillin, codeine, dobutamine, erythromycin gluceptate, erythromycin lactobionate, gentamicin, haloperidol, hyaluronidase, hydrocortisone sodium succinate, hydroxyzine, kanamycin, levorphanol, meperidine, methadone, morphine, oxytetracycline, penicillin G sodium, polymyxin B, prochlorperazine edisylate, promethazine, 1/6 M sodium lactate, streptomycin, tetracycline, and vancomycin.

Heparin also may be incompatible with solutions containing a phosphate buffer, sodium carbonate, or sodium oxalate.

Administration

- *Direct injection:* Inject the diluted or undiluted drug through an intermittent infusion device or into I.V. tubing containing a free-flowing, compatible solution.
- *Intermittent infusion:* Using an infusion pump, administer the drug through a peripheral or central venous line over the prescribed time.
- *Continuous infusion:* Using an infusion pump, give the diluted heparin solution over a 24-hour period.
- *S.C. injection:* First, grasp some fatty tissue, such as that above the iliac crest, and hold it away from the deeper tissues. Using a small needle, inject the ordered dose deep into the fatty tissue. Don't aspirate to check for blood or massage the area after the injection. Apply gentle pressure over the injection site for 2 minutes. To prevent hematoma formation, rotate the injection sites.

Adverse reactions

- *Life-threatening:* acute thrombocytopenia, anaphylaxis, gasping syndrome in neonates, new thrombus formation (white clot syndrome), severe hemorrhage with excessive dosage.
- *Other:* allergic vasospastic reac-

EMERGENCY INTERVENTION

Managing a heparin overdose

Signs of an overdose include exaggerated effects of the drug and, sometimes, uncontrollable bleeding. For a mild overdose, withdraw the drug and monitor the patient.

If you note a more severe overdose, also give a 1% solution of protamine sulfate by slow infusion, as ordered. Typically, 1 mg of protamine sulfate will neutralize about 100 units of heparin. Within 30 minutes, only half as much protamine will neutralize the same amount of heparin. Don't infuse more than 50 mg of protamine in any 10-minute period.

tion, alopecia (delayed, transient), arthralgia, asthma (rare), chest pain, chills, cutaneous necrosis, fever, headache, hypertension, lacrimation, nausea, priapism, rebound hyperlipidemia, rhinitis, suppressed aldosterone synthesis and renal function, urticaria, vomiting.

Interactions

- *Antihistamines, cardiac glycosides, nicotine, tetracyclines:* diminished anticoagulant effect.
- *Aspirin, chloroquine, dextran, dipyridamole, hydrochloroquine, ibuprofen and other nonsteroidal anti-inflammatory drugs, indomethacin, penicillins (in high doses), phenylbutazone:* impaired platelet aggregation and possible heightened risk of bleeding.
- *Cefamandole, cefoperazone, moxalactam, plicamycin:* possible platelet inhibition or damage and enhanced risk of bleeding.
- *Corticosteroids, corticotropin, insulin:* possible antagonized action.
- *Coumarin or indanedione anticoagulants:* possible prolonged prothrombin time (PT).
- *Dihydroergotamine mesylate:* potentiated heparin effects.
- *Nitroglycerin I.V.:* possible diminished heparin effects.
- *Probenecid:* possible increased and prolonged anticoagulant effect.
- *Streptokinase, urokinase:* heightened risk of hemorrhage.

Special considerations

Keep in mind that some preparations contain benzyl alcohol.

Give all doses on time. If the infusion rate falls behind, don't increase it to catch up. If the solution runs out, restart the infusion as soon as possible, and administer a bolus dose immediately, if necessary.

Limit or eliminate I.M. injections for patients receiving heparin therapy. This reduces the risk of hematoma formation and bleeding into I.M. injection sites.

Monitor the patient for bleeding, which may occur at any site and is often difficult to detect. Regularly inspect the skin and I.V. and wound sites, test all exudate for blood, and promote safety. Teach the patient to recognize and report signs and symptoms of bleeding. Frequently monitor hematocrit and check stools for occult blood to detect asymptomatic bleeding. Major bleeding episodes occur more frequently with intermittent infusions than with continuous infusions. Uncontrollable bleeding and exaggerated drug effects may indicate an overdose. Keep in mind that hemodialysis doesn't remove the drug. (See *Managing a heparin overdose.*)

Frequently monitor the patient's platelet count and coagulation tests, such as PT, activated partial thromboplastin time (APTT), and activated clotting time (ACT). The therapeutic range for APTT is 1½ to 2½ times the control value; for ACT, 2 to 3 times the control value.

You can draw blood for an APTT 8 hours after starting continuous I.V. heparin therapy. Never draw blood for an APTT from the I.V. tubing used for the heparin infusion or from the vein receiving the infusion because the results will be falsely elevated. Always draw blood from the opposite arm. With intermittent I.V. therapy, draw blood ½ hour before the next scheduled dose to avoid falsely elevated results.

Use caution when transfusing blood collected in heparin sodium and later converted to acid-citrate-dextrose blood; it may alter clotting.

If you detect acute adrenal hemorrhage and insufficiency, discontinue the heparin, give I.V. corticosteroids, and draw samples for plasma cortisol determinations. If white clot syndrome or severe thrombocytopenia occurs, promptly discontinue the heparin and substitute a coumarin anticoagulant, as ordered.

Heparin affects many diagnostic tests. Partial pressure of carbon dioxide ($PaCO_2$) and bicarbonate concentration measurements will be inaccurate as will base excess if heparin makes up 10% or more of the sample. Also, ACT, APTT, plasma recalcification time, PT, thrombin time, and whole blood clotting times will be prolonged.

Levels of free fatty acids; serum alkaline phosphatase; bilirubin; lactate dehydrogenase; aspartate aminotransferase (AST), formerly SGOT; and alanine aminotransferase (ALT), formerly SGPT, may be elevated. Serum cholesterol and triglyceride levels may be reduced. Serum thyroxine levels will be elevated if competitive protein-binding methods are used. Tests for ^{125}I fibrinogen uptake will be false-negative; tests for sulfobromophthalein will be false-positive.

Hydralazine hydrochloride

(Apresoline)

Indicated for the emergency treatment of hypertension and pregnancy-induced hypertension, hydralazine hydrochloride—a phthalazine-derivative antihypertensive—directly relaxes arteriolar smooth muscle, reducing peripheral vascular resistance. It also increases heart rate and cardiac output, possibly as a compensatory response to the reduced peripheral resistance. Hydralazine has little effect on the veins. (See *Hydralazine's cardiovascular effects,* page 99.)

The drug takes effect in 10 to 20 minutes. The duration of action lasts 3 to 8 hours.

Distributed throughout the body tissues, hydralazine is most concentrated in the plasma, liver, kidneys, and arterial walls and is least concentrated in the heart, lungs, brain, muscle, and fat. About 85% of the drug binds to plasma proteins. Hydralazine crosses the placenta. Metabolized in the liver and GI tract mucosa by acetylation, hydroxylation, and conjugation, hydralazine is rapidly removed in urine—primarily as metabolites, which have no therapeutic effect. Small amounts appear in breast milk. (See *Hydralazine: Indications and dosages,* page 98.)

Contraindications and cautions

Hydralazine is contraindicated for patients with a known hypersensitivity to the drug. It's also contraindicated for patients with dissecting aortic aneurysm and rheumatic disease affecting the mitral valve because the drug may exacerbate

DOSAGE FINDER

Hydralazine: Indications and dosages

Treatment of hypertension

▶ For adults, give 10 to 20 mg I.V. or 20 to 40 mg I.M., as needed, usually every 4 to 6 hours.

▶ For children, give 1.7 to 3.5 mg/kg I.V. or I.M. every 4 to 6 hours. Don't exceed the maximum initial dose of 20 mg.

Treatment of pregnancy-induced hypertension

▶ For adults, give 5 mg I.V. or I.M. initially, then 5 to 10 mg every 20 to 30 minutes, as needed.

these conditions.

Give hydralazine cautiously to patients with coronary artery disease (CAD) because of possible myocardial ischemia, and to patients with cerebrovascular accident or increased intracranial pressure (ICP) because cerebral ischemia may occur or worsen. Also give hydralazine carefully and in reduced amounts to patients with renal impairment.

Give hydralazine, a pregnancy risk category C drug, carefully to pregnant patients.

Preparation

Hydralazine is available in 1-ml ampules with a concentration of 20 mg/ml. Store the ampules at room temperature and prevent freezing.

Avoid contact with metal syringe parts because discoloration and a change in the drug's stability may result. Prepare the drug just before use and discard any unused portion.

Incompatibilities

Avoid mixing hydralazine in the same container with another drug. Hydralazine is incompatible with these drugs and solutions: aminophylline, ampicillin, chlorothiazide, dextrose 10% in lactated Ringer's, dextrose 10% in 0.9% sodium chloride, edetate calcium disodium, ethacrynate sodium, fructose 10% in water, hydrocortisone sodium succinate, mephentermine, methohexital, nitroglycerin, phenobarbital, and verapamil.

Administration

- *Direct injection:* Inject the undiluted drug directly into the vein. Or inject it into an I.V. line as close to the insertion site as possible. Give the drug at a rate of 10 mg/minute.
- *I.M. injection:* Inject the ordered dose into any I.M. injection site.

Adverse reactions

- *Life-threatening:* anaphylaxis, cerebral ischemia (in patients with elevated ICP), myocardial ischemia.
- *Other:* ***angina pectoris,*** anorexia, anxiety, ***arrhythmias,*** arthralgia, asthenia, blood dyscrasias (agranulocytosis, leukopenia, thrombocytopenia with or without purpura), chills, conjunctivitis, constipation, depression, ***diarrhea,*** disorientation, dizziness, dyspnea, edema, eosinophilia, fever, flushing, ***headache,*** hypotension, lacrimation, lymphadenopathy, malaise, muscle cramps, myalgia, nasal congestion, ***nausea,*** orthostatic hypotension, ***palpitations,*** paralytic ileus, peripheral neuritis, pleuritic chest pain, pruritus, rash, ***sodium retention,*** splenomegaly, ***systemic lupus erythematosus (SLE)-like syndrome, tachycardia,*** tremor, urticaria, ***vomiting,*** weakness, ***weight gain.***

Interactions

- *Diazoxide, diuretics, monoamine oxidase inhibitors:* potentiated hypotensive effects.
- *Epinephrine:* orthostatic hypoten-

MECHANISM OF ACTION

Hydralazine's cardiovascular effects

Hydralazine's exact mechanism of action isn't known. But the drug probably interferes with normal calcium movement within arteriolar smooth muscle, causing vasodilation. Increased blood flow through the peripheral vessels results from the decreased peripheral vascular resistance. The drug also acts on renal vessels, increasing blood flow there as well.

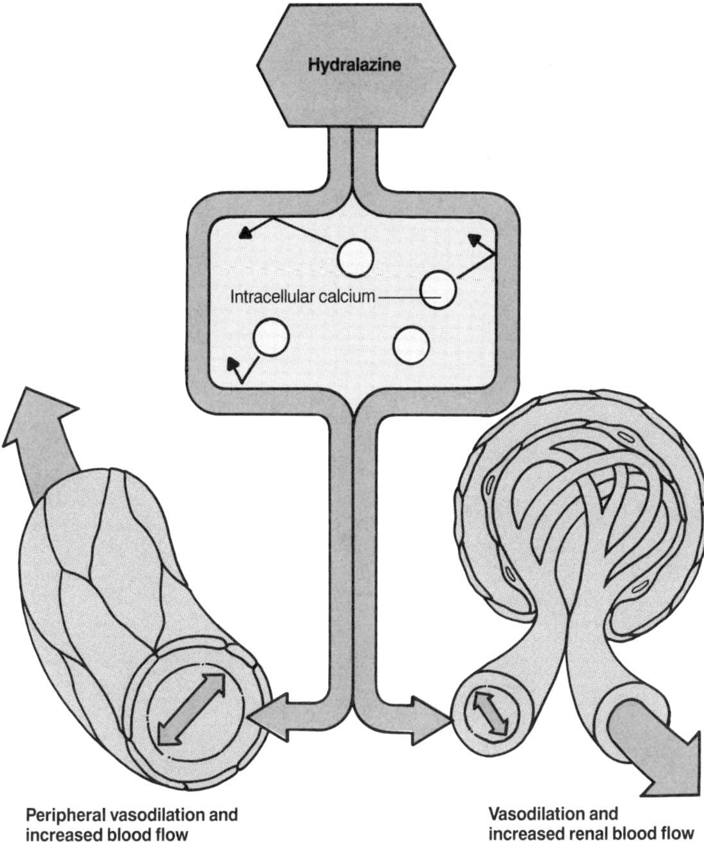

sion resulting from reduced pressor response.

- *Estrogens, nonsteroidal anti-inflammatory drugs (especially indomethacin), sympathomimetics:* antagonized hydralazine effects.

Special considerations

Using a beta-adrenergic blocker and a diuretic may prevent myocardial ischemia in CAD patients who must receive hydralazine.

To control sodium retention and weight gain, use a thiazide diuretic.

After an injection, check vital signs every 5 to 10 minutes for 1 hour, every hour for the next 2 hours, and then every 4 hours. Continuously monitor fluid and electrolyte status and the cardiac rhythm strip. Have the patient sit up slowly to prevent postural hypotension.

Tell the patient to report a headache or chest pain. Headache and tachycardia commonly occur; they can be minimized by starting with a small dose and gradually increasing the dosage. If they do occur, reducing the dosage or discontinuing the drug usually reverses them. Keep in mind that patients with slower acetylation run a higher risk of developing such reactions.

Monitor the patient's complete blood count, lupus erythematosus cell preparation, and antinuclear antibody titer before therapy and regularly during prolonged therapy to detect SLE-like syndrome. Discontinue the drug if this syndrome occurs. Also discontinue it if blood dyscrasias occur. Withdraw the drug gradually in patients with a markedly reduced blood pressure to avoid rebound hypertension.

Be alert for signs of a hydralazine overdose, including arrhythmias, headache, hypotension, shock, and tachycardia. As indicated, give volume expanders to support blood pressure and treat shock. If a vasopressor is needed, give one that doesn't aggravate arrhythmias.

This drug affects some diagnostic studies. The antinuclear antibody test and Coombs' test may falsely indicate a rheumatic disorder. Also, the hemoglobin level and red blood cell and white blood cell counts will be reduced.

Hydrocortisone sodium phosphate

(Hydrocortone Phosphate)

Hydrocortisone sodium succinate

(A-hydroCort, Solu-Cortef)

Hydrocortisone suspension

A naturally occurring corticosteroid, hydrocortisone affects virtually all body systems. Given systemically, it decreases inflammation by stabilizing leukocyte lysosomal membranes. It also suppresses the pituitary release of corticotropin, so the adrenal cortex stops secreting corticosteroids. Hydrocortisone is used to treat shock, severe inflammation, and adrenal insufficiency.

The drug takes effect rapidly. Its duration of action varies with the dosage and the length of therapy.

Rapidly dispersed to the muscles, liver, skin, intestines, and kidneys, hydrocortisone is bound to plasma proteins. The drug is metabolized in the liver, kidneys, and most tissues. The kidneys remove inactive metabolites; small amounts of unmetabolized drug are excreted in urine and negligible amounts in bile. The drug appears in breast milk. (See *Hydrocortisone: Indications and dosages.*)

Contraindications and cautions

Don't give this drug to patients with a known hypersensitivity to hydrocortisone or other corticosteroids.

Give hydrocortisone cautiously to patients with hypothyroidism or cirrhosis because an exaggerated response can occur. Also give it cautiously to patients with seizure disorders because of an increased risk of seizures; to patients with renal insufficiency because of a greater risk of edema; to patients with osteoporosis because of possible exacerbation; and to patients with a history of tuberculosis because of possible reactivation.

Because hydrocortisone may mask the signs of an infection, give it cautiously to patients with recent intestinal anastomosis or diverticulitis. Also use caution if the patient has nonspecific ulcerative colitis and is at risk for perforation, abscess, or other pyogenic infection.

Use the drug cautiously in patients with uncontrolled viral or bacterial infection; it may mask signs and increase susceptibility.

Give it cautiously to children because of possible bone growth retardation, pancreatitis and pancreatic destruction, and increased intracranial pressure (ICP). Increased ICP can cause headache, papilledema, oculomotor or abducens nerve paralysis, and vision loss.

Hydrocortisone, a pregnancy risk category C drug, should be given cautiously to pregnant patients.

Preparation

Hydrocortisone sodium phosphate comes in 2-ml and 10-ml multidose vials and 2-ml disposable syringes with concentrations of 50 mg/ml.

Hydrocortisone sodium succinate comes in 100-mg vials that require reconstitution with no more than 2 ml of bacteriostatic water or bacteriostatic 0.9% sodium chloride solution for injection. It also comes in 100-mg, 250-mg, 500-mg, and 1-g containers that require dilution with dextrose 5% in water, 0.9% sodium chloride solution, or dextrose 5% in 0.9% sodium chloride solution to a concentration of 0.1 to 1 mg/ml.

Hydrocortisone suspension comes in vials containing 25 or 50 mg/ml.

Store reconstituted hydrocortisone solutions at 77° F (25° C) or below for up to 3 days. Discard a solution that doesn't look clear or that's been stored for longer than 3 days.

DOSAGE FINDER

Hydrocortisone: Indications and dosages

Treatment of shock

▶ For adults, give 50 mg/kg of hydrocortisone sodium succinate I.M. or I.V.; repeat this dose every 4 hours or every 24 hours. Or give 0.5 to 2 g I.M. or I.V.; repeat this dose every 2 to 6 hours, as required.

Treatment of severe inflammation or adrenal insufficiency

▶ For adults, give 15 to 240 mg of hydrocortisone sodium phosphate I.V. or I.M. daily. Or give 100 to 500 mg of hydrocortisone sodium succinate I.V. or I.M., then repeat the dose every 2 to 10 hours, as needed. Or give 15 to 240 mg of hydrocortisone suspension I.M. daily.

▶ For children, give 0.16 to 1 mg/kg or 6 to 30 mg/m^2 of hydrocortisone sodium succinate or hydrocortisone sodium phosphate I.M. or I.V. Or give 186 to 240 mcg/kg or 10 to 12.5 mg/m^2 of hydrocortisone suspension I.M.

Incompatibilities

Hydrocortisone is incompatible with ampicillin and cephalothin. But because the reaction doesn't occur for 4 hours, you can infuse hydrocortisone along with these drugs.

Hydrocortisone is incompatible with the following drugs: amobarbital; bleomycin; colistimethate; diazepam; dimenhydrinate; diphenhydramine; doxorubicin; ephedrine; ergotamine; fructose 10% in 0.9% sodium chloride solution; heparin sodium; hydralazine; Ionosol B, D, or G with invert sugar 10%; kanamycin; metaraminol; methicillin; nafcillin; oxytetracycline; pentobarbital; phenobarbital; prochlorperazine; promethazine; secobarbital sodium; tetracycline; vancomycin; and vitamin B complex with C.

Administration

- *Direct injection:* Over a period of 30 seconds to several minutes, inject the drug directly into a vein or into an I.V. line containing a free-flowing, compatible solution.
- *Intermittent infusion:* Give the diluted solution over the prescribed duration.
- *Continuous infusion:* Infuse the diluted solution over 24 hours.
- *I.M. injection:* Inject the ordered dose deep into the gluteal muscle.

Adverse reactions

- *Life-threatening:* anaphylaxis, congestive heart failure.
- *Other:* acne, adrenal insufficiency, anorexia, cataracts, delayed wound healing, ***edema, euphoria,*** fever, fluid and electrolyte disturbances, glaucoma, headache, ***hyperglycemia,*** hypertension, ***hypokalemia,*** hypotension, infection, joint pain, lethargy, nausea, ***peptic ulcer,*** psychotic behavior, vomiting, weakness, weight loss.

Interactions

- *Alcohol, nonsteroidal anti-inflammatory drugs, ulcerogenic drugs:* heightened risk of GI ulcers.
- *Amphotericin B, carbonic anhydrase inhibitors, potassium-depleting diuretics, other potassium-depleting drugs:* possible enhanced potassium loss.
- *Anabolic steroids, androgens:* increased risk of edema.
- *Anticholinesterase drugs:* severe weakness in myasthenia gravis patients.
- *Anticoagulants, thrombolytics:* altered effects and increased risk of GI ulcers or hemorrhage.
- *Antithyroid drugs, thyroid hormones:* altered hydrocortisone removal. Adjust antithyroid or thyroid dosage.
- *Cardiac glycosides:* heightened risk of toxicity or arrhythmias.
- *Drugs and foods containing sodium:* hypernatremia.
- *Drugs that induce hepatic microsomal enzymes, such as phenytoin and barbiturates:* possible enhanced hydrocortisone metabolism.
- *Ephedrine:* increased hydrocortisone metabolism.
- *Estrogens, oral contraceptives:* enhanced therapeutic and toxic effects of hydrocortisone.
- *Immunosuppressants:* magnified risk of infection, lymphomas, and lymphoproliferative disorders.
- *Mexiletine:* reduced serum levels of mexiletine.
- *Mitotane:* suppressed adrenocortical function. Give higher hydrocortisone doses if necessary.
- *Nondepolarizing neuromuscular blocking drugs:* enhanced neuromuscular blockade.
- *Potassium-sparing diuretics, potassium supplements:* diminished hypokalemic effects of hydrocortisone.
- *Streptozocin:* heightened risk of hyperglycemia.
- *Toxoids, vaccines:* diminished response.

Special considerations

Find out if the patient is sensitive to sulfites or benzyl alcohol. Hydrocortone Phosphate contains sulfites, whereas A-hydroCort and Solu-Cortef contain benzyl alcohol.

Before long-term therapy, evaluate the patient's baseline electrocardiogram, blood pressure, chest and spinal X-rays, glucose tolerance, serum potassium levels, and hypothalamic and pituitary function.

As ordered, adjust a diabetic patient's antidiabetic drug dosage to compensate for hydrocortisone's hyperglycemic effects.

As needed, increase your patient's protein intake to keep pace with drug-induced protein catabolism.

During therapy, monitor the patient's weight, blood pressure, and serum electrolytes. Also be sure to monitor his mental status. Administer a phenothiazine or lithium, as ordered, for depression or psychotic behavior.

Don't halt short-term, high-dose therapy abruptly. Expect adrenal recovery to occur within 1 week.

This drug can affect diagnostic test results. Basophil, eosinophil, lymphocyte, and monocyte counts may decline. The corticotropin stimulation test may show decreased levels. Protein-bound iodine, plasma cortisol, and serum calcium, potassium, and thyroxine levels may be decreased. Also, urine 17-hydroxycorticosteroid and 17-ketosteroid levels may be diminished.

The polymorphonuclear leukocyte count may rise. Serum cholesterol, fatty acid, sodium, and uric acid levels may be elevated. Both serum and urine glucose levels may rise.

Platelet counts may be increased or decreased. Skin tests may show a suppressed reaction. The gonadorelin test will show altered results. And the nitroblue tetrazolium test may show false-negative results.

A radioactive iodine test will show a reduced uptake of ^{123}I or ^{131}I. Radionuclide brain and bone scans will show diminished uptake of sodium pertechnetate Tc 99m, and of technetium Tc 99m gluceptate, medronate, oxidronate, pentetate, or pyrophosphate.

Insulin, regular

(Humulin R, Novolin R, Regular, Regular Iletin I, Regular Iletin II, Velosulin, Velosulin Human)

Used to counteract the effects of severe ketoacidosis and diabetic coma, insulin – a naturally occurring hormone – aids the transport of glucose into cells. The drug also controls the storage and metabolism of carbohydrates, proteins, and fats in the liver, muscle, and adipose tissue. Plus, insulin stimulates protein synthesis and lipogenesis, inhibits lipolysis and the release of free fatty acids from adipose tissue, and promotes intracellular shifts of potassium and magnesium, temporarily reducing elevated serum levels of electrolytes. (See *How insulin aids glucose uptake,* page 105.)

Although customarily given S.C., insulin is administered I.V. in an emergency. It takes effect right after injection, and its action lasts 30 to 60 minutes.

Distribution occurs rapidly throughout extracellular fluids. The drug is rapidly metabolized, mainly in the liver and, to a lesser extent, in the kidneys and muscles, with only a small amount excreted unchanged in urine. (See *Insulin: Indications and dosages,* page 104.)

Contraindications and cautions

Avoid giving the beef or pork forms of insulin to patients hypersensitive to beef or pork.

Use insulin cautiously in pregnant patients. The drug has a pregnancy risk category of B.

Preparation

Insulin comes in concentrations of 40 and 100 units/ml in 10-ml vials.

DOSAGE FINDER

Insulin: Indications and dosages

Treatment of severe ketoacidosis and diabetic coma

▶ For adults, give 50 to 100 units of insulin by direct injection, usually along with the same S.C. dose. Base further doses on the patient's response and serum glucose level.

As an alternative, administer 2.4 to 7.2 units by direct injection initially, then give 2.4 to 7.2 units/hour by continuous infusion. Base the dosage on the patient's response and his serum glucose level.

▶ For children, give 0.5 to 1 unit/kg by direct injection initially, along with the same dose S.C. Base further doses on the child's response and serum glucose level.

As an alternative, give 0.1 unit/kg by direct injection initially, and then 0.1 unit/kg/hour by continuous infusion.

You can safely add it to most I.V. and total parenteral nutrition solutions.

Store insulin at 36° to 46° F (2.2° to 7.8° C), making sure it doesn't freeze. Discard any cloudy, discolored, or unusually viscous preparation. To mix the drug, roll the vial between your palms. Don't shake it, or the drug may froth. Use only a syringe calibrated for the specific insulin concentration ordered.

Incompatibilities
Insulin is incompatible with aminophylline, amobarbital sodium, chlorothiazide sodium, cytarabine, dobutamine hydrochloride, methylprednisolone sodium succinate, pentobarbital sodium, phenobarbital sodium, phenytoin sodium, secobarbital sodium, sodium bicarbonate, and thiopental sodium.

Administration
- *Direct injection:* Inject the drug at the ordered rate directly into a vein, through an intermittent infusion device, or into an I.V. line close to the I.V. site.
- *Continuous infusion:* Infuse the drug diluted in 0.9% sodium chloride solution at a rate sufficient to reverse ketoacidosis.
- *S.C. injection:* Inject the ordered dose into any S.C. site.

Adverse reactions
- *Life-threatening:* hypoglycemia.
- *Other:* anxiety, aphasia, blurred vision, chills, cold sweats, concentration difficulty, confusion, cool and pale skin, drowsiness, excessive hunger, fatigue, headache, irritability, maniacal behavior, nausea, pallor, paresthesia, personality changes, shallow breathing, tachycardia, tremor, unconsciousness, unusual tiredness or weakness, yawning.

Interactions
- *Adrenocorticosteroids, amphetamines, baclofen, corticotropin, danazol, dextrothyroxine, epinephrine, estrogen-containing oral contraceptives, estrogens, ethacrynic acid, furosemide, glucagon, and glucocorticoids:* decreased hypoglycemic effects, requiring a dosage adjustment of insulin.
- *Alcohol, anabolic steroids, androgens, disopyramide, guanethidine, and monoamine oxidase inhibitors:* increased hypoglycemic effect of insulin.
- *Appetite suppressants:* alteration in serum glucose levels.
- *Beta-adrenergic blockers including propranolol:* increased risk of hypoglycemia or hyperglycemia.
- *Carbonic anhydrase inhibitors:* reduced hypoglycemic response.
- *Molindone, phenytoin, thiazide-like*

MECHANISM OF ACTION

How insulin aids glucose uptake

Normally produced by the beta cells of the pancreas, insulin binds to receptors on the surface of a target cell. There, it helps transport glucose across the cell membrane. How the cell uses the glucose isn't known.

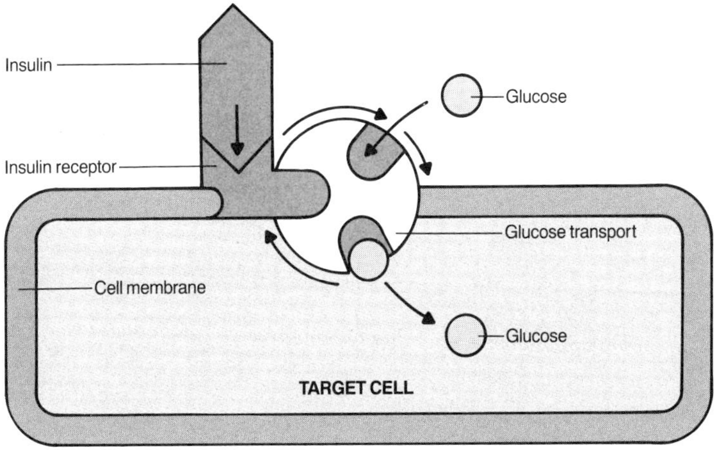

diuretics, thiazides, thyroid hormones, and triamterene: enhanced hyperglycemic effects, requiring an adjustment of the patient's insulin dosage.
- *Nicotine resin complex and smoking deterrents such as lobeline sulfate:* increased effect of insulin.
- *Nonsteroidal anti-inflammatory drugs, oral antidiabetic agents, and large doses of salicylates:* increased hypoglycemic effect of insulin.
- *Parenteral diazoxide:* reversed hypoglycemic effect.

Special considerations

Because of insulin's short serum half-life, it's rarely given in a large single dose. The dosage will be adjusted according to the patient's clinical condition. Before administering insulin, obtain baseline serum and urine glucose and ketone levels. During therapy, monitor the patient for signs and symptoms of hypoglycemia. (See *Managing an insulin overdose,* page 106.) Also, check serum glucose levels every hour using a reflectance meter. And measure serum acetone or ketone levels every 1 to 2 hours.

Expect a patient with a high fever, hyperthyroidism, severe infection, or trauma—or one who has undergone or is about to undergo surgery—to need a larger dosage. A patient with diarrhea, hepatic or renal impairment, hypothyroidism, or nausea and vomiting may need a smaller dosage.

Insulin may reduce serum magnesium, phosphate, and potassium levels. So for a hyperkalemic patient, regular insulin may be added to a dextrose infusion to promote intracellular potassium shift.

EMERGENCY INTERVENTION

Managing an insulin overdose

An overdose of insulin causes hypoglycemia. Left untreated, severe hypoglycemia can cause irreversible brain damage. If you note such signs and symptoms as anxiety, blurred vision, changes in level of consciousness, chills, cold sweats, cool and pale skin, drowsiness, excessive hunger, headache, lethargy, nausea, shakiness, and tachycardia, take the following actions, as ordered:

- Give a conscious patient orange juice, sugar, or candy.
- If a patient develops severe hypoglycemia or lapses into a coma, administer 10 to 30 ml of dextrose 50% I.V. Or, as an alternative, you can give a patient with sufficient hepatic stores of glycogen 1 unit of glucagon.

Isoproterenol hydrochloride

(Isuprel)

A sympathomimetic amine, isoproterenol hydrochloride works as both a cardiac stimulant and a smooth-muscle relaxant. Acting on $beta_1$ receptors in the heart, isoproterenol produces positive chronotropic and inotropic effects that increase myocardial contractility, cardiac output, and systolic pressure. The drug's action on $beta_2$ receptors in vascular smooth muscle results in arteriolar dilation, which decreases peripheral vascular resistance and diastolic pressure. Isoproterenol also works on $beta_2$ receptors in the bronchi to relax bronchial smooth muscle. This relieves bronchospasm, increases vital capacity, reduces residual lung volume, and eases the passage of pulmonary secretions.

Isoproterenol is indicated for cardiac arrhythmias, including atropine-resistant, hemodynamically significant bradycardia and complete heart block after closure of a ventricular septal defect. The drug is also used to relieve bronchospasm and acute asthma. Plus, isoproterenol serves as an adjunct in the treatment of shock.

When administered by the I.V. or intracardiac route, isoproterenol starts working at once; when inhaled, it works in 2 to 5 minutes. The drug's duration of action is less than an hour when given by the I.V. or intracardiac route, and less than 2 hours when inhaled.

The drug is distributed throughout the body and metabolized in the liver, lungs, and other tissues by the enzyme catechol-O methyltransferase. Distribution and metabolism occur more rapidly and extensively in children than adults. Isoproterenol is excreted in urine. About 40% to 50% of an I.V. dose and 5% to 15% of an inhaled dose is excreted unchanged; the rest, as the metabolite 3-O-methylisoproterenol. In children, small amounts of unidentified metabolites also appear in feces. The body excretes about 75% of the drug within 15 hours. Whether the drug appears in breast milk isn't known. (See *Isoproterenol: Indications and dosages*.)

Contraindications and cautions

Don't give isoproterenol to patients with a known hypersensitivity to it or other sympathomimetics, or to patients with tachyarrhythmias, especially ventricular tachycardia and arrhythmias that require increased inotropic activity. The drug is also contraindicated for patients with un-

DOSAGE FINDER

Isoproterenol: Indications and dosages

Treatment of cardiac arrhythmias and cardiac standstill

▶ For adults, give an I.V. bolus of 0.02 to 0.06 mg. Then give either 0.01 to 0.02 mg I.V., as needed, or start a continuous infusion of 5 mcg/minute and titrate the infusion to the patient's response. The rate may range from 2 to 20 mcg/minute.

Alternatively, give 0.2 mg I.M. or S.C. initially. Then give 0.02 to 1 mg I.M. or 0.15 to 0.2 mg S.C., as needed. In extreme cases, the doctor may give an intracardiac injection of 0.02 mg (0.1 ml of a 1:5,000 dilution).

▶ For children, administer half the adult dosage.

Immediate temporary control of atropine-resistant, hemodynamically significant bradycardia

▶ For adults, give a continuous infusion of 2 to 10 mcg/minute titrated to the patient's response.

▶ For children, give a continuous infusion of 0.1 mcg/kg/minute titrated to the patient's response. Don't exceed 1 mcg/kg/minute.

Treatment of complete heart block after closure of ventricular septal defect

▶ For adults, give an I.V. bolus of 0.04 to 0.06 mg (2 to 3 ml of a 1:50,000 dilution).

▶ For children, give an I.V. bolus of 0.01 to 0.03 mg (0.5 to 1.5 ml of a 1:50,000 dilution).

Relief of bronchospasm in acute asthma

▶ For adults and children, administer one inhalation initially with a metered-dose inhaler. Repeat the dose after 1 to 5 minutes if necessary, up to six inhalations daily.

With a hand-held nebulizer, give 5 to 15 deep inhalations of a 0.5% solution. Repeat as needed after 5 to 10 minutes, up to five times daily. Or, give 3 to 7 inhalations of a 1% solution. Repeat once in 5 to 10 minutes if needed, up to five times daily.

With a compressed air nebulizer or an intermittent positive pressure breathing (IPPB) device, give 6 to 12 inhalations of a 0.025% nebulized solution. Repeat at 15-minutes intervals to a maximum of three treatments per attack. Don't exceed eight treatments in 24 hours.

Relief of bronchospasm in chronic obstructive pulmonary disease

▶ For adults and children, give 5 to 15 deep inhalations of a 0.5% solution with a hand-held nebulizer—or 3 to 7 deep inhalations of a 1% solution—no more than every 3 to 4 hours.

With a compressed air nebulizer, give 6 to 12 inhalations of a 0.025% nebulized solution. Repeat at 15-minute intervals to a maximum of three treatments per attack. Don't exceed eight treatments in 24 hours.

▶ For adults, give 2 ml of a 0.125% solution or 2.5 ml of a 0.1% solution with an IPPB device. Deliver the dose over 10 to 20 minutes, and repeat the dose if needed up to five times daily.

▶ For children, give 2 ml of a 0.0625% solution or 2.5 ml of a 0.05% solution with an IPPB device over 10 to 15 minutes. Repeat the dose as necessary up to five times daily.

Relief of acute asthma unresponsive to inhalation therapy and control of bronchospasm during anesthesia

▶ For adults, give an I.V. bolus of 0.01 to 0.02 mg (0.5 to 1 ml of a 1:50,000 dilution). Repeat as needed.

Adjunctive treatment of shock

▶ For adults and children, give a continuous infusion of 0.5 to 5 mcg/minute titrated to the patient's response.

Drip rates for isoproterenol infusions

A doctor's order for isoproterenol may be in micrograms per minute or micrograms per kilograms per minute. Using this chart, you can convert either to the drip rate you need for a standard concentration of 2 mg in 500 ml (4 mcg/ml).

For an order in micrograms per minute, use the first column of the chart on this page. Find the number that's closest to the ordered number of micrograms per minute. Then look to the right to find the appropriate drip rate. For example, for an order of 2 mcg/minute, you'd scan down the first column to the line for 2.0 mcg/minute. Looking to the right, you'd find the corresponding drip rate is 30 microdrops/minute.

PRESCRIBED DOSAGE (mcg/minute)	DRIP RATE (microdrops/ minute)	PATIENT'S WEIGHT kg 35 / lb 77	kg 40 / lb 88	kg 45 / lb 99	kg 50 / lb 110	kg 55 / lb 121	kg 60 / lb 132	kg 65 / lb 143
		PRESCRIBED DOSAGE (mcg/kg/minute)						
0.333	5	0.010	0.008	0.007	0.007	0.006	0.006	0.005
0.667	10	0.019	0.017	0.015	0.013	0.012	0.011	0.010
1.000	15	0.029	0.025	0.022	0.020	0.018	0.017	0.015
1.333	20	0.038	0.033	0.030	0.027	0.024	0.022	0.021
1.667	25	0.048	0.042	0.037	0.033	0.030	0.028	0.026
2.000	30	0.057	0.050	0.044	0.040	0.036	0.033	0.031
2.333	35	0.067	0.058	0.052	0.047	0.042	0.039	0.036
2.667	40	0.076	0.067	0.059	0.053	0.048	0.044	0.041
3.000	45	0.086	0.075	0.067	0.060	0.055	0.050	0.046
3.333	50	0.095	0.083	0.074	0.067	0.061	0.056	0.051
3.667	55	0.105	0.092	0.081	0.073	0.067	0.061	0.056
4.000	60	0.114	0.100	0.089	0.080	0.073	0.067	0.062
4.333	65	0.124	0.108	0.096	0.087	0.079	0.072	0.067
4.667	70	0.133	0.117	0.104	0.093	0.085	0.078	0.072
5.000	75	0.143	0.125	0.111	0.100	0.091	0.083	0.077
5.333	80	0.152	0.133	0.119	0.107	0.097	0.089	0.082
5.667	85	0.162	0.142	0.126	0.113	0.103	0.094	0.087
6.000	90	0.171	0.150	0.133	0.120	0.109	0.100	0.092
6.333	95	0.181	0.158	0.141	0.127	0.115	0.106	0.097
6.667	100	0.190	0.167	0.148	0.133	0.121	0.111	0.103

corrected hypoxia, acidosis, hypokalemia, hyperkalemia, or hypercapnia because its effects may be reduced or the risk of adverse reactions increased.

Use the drug cautiously in elderly patients and in those with cardiovascular disease, hyperthyroidism, or cardiac glycoside-induced tachycardia because of the increased risk of adverse cardiovascular effects. In patients with Parkinson's disease, the drug may temporarily worsen symptoms, and in those with diabetes mellitus, the dosage of insulin or a hypoglycemic agent may need adjustment. Use the drug cautiously in those with a hypersensitivity to sulfites because some preparations contain a sulfite preservative.

Administer this pregnancy risk category C drug carefully to pregnant patients.

Preparation

Isoproterenol comes in a dilution of

For an order in micrograms per kilograms per minute, first find the number closest to the patient's weight (in kilograms or pounds). Follow that column down until you find the number closest to the prescribed dosage. Follow that line across to the drip rate column to find the appropriate rate. For example, if a doctor ordered 0.05 mcg/kg/minute for a 230-lb patient, you'd locate the column for 231 lb. Then you'd follow that column down to the line for 0.051 mcg/kg/minute. Finally, you'd follow this line across to the left and learn that you need a drip rate of 80 microdrops/minute.

DRIP RATE (microdrops/minute)	PATIENT'S WEIGHT								
kg	70	75	80	85	90	95	100	105	110
lb	154	165	176	187	198	209	220	231	242
	PRESCRIBED DOSAGE (mcg/kg/minute)								
5	0.005	0.004	0.004	0.004	0.004	0.004	0.003	0.003	0.003
10	0.010	0.009	0.008	0.008	0.007	0.007	0.007	0.006	0.006
15	0.014	0.013	0.013	0.012	0.011	0.011	0.010	0.010	0.009
20	0.019	0.018	0.017	0.016	0.015	0.014	0.013	0.013	0.012
25	0.024	0.022	0.021	0.020	0.019	0.018	0.017	0.016	0.015
30	0.029	0.027	0.025	0.024	0.022	0.021	0.020	0.019	0.018
35	0.033	0.031	0.029	0.027	0.026	0.025	0.023	0.022	0.021
40	0.038	0.036	0.033	0.031	0.030	0.028	0.027	0.025	0.024
45	0.043	0.040	0.038	0.035	0.033	0.032	0.030	0.029	0.027
50	0.048	0.044	0.042	0.039	0.037	0.035	0.033	0.032	0.030
55	0.052	0.049	0.046	0.043	0.041	0.039	0.037	0.035	0.033
60	0.057	0.053	0.050	0.047	0.044	0.042	0.040	0.038	0.036
65	0.062	0.058	0.054	0.051	0.048	0.046	0.043	0.041	0.039
70	0.067	0.062	0.058	0.055	0.052	0.049	0.047	0.044	0.042
75	0.071	0.067	0.063	0.059	0.056	0.053	0.050	0.048	0.045
80	0.076	0.071	0.067	0.063	0.059	0.056	0.053	0.051	0.048
85	0.081	0.076	0.071	0.067	0.063	0.060	0.057	0.054	0.052
90	0.086	0.080	0.075	0.071	0.067	0.063	0.060	0.057	0.055
95	0.090	0.084	0.079	0.075	0.070	0.067	0.063	0.060	0.058
100	0.095	0.089	0.083	0.078	0.074	0.070	0.067	0.063	0.061

1:5,000 in 1-ml (0.2-mg) and 5-ml (1-mg) ampules, and in 5-ml (1-mg) and 10-ml (2-mg) vials. Keep the drug in an opaque container to protect it from light, and store it in a cool place.

To prepare a direct I.V. or intracardiac injection, add 1 ml of the drug to 10 ml of 0.9% sodium chloride solution or dextrose 5% in water (D_5W) to yield a 1:50,000 dilution (20 mcg/ml). For an infusion, dilute 10 ml (2 mg) of isoproterenol with 500 ml of D_5W to yield a dilution of 1:250,000 (4 mcg/ml). (See *Drip rates for isoproterenol infusions.*) You can also combine the drug with lactated Ringer's solution and dextrose 5% in lactated Ringer's solution.

Don't use the drug if it appears pink or brown or if a precipitate forms.

Incompatibilities

Isoproterenol is incompatible with

alkalies, aminophylline, metals, and sodium bicarbonate.

Administration

- *Direct injection:* Inject the diluted solution (1:50,000) directly into a vein or into an I.V. line of a free-flowing, compatible solution.
- *Continuous infusion:* Using an infusion pump, administer the diluted drug (1:250,000) at the ordered rate.
- *I.M. injection:* Inject the ordered dose into any I.M. site.
- *S.C. injection:* Inject the ordered dose into any S.C. site.
- *Intracardiac injection:* The doctor will inject the diluted drug (1:50,000) directly into the ventricle.
- *Inhalation:* Use a hand-held nebulizer, a compressed air or oxygen nebulizer, an intermittent positive pressure breathing device, or a metered-dose inhaler to deliver the ordered dose.

Adverse reactions

- *Life-threatening:* anaphylaxis, arrhythmias.
- *Other:* ***angina,*** anxiety, asthenia, ***blood pressure that rises and then falls,*** diaphoresis, dizziness, excitement, fear, flushed face, ***headache,*** hypotension, insomnia, light-headedness, nausea, ***palpitations,*** restlessness, ***tachycardia,*** tinnitus, trembling, vomiting, weakness.

Interactions

- *Antihypertensives:* reduced effects of these drugs.
- *Beta blockers:* inhibited effects of both drugs.
- *Cardiac glycosides:* increased risk of arrhythmias.
- *Central nervous system (CNS) stimulants:* excessive stimulation.
- *Epinephrine and other sympathomimetics:* severe arrhythmias. Administer isoproterenol and sympathomimetics at least 4 hours apart.
- *Inhalation hydrocarbon anesthetics:* severe arrhythmias.
- *Levodopa:* arrhythmias.
- *Monoamine oxidase inhibitors and tricyclic antidepressants:* arrhythmias, severe hypertension, and tachycardia.
- *Nitrates:* reduced effects of these drugs.
- *Oxytocic drugs:* severe persistent hypertension and risk of cerebral hemorrhage.
- *Thyroid hormones:* increased effects of both drugs and increased risk of coronary insufficiency in patients with coronary artery disease.
- *Xanthines:* risk of enhanced CNS effects.

Special considerations

Before administering isoproterenol, check the patient's peripheral vascular beds. If you detect dilation, the drug won't be useful. Make sure a patient in shock has received fluid replacement to treat volume deficit before he receives isoproterenol. And before giving the drug to an elderly patient, double-check the dosage. Usually, he'll need less drug than a younger adult.

During therapy, monitor the bicarbonate level, the partial pressure of carbon dioxide, and the pH of the patient's blood. Also observe him for ventilation-perfusion abnormalities because the drug reduces arterial oxygen tension even as breathing improves.

Closely monitor the cardiac rhythm strip of a patient in cardiac arrest or shock or a patient with arrhythmias, including heart block. For a patient in shock, also monitor central venous pressure, heart rate, blood pressure, and urine output.

Adjust the infusion rate according

to the patient's heart rate and blood pressure. If an adult's heart rate exceeds 110 beats per minute, you may need to decrease the infusion rate or temporarily stop the infusion. (The heart rate will be higher in children.) Doses that increase the heart rate to more than 130 beats per minute may induce ventricular arrhythmias. You should see a systolic blood pressure drop in a patient receiving a high dosage of the drug because of the marked reduction in peripheral vascular resistance isoproterenol causes. If blood pressure rises, temporarily stop the infusion.

You should also stop the infusion until the patient's condition stabilizes if you note severe and persistent chest pain, an irregular heartbeat, headache, or dizziness.

If ordered, give a sedative to reduce CNS stimulation.

Isoproterenol increases serum bilirubin, urine catecholamines, and vanillylmandelic acid levels.

Labetalol hydrochloride

(Normodyne, Trandate)

Indicated for severe hypertension and hypertensive crisis, labetalol hydrochloride competitively blocks the stimulation of myocardial beta$_1$ receptors, bronchial beta$_2$ receptors, and alpha and beta$_2$ receptors of the vascular smooth muscle. The drug, which also depresses renin secretion, reduces blood pressure in 5 to 10 minutes.

Labetalol has an onset of action of 2 to 5 minutes. The duration of action lasts from 2 to 4 hours.

The drug is distributed rapidly throughout the extravascular space, with the highest concentrations occurring in the lungs, liver, and kidneys. Distribution declines in patients with hepatic impairment. About 50% of the drug binds to plasma proteins, and a small amount crosses the placenta and blood-brain barrier. In the liver, labetalol undergoes conjugation, emerging as glucuronide metabolites such as O-alkylglucuronide. From 55% to 60% of the drug is eliminated in urine within 24 hours; within 4 days, another 30% passes from the body in feces. Less than 5% of the drug is excreted unchanged. A small amount is excreted in breast milk. (See *Labetalol: Indications and dosages.*)

DOSAGE FINDER

Labetalol: Indications and dosages

Treatment of severe hypertension and hypertensive crisis

▶ For adults, give 20 mg by direct injection, followed by 20 to 80 mg every 10 minutes. As an alternative, start an infusion of 2 mg/minute, and titrate the dosage to the patient's response. When the patient's blood pressure reaches the desired level, stop the infusion. If necessary, repeat the infusion in 6 to 8 hours.

For either administration method, don't exceed a total dose of 300 mg.

Contraindications and cautions

Labetalol is contraindicated for patients with a known hypersensitivity to it. Don't give the drug to patients with second- or third-degree heart block, overt congestive heart failure, cardiac ischemia, cardiogenic shock, or severe bradycardia because of the risk of further myocardial depression. The drug is also contraindicated for those with asthma or bronchospastic disease because it can inhibit bronchodilation. Don't give this drug to children.

Use labetalol cautiously in patients with diabetes mellitus controlled by a hypoglycemic agent because it can mask signs of hypoglycemia, and in those with myasthenia gravis, depression, or psoriasis because the drug may worsen these conditions. Also give it carefully to those with pheochromocytoma because of the risk of paradoxical hypertension, and to those with hepatic impairment because of the increased risk of toxicity.

Use caution when giving this pregnancy risk category C drug to a pregnant woman.

Preparation

Labetalol is available as a clear, colorless to light yellow solution in 20-ml ampules that contain 5 mg/ml. Store the undiluted drug at room temperature.

To prepare a concentration of 1 mg/ml for infusion, add two 20-ml ampules to 160 ml of dextrose 5% in water, 0.9% sodium chloride solution, dextrose 2.5% in 0.45% sodium chloride solution, dextrose 5% in lactated Ringer's solution, or lactated Ringer's solution. For a concentration of 2 mg/3 ml, increase the diluent to 260 ml. The solutions will remain stable for at least 24 hours at room temperature or when refrigerated.

Incompatibility

Labetalol is incompatible with sodium bicarbonate.

Administration

- *Direct injection:* Over a 2-minute period, inject the drug directly into a vein or into an I.V. line with a free-flowing, compatible solution.
- *Continuous infusion:* Initially administer 2 mg/minute, then titrate the dose until the patient's blood pressure reaches the desired level.

Adverse reactions

- *Life-threatening:* agranulocytosis, intensified atrioventricular block, severe hypotension.
- *Other:* atrioventricular conduction delay, bradycardia, bronchospasm, chest pain, decreased libido, diaphoresis, diarrhea, ***dizziness,*** dyspepsia, dyspnea, facial erythema, fatigue, fever, headache, impotence, increased airway resistance, infusion site pain, laryngospasm, lethargy, leukopenia, memory loss, mild hyperglycemia, muscle cramps, nasal congestion, nausea, ***orthostatic hypotension,*** Peyronie's disease, pruritus, rash, reversible alopecia, skin or scalp tingling, systemic lupus erythematosus-like illness, urinary difficulty, urine retention, ventricular arrhythmias, vivid dreams, vomiting, wheezing.

Interactions

- *Antihypertensives:* potentiated antihypertensive effects.
- *Anti-inflammatory drugs:* reduced effects of labetalol.
- *Cardiac glycosides:* extreme bradycardia.
- *Estrogens:* reduced antihypertensive effect.
- *Halothane anesthetics:* synergistic hypotensive effects.
- *Insulin and oral hypoglycemics:* altered dosage requirements of these drugs.
- *Lidocaine:* possible prolonged lidocaine metabolism and increased risk of toxicity.
- *Monoamine oxidase inhibitors:* severe hypertension for up to 2 weeks after this drug has been discontinued.
- *Nitroglycerin:* reduced reflex tachycardia and potentiated hypotension.

EMERGENCY INTERVENTION

Managing a labetalol overdose

An overdose of labetalol can cause severe bradycardia and hypotension, premature ventricular contractions (PVCs), heart failure, bronchospasm, and seizures.

If your patient develops signs of an overdose, stop the drug and provide the following symptomatic treatment, as ordered:

- For severe bradycardia and hypotension, administer atropine. If the patient doesn't respond, cautiously administer isoproterenol or dobutamine. He may need epinephrine or a temporary pacemaker.
- For PVCs, give him phenytoin or lidocaine.
- For heart failure, administer oxygen, digitalis, and a diuretic. The patient may also need fluids and a vasopressor such as epinephrine, norepinephrine, dopamine, or dobutamine.
- To relieve bronchospasm, give the patient a $beta_2$ agonist, such as isoproterenol or a theophylline derivative.
- To control seizures, give phenytoin.

- *Nondepolarizing neuromuscular blockers:* possible prolonged action of these drugs.
- *Phenothiazines:* increased serum levels of both drugs.
- *Phenoxybenzamine and phentolamine:* enhanced alpha-adrenergic blocking action.
- *Sympathomimetics and xanthine derivatives:* inactivation of these drugs and labetalol.

Special considerations

Before administering the drug, warn the patient that he may feel transient scalp tingling when therapy starts.

A patient who needs a high initial dose may experience severe hypotension, along with nausea. If the patient has severe renal impairment, he'll need a reduced dosage. Dialysis removes less than 1% of the drug.

During therapy, monitor blood pressure with the patient supine and adjust the dosage accordingly. Make sure his blood pressure doesn't drop too rapidly. A steady-state plasma level won't be achieved during the infusion because of the drug's short half-life. (See *Managing a labetalol overdose*.)

While monitoring the patient, you probably won't see a drop in heart rate or cardiac output as you might with other beta blockers. Keep in mind that labetalol masks the common signs of shock and hypoglycemia.

After discontinuing the infusion, keep the patient supine for 3 hours to prevent severe orthostatic hypotension. With the patient in this position, his blood pressure will eventually start to rise again. When it does, you should begin oral labetalol therapy.

Labetalol affects several laboratory tests. Blood urea nitrogen and serum creatinine levels will rise. Labetalol also falsely increases urine catecholamine levels when they're measured by nonspecific trihydroxyindole reaction. The antinuclear antibody test will show a positive titer, and radionuclide ventriculography may reveal bradycardia. Intraocular pressure may also be altered.

Lidocaine hydrochloride

(LidoPen, Xylocaine, Xylocard)

This Class Ib antiarrhythmic – a fast sodium channel blocker – suppresses ventricular arrhythmias. Lidocaine hydrochloride works by reducing electrical conduction in ischemic or injured cardiac muscle, especially in the His-Purkinje system. The drug achieves this effect without involving the autonomic nervous system or adversely affecting normal cardiac tissue or the sinoatrial or atrioventricular nodes. (See *How lidocaine suppresses ventricular arrhythmias.*)

Indications include the suppression of acute ventricular arrhythmias – premature ventricular contractions (PVCs) and ventricular tachycardia – associated with acute myocardial infarction (MI), digitalis toxicity, cardioversion, cardiac manipulation from trauma or surgery, or adverse effects of drugs. The drug is particularly useful in treating ventricular arrhythmias in the first 24 to 48 hours after an MI, when ischemic or injured tissue is most irritable. Lidocaine can also be used as a last resort in the treatment of status epilepticus.

The onset of action occurs within 45 to 90 seconds; the duration of action lasts 10 to 20 minutes. Lidocaine has an initial phase half-life of 7 to 30 minutes and a terminal phase half-life of 1½ to 2 hours.

The drug is distributed rapidly to the kidneys, lungs, liver, and heart, and more slowly to skeletal muscle and fat. It crosses the placenta and the blood-brain barrier. Between 60% and 80% binds to plasma proteins. About 90% is metabolized in the liver. The drug is excreted mainly in urine, primarily as metabolites; it's also excreted in breast milk. (See *Lidocaine: Indications and dosages.*)

Contraindications and cautions

Patients with a hypersensitivity to lidocaine or amidelike anesthetics shouldn't receive this drug. It's also contraindicated for patients with

DOSAGE FINDER

Lidocaine: Indications and dosages

Treatment of acute ventricular arrhythmias associated with acute myocardial infarction, digitalis toxicity, cardioversion, cardiac manipulation from trauma or surgery, or adverse effects of drugs

▶ For adults, administer 50 to 100 mg in an I.V. bolus or endotracheally. If the arrhythmias don't stop within 5 minutes, repeat the dose. Start a maintenance infusion of 20 to 50 mcg/kg/minute (1 to 4 mg/minute for a 155-lb [70-kg] adult). Don't administer more than 300 mg in 1 hour. In a patient with congestive heart failure or liver disease, don't exceed 30 mcg/kg/minute.

If you can't use the I.V. or endotracheal route, administer 300 mg (for a 155-lb adult) by I.M. injection initially. If necessary, repeat the dose in 60 to 90 minutes.

▶ For children, give 0.5 to 1 mg/kg in an I.V. bolus or endotracheally. Repeat the dose as necessary, and start an infusion of 10 to 50 mcg/kg/minute. Don't exceed a total dose of 5 mg/kg.

Treatment of status epilepticus unresponsive to all other measures

▶ For adults and children, administer an initial bolus of 1 mg/kg by direct injection. If the seizure doesn't stop after 2 minutes, administer another 0.5 mg/kg and start a maintenance infusion of 30 mcg/kg/minute.

MECHANISM OF ACTION

How lidocaine suppresses ventricular arrhythmias

Lidocaine works in injured or ischemic myocardial cells to retard sodium influx and restore cardiac rhythm. Normally, the ventricles contract in response to impulses from the sinoatrial (SA) node. But when tissue damage occurs in the ventricles, ischemic cells can create an ectopic pacemaker (shown directly below), which can trigger ventricular arrhythmias. How these arrhythmias develop at the cellular level—and how lidocaine suppresses them—is depicted in the two illustrations at the bottom of the page.

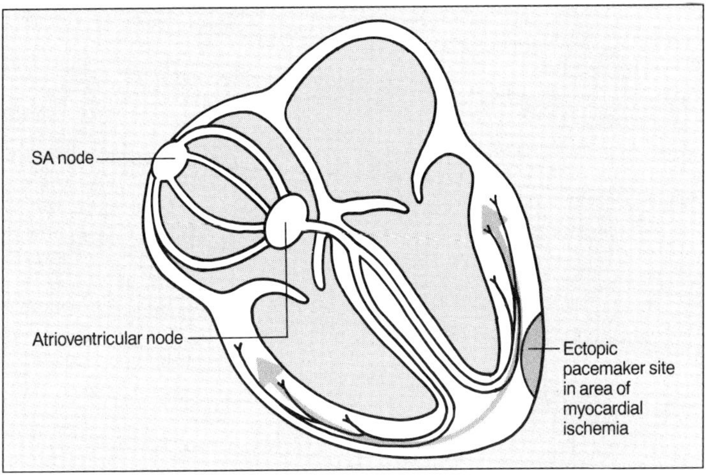

Ischemic myocardial cells allow a rapid infusion of sodium ions (Na^+). This causes the cells to depolarize much more quickly than normal and then begin firing spontaneously. The result: a ventricular arrhythmia.

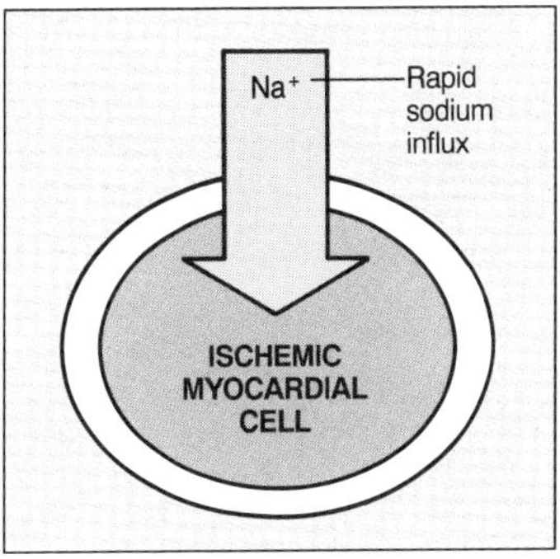

By slowing sodium's influx, lidocaine raises the cells' electrical stimulation threshold (EST). The increased EST prolongs depolarization in the ischemic cells and returns control to the SA node, the heart's main pacemaker.

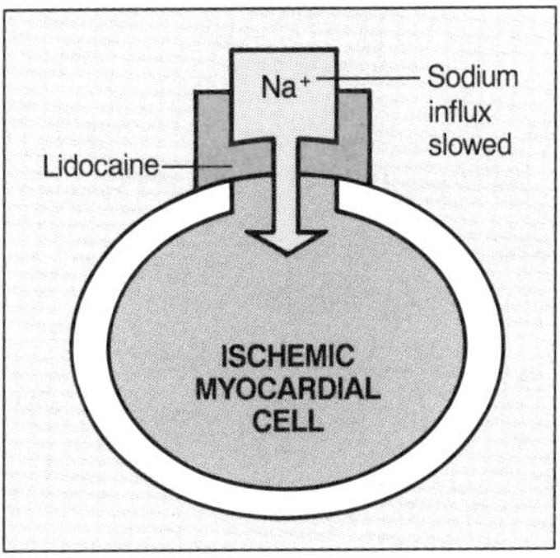

Adams-Stokes disease, Wolff-Parkinson-White syndrome, or second- or third-degree heart block.

Use the drug cautiously in patients with sinus bradycardia or incomplete heart block who haven't received isoproterenol or a pacemaker because lidocaine may increase PVCs and ventricular escape beats, leading to ventricular tachycardia. And because the drug may accumulate, give lidocaine cautiously to children, elderly patients, and patients with severe kidney or liver disease, congestive heart failure, or shock. Controlled studies haven't determined the dosage ranges and drug efficacy in children.

A pregnancy risk category B drug, lidocaine should be given cautiously to pregnant patients.

Preparation

For injection, lidocaine comes in 5-ml ampules and prefilled syringes of 10 or 20 mg/ml.

For continuous infusion, the drug comes in 25-ml and 50-ml single-use vials containing 40 mg, 1 g, or 2 g. And it comes in 5-ml and 10-ml syringes that require mixing with dextrose 5% in water (D_5W). To obtain a 0.4% solution (4 mg/ml) for infusion, dilute 2 g of lidocaine in 500 ml of D_5W. The drug also comes in premixed 250-ml bottles of 0.4% or 0.8% solution, and in 500-ml bottles of 0.2%, 0.4%, or 0.8% solution.

Store lidocaine at room temperature.

Incompatibilities

Lidocaine is incompatible with amphotericin B, ampicillin sodium, cefazolin sodium, methohexital sodium, and phenytoin sodium.

Administration

- *Direct injection:* Inject the undiluted drug through a free-flowing I.V. line at a rate of 25 to 50 mg/minute.
- *Continuous infusion:* Using an infusion pump and microdrip tubing, titrate the dose to effectively control ventricular arrhythmias.
- *I.M. injection:* Inject the ordered dose into the deltoid muscle. To make sure you're not injecting the drug into a vein, frequently aspirate the drug during injection.
- *Endotracheal route:* Deliver several breaths with a manual resuscitation bag. Then, using a syringe or endotracheal medication administration device, administer a loading dose of lidocaine diluted in 5 to 10 ml of sterile 0.9% sodium chloride solution deep into the endotracheal tube. Follow this with several more breaths to distribute the drug into the alveoli.

Adverse reactions

- *Life-threatening:* anaphylaxis, bradycardia, cardiac arrest, coma, ***hypotension,*** respiratory arrest, seizures.
- *Other:* agitation, anxiety, apprehension, ***blurred or double vision, confusion,*** dizziness, drowsiness, dysphagia, dyspnea, euphoria, lethargy, ***light-headedness,*** nausea, paresthesia, psychosis, restlessness, ***seizures,*** slurred speech, ***stupor,*** thrombophlebitis, ***tinnitus, tremor,*** twitching, unconsciousness, vomiting.

Interactions

- *Aminoglycosides and polymyxin B:* enhanced neuromuscular blockade.
- *Beta blockers and cimetidine:* reduced metabolism and increased risk of lidocaine toxicity.
- *Hydantoin anticonvulsants:* excessive respiratory depression.
- *Phenytoin, procainamide, propranolol, and quinidine:* potentiated or antagonized antiarrhythmic effects.

EMERGENCY INTERVENTION

Managing a lidocaine overdose

When serum levels of lidocaine reach 6 to 8 mcg/ml, the patient may experience blurred or double vision, nausea and vomiting, tinnitus, or tremor and twitching. If levels pass 8 mcg/ml, he may have trouble breathing and develop severe dizziness or syncope, seizures, or bradycardia.

If such signs and symptoms develop, stop the infusion at once and notify the doctor. Make sure the patient has an adequate airway, and administer oxygen by nasal cannula if necessary. You may have to start cardiopulmonary resuscitation. Also, take these steps, as ordered:

- Continue to monitor the cardiac rhythm strip for underlying ventricular arrhythmias, and prepare to administer a different antiarrhythmic, such as procainamide.
- Assess the patient's respirations and blood pressure every 5 minutes for 20 minutes.
- If bradycardia develops, administer atropine and monitor for tachycardia.
- If circulatory depression develops, give a vasopressor – such as ephedrine or metaraminol – and I.V. fluids.
- For seizures, administer diazepam and monitor the patient carefully for respiratory depression.

Special considerations

Before administering the drug, read the label carefully. Make sure you have lidocaine for arrhythmias – not for local anesthesia. Administering the local anesthetic form of lidocaine could exacerbate the patient's condition.

As soon as possible, obtain the patient's weight to use in your dosage calculations. To avoid an overdose, use the smallest dose possible that controls the arrhythmia. Therapeutic serum levels range from 1.5 to 5 mcg/ml; levels above that may result in toxicity.

Use an infusion control device to ensure accurate delivery of the drug.

Instruct an alert patient to report symptoms of toxicity during the infusion. These include blurred or double vision, nausea, and ringing in the ears. Also, assess the patient frequently for signs of toxicity. (See *Managing a lidocaine overdose*.)

Carefully monitor his alanine aminotransferase (ALT), formerly SGOT; aspartate aminotransferase (AST), formerly SGPT; blood urea nitrogen; serum creatinine; and electrolyte levels. Report any abnormalities to the doctor.

Also, closely monitor the patient's cardiac rhythm strip so you can titrate the dosage appropriately. Note such changes as a prolonged PR interval (more than 0.2 second), widened QRS complex (more than 0.12 second), or worsened ventricular arrhythmias. If you see any of these changes, notify the doctor and prepare to switch to a different antiarrhythmic. Keep resuscitation equipment, including a defibrillator, nearby.

If the patient received the lidocaine I.M., his level of serum creatine phosphokinase – an enzyme that originates in skeletal muscle – will increase sevenfold. To avoid misleading results, test for cardiac-specific enzymes by measuring isoenzyme levels.

Treat the underlying cause of the arrhythmia, as ordered.

Magnesium sulfate

Magnesium sulfate has several emergency indications. It's used to treat eclampsia and preeclampsia; to prevent or control seizures associated with those disorders as well as with epilepsy, glomerulonephritis, hypothyroidism, severe hypertension, and encephalopathy; and to treat severe magnesium deficiency, barium poisoning, and paroxysmal atrial tachycardia.

The drug produces its anticonvulsant effects by depressing the central nervous system (CNS). Magnesium sulfate achieves this depression by reducing the release of acetylcholine at the myoneural junction, diminishing the motor end plate's sensitivity to acetylcholine, and depressing the motor end plate's excitability.

The onset of action occurs immediately after I.V. administration and about an hour after I.M. administration. The duration of action is 30 minutes.

Magnesium sulfate is widely distributed and readily crosses the placenta. It's not metabolized. Instead, it's filtered in the kidneys and excreted in urine at a rate directly related to the drug's serum concentration and the glomerular filtration

DOSAGE FINDER

Magnesium sulfate: Indications and dosages

Treatment of preeclampsia or eclampsia

▶ For adults, give an initial dose of 4 g by direct injection. Follow this with either 1 to 2 g/hour by continuous infusion, or 4 to 11 g by I.M. injection. The dosage over the next 24 hours depends on the patient's serum magnesium levels and urine output. Don't exceed 40 g over 24 hours; in patients with renal disease, don't exceed 20 g over 48 hours.

Prevention and control of seizures in severe preeclampsia, eclampsia, epilepsy, glomerulonephritis, hypothyroidism, severe hypertension, or encephalopathy

▶ For adults, give 1 to 4 g (8 to 32 mEq of magnesium) of 10% to 20% solution by direct injection. Follow this with an infusion of 1 to 4 g hourly. As an alternative, infuse 4 g in 250 ml of dextrose 5% in water and give 4 g by deep I.M. injection—2 g in each buttock. Follow this with 4 g by deep I.M. injection into alternate buttocks every 4 hours, as needed.

Control of seizures

▶ For children, give 20 to 40 mg/kg of 20% solution I.M. Or give 100 to 200 mg/kg of a 10% solution by continuous infusion. Give the whole infusion within an hour—half over the first 15 to 20 minutes, and the rest over the remainder of the hour.

Treatment of severe magnesium deficiency

▶ For adults, administer 5 g by continuous infusion.

Treatment of barium poisoning

▶ For adults, administer 1 to 2 g by direct injection.

Treatment of paroxysmal atrial tachycardia

▶ For adults, administer 3 to 4 g by direct injection.

rate. The drug is also excreted in breast milk. (See *Magnesium sulfate: Indications and dosages.*)

Contraindications and cautions

Don't give magnesium sulfate to patients with myocardial damage or heart block because the drug depresses cardiac muscle. The drug is also contraindicated within 2 hours of an expected delivery because it can cause magnesium toxicity in neonates.

Use the drug cautiously in patients with renal impairment. Also use caution with pregnant patients because magnesium sulfate is a pregnancy risk category B drug.

Preparation

Magnesium sulfate is available as a 10% concentration in 20-ml vials (1 g/10 ml), a 12.5% concentration in 8-ml vials (1.25 g/10 ml), and a 50% concentration in 5-ml vials (5 g/10 ml).

Store the drug at room temperature, and don't let it freeze.

To prepare the drug for I.V. administration to treat seizures, dilute the ordered dose in 250 ml of dextrose 5% in water (D_5W). For magnesium deficiency, dilute the dose in 1 liter of D_5W or dextrose 5% in 0.9% sodium chloride solution. Never infuse a concentration over 20% (200 mg/ml).

For I.M. injection, use a 25% or 50% solution. For children, dilute the drug to a 20% concentration.

Incompatibilities

Magnesium sulfate is incompatible with alcohol, alkali carbonates or bicarbonates, barium, calcium gluceptate, calcium gluconate, clindamycin phosphate, dobutamine hydrochloride, hydrocortisone sodium succinate, 10% I.V. fat emulsion, polymyxin B sulfate, procaine hydrochloride, and soluble phosphates.

EMERGENCY INTERVENTION

Managing a magnesium sulfate overdose

The signs and symptoms of magnesium toxicity depend on the patient's serum magnesium level:

- A level of 7 to 10 mEq/ml causes hypotension, a loss of deep tendon reflexes, and narcolepsy.
- A level of 12 to 15 mEq/ml causes respiratory paralysis.
- A level above 15 mEq/ml alters cardiac conduction.
- A level above 25 mEq/ml can cause cardiac arrest.

To reverse heart block or respiratory depression, administer 5 to 10 mEq of calcium (usually as 10 to 20 ml of a 20% solution of calcium gluconate), as ordered. If a patient develops respiratory paralysis, he'll need mechanical ventilation. A patient with severe toxicity may need peritoneal dialysis or hemodialysis.

Administration

- *Direct injection:* Slowly inject the drug directly into a vein at a rate not exceeding 1.5 ml/minute.
- *Continuous infusion:* Using an infusion pump if possible, administer the diluted drug at a rate not exceeding 3 ml/minute.
- *I.M. injection:* Inject the ordered dose into the gluteal muscle. Alternate buttocks with each dose.

Adverse reactions

- *Life-threatening:* cardiac arrest, hypermagnesemia (serum level greater than 4 mEq/liter), respiratory paralysis, severe bradycardia, severe hypotension.
- *Other:* ***depressed reflexes,*** diaphoresis, ***flushing,*** hypotension, hypothermia, hypotonia, prolonged PR

interval, ***sweating,*** widened QRS complex.

Interactions

- *Calcium salts:* possible neutralization of magnesium sulfate.
- *CNS depressants:* additive CNS depression.
- *Neuromuscular blocking agents:* possible excessive neuromuscular blockade.
- *Streptomycin, tetracycline, and tobramycin:* reduced antibiotic action.

Special considerations

Before starting therapy, make sure you have I.V. calcium gluconate on hand to treat an overdose. If you're treating a patient undergoing digitalization, use the drug cautiously because it can cause arrhythmias. (See *Managing a magnesium sulfate overdose,* page 119.)

Don't administer magnesium sulfate too rapidly or the patient will feel an uncomfortable sensation of heat. Remember that the I.M. route is usually preferred for an infant or a child with hypertension or encephalopathy.

During therapy, assess the patient's vital signs every 15 minutes and monitor his serum magnesium levels. Watch for respiratory depression and monitor his cardiac rhythm strip for signs of heart block. Monitor his fluid intake and output. Before each dose, his respiratory rate should be about 16 breaths per minute. His urine output should be 100 ml or more over 4 hours.

If a neonate's mother received magnesium sulfate before delivery—especially less than 24 hours before delivery—assess the neonate for signs of magnesium toxicity, including neuromuscular or respiratory depression.

Magnesium sulfate results in unreliable reticuloendothelial cell imaging when technetium Tc 99m sulfur colloid is used.

Mannitol

(Osmitrol)

Mannitol produces diuresis by increasing the osmotic pressure of the glomerular filtrate, which in turn inhibits renal tubular reabsorption of water and solutes and facilitates the excretion of sodium, potassium, chloride, calcium, phosphates, lithium, magnesium, and some toxins. Besides its diuretic action, mannitol also elevates plasma osmolality, increasing the flow of water from the brain, cerebrospinal fluid, and eyes into the interstitial fluid and plasma—thus reducing intracranial pressure (ICP) and intraocular pressure (IOP). (See *How mannitol promotes osmotic activity,* page 122.)

Mannitol has several indications. It can prevent or treat the oliguric phase of acute renal failure, treat oliguria, reduce ICP and IOP, reduce the nephrotoxic effects of amphotericin B, and serve as an adjunct in the treatment of drug intoxication (by promoting diuresis), edema, and ascites.

The onset of action begins in 15 minutes when the drug is given to reduce ICP or IOP and in 1 to 3 hours when it's used for diuresis. The duration of action ranges from 3 to 8 hours for ICP or IOP. The serum half-life is 100 minutes.

The drug is distributed only to the extracellular spaces. It doesn't cross the blood-brain barrier unless there is a high drug concentration or the patient has acidosis. Mannitol doesn't reach the eyes, either. Whether it crosses the placenta isn't known. A small amount may be me-

DOSAGE FINDER

Mannitol: Indications and dosages

Prevention or treatment of oliguric phase of acute renal failure

▶ For adults, give 50 to 100 g as a concentrated solution (20% or 25%). Follow this with a 5% or 10% solution.

Treatment of oliguria

▶ For adults, infuse a test dose of 200 mg/kg or 12.5 g of 15% to 25% solution over 3 to 5 minutes. If at least 30 ml of urine/hour is excreted by the patient over the next 2 to 3 hours, infuse 100 g of a 15% or 20% solution over a period of 90 minutes to several hours.

▶ For children age 12 and under, infuse 200 mg/kg or 6 g/m² as a test dose over 3 to 5 minutes. If urine output is adequate, infuse 2 g/kg or 60 g/m² over 2 to 6 hours.

Reduction of intracranial and intraocular pressure

▶ For adults, infuse 1.5 to 2 g/kg of a 15%, 20%, or 25% solution over 30 to 60 minutes.

▶ For children age 12 and under, infuse 1 to 2 g/kg of a 15% or 20% solution over 30 to 60 minutes.

Reduction of nephrotoxic effects of amphotericin B

▶ Give adults 12.5 g immediately before and after each dose of amphotericin B.

Adjunctive treatment for drug intoxication

▶ For adults, give 50 to 200 g of a 5% to 25% solution. Then infuse mannitol at a rate that maintains urine output at 100 to 500 ml/hour.

▶ For children, infuse up to 2 g/kg of a 5% or 10% solution.

Adjunctive treatment for edema and ascites

▶ For adults, infuse 100 g of a 10% or 20% solution over 2 to 6 hours.

▶ For children age 12 and under, infuse 2 g/kg of a 15% or 20% solution over 2 to 6 hours.

tabolized in the liver to glycogen. About 80% is eliminated unchanged in urine within 3 hours, although clearance will be decreased in a patient with renal disease. Whether the drug appears in breast milk isn't known. (See *Mannitol: Indications and dosages.*)

Contraindications and cautions

Don't give mannitol to patients with anuria because it may cause circulatory overload. The drug is also contraindicated for patients with intracranial bleeding (except during a craniotomy) because it can increase bleeding, for those with severe dehydration because it worsens the condition, and for those with severe pulmonary congestion or congestive heart failure (CHF) because the increased circulating volume mannitol produces aggravates these conditions.

Use the drug cautiously in patients with a known hypersensitivity to mannitol. Use it cautiously in patients with cardiopulmonary impairment because of the risk of CHF, and in those with hyperkalemia or hyponatremia because it may worsen their electrolyte imbalance. Also, use mannitol cautiously in patients with hypovolemia because the drug may mask signs and symptoms of the condition and enhance hemoconcentration. In those with severe renal impairment, it can increase

MECHANISM OF ACTION

How mannitol promotes osmotic activity

When administered I.V., mannitol, an inert sugar molecule, can't be absorbed. The drug's presence increases osmotic pressure, which promotes diuresis in the kidneys and helps reduce edema in the tissues.

Without mannitol, sodium and water in the proximal tubule are reabsorbed in the same ratio as exists in the glomerular filtrate.

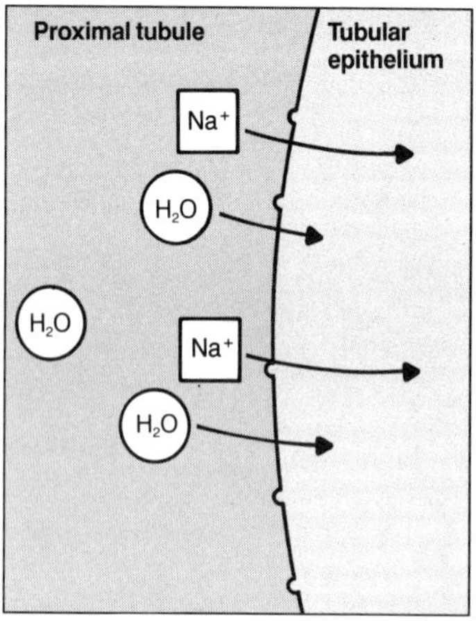

When the nonreabsorbable mannitol reaches the proximal tubule, the drug becomes part of the glomerular filtrate. The increased osmotic pressure produces a counterforce to the normal reabsorption of water, promoting diuresis.

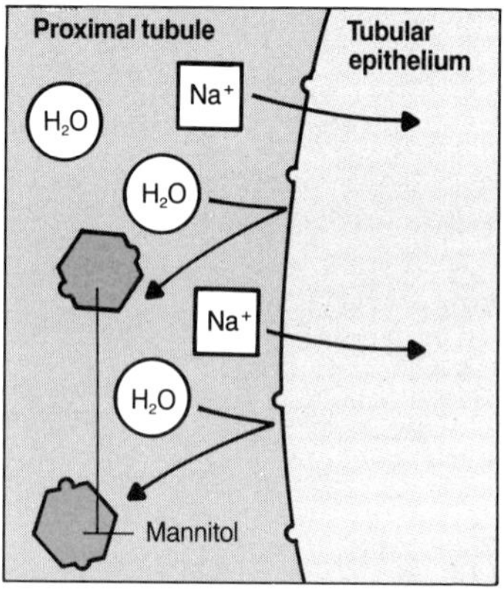

Similarly, when mannitol reaches the bloodstream, the increased osmotic pressure enhances water flow from the tissues into intravascular fluid and plasma, reducing edema.

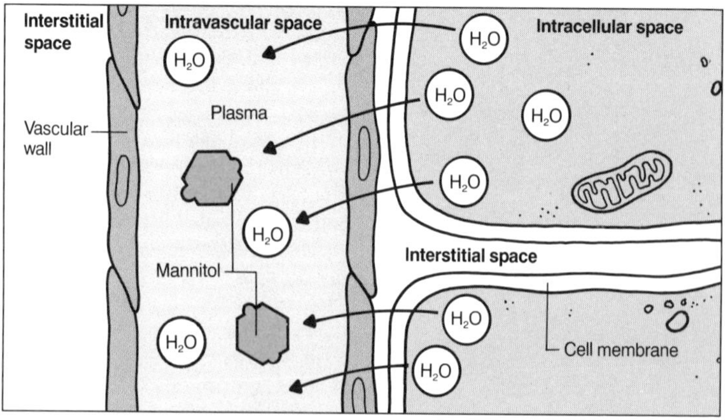

the risk of circulatory overload.

Mannitol's safety and efficacy in children haven't been established. Use this pregnancy risk category C drug cautiously in pregnant patients.

Preparation
Available in concentrations of 5%, 10%, 15%, 20%, and 25%, mannitol comes in glass or plastic I.V. containers that hold 150, 250, 500, or 1,000 ml.

Store the drug at room temperature, and make sure it doesn't freeze. Mannitol can crystallize, especially if chilled. If crystals form, dissolve them according to the manufacturer's directions. Don't use any solution that contains undissolved crystals.

Incompatibilities
Mannitol is incompatible with imipenem-cilastatin sodium and blood products. If the patient must receive blood and mannitol, add 20 mEq of sodium chloride to each liter of mannitol before administration.

Administration
- *Intermittent or continuous infusion:* Give the appropriate dose and concentration at the ordered rate.

Adverse reactions
- *Life-threatening:* acute renal failure, arrhythmias, vacuolar nephrosis.
- *Other:* acidosis, arm pain, backache, blurred vision, ***cellular dehydration,*** chest pain, chills, confusion, dizziness, dry mouth, extravasation (localized edema and necrosis), fever, ***fluid and electrolyte imbalance,*** headache, hypertension, hypotension, muscle rigidity, nausea, paresthesia, pulmonary congestion (dyspnea and wheezing), rhinitis, seizures, tachycardia, thirst, thrombophlebitis, uricosuria, urine retention, urticaria, vomiting, ***water intoxication,*** weakness in extremities.

Interactions
- *Cardiac glycosides:* increased risk of hypokalemia-induced toxicity.
- *Diuretics, including carbonic anhydrase inhibitors:* risk of potentiated diuretic and intraocular effects.
- *Lithium:* decreased lithium effects.

Special considerations
Before infusing mannitol concentrations of 15% or more, make sure the administration set has a filter.

If the patient receives a rapid infusion of a large dose, the drug may accumulate and cause circulatory overload. Also, take steps to prevent extravasation, or the drug may cause edema and necrosis.

Before giving a therapeutic dose to a patient who has marked oliguria or may have inadequate renal function, give him a test dose to determine his response. After the test dose, his urine flow should increase to at least 30 ml/hour for 2 to 3 hours. A small or debilitated patient receiving mannitol for any reason may need a lower dose.

Right before administration, obtain a baseline blood pressure reading and cardiac rhythm strip, and assess the patient's heart and lung sounds. For a comatose or bedridden patient, insert an indwelling urinary catheter. This allows a careful evaluation of fluid intake and output for use in calculating the mannitol dosage. If necessary, you can use an hourly urimeter collection device to assess the patient's urine output. (*Note:* If the drug is effective, you need to check the urimeter more frequently than every hour.)

During the first hour of infusion, monitor vital signs frequently, then check them hourly or as needed. Throughout therapy, monitor the fluid intake and output, blood urea nitrogen level, and serum electrolytes, especially sodium and potassium. You can reduce the risk of dehydration and electrolyte depletion by administering a lower mannitol concentration or a solution that contains sodium chloride. Provide adequate hydration and electrolyte therapy to maintain hemostasis.

Monitor a patient receiving a large dose for signs of decreased ICP, tissue dehydration, and fluid and electrolyte imbalance. A large dose may cross the blood-brain barrier and cause central nervous system damage—even death—especially if the patient has acidosis.

A patient receiving mannitol as an adjunct for salicylate or barbiturate poisoning may need sodium bicarbonate to help alkalinize his urine.

About 12 hours after receiving mannitol, the patient's ICP and IOP may rebound.

Mannitol alters blood ethylene glycol results and levels of inorganic phosphorus and serum electrolytes.

Meperidine hydrochloride

(Demerol)

A morphinelike agonist, meperidine hydrochloride binds with opiate receptors in the central nervous system (CNS) to alter the patient's perception of and emotional response to pain. This schedule II controlled substance is used to control moderate to severe pain and as an adjunct to anesthesia. (See *How meperidine controls pain,* page 126.)

The drug's onset of action occurs within 1 minute of I.V. administration and within 10 to 15 minutes of I.M. or S.C. injection. The peak action occurs in 5 to 7 minutes when the drug is given I.V., in 30 to 50 minutes when it's given I.M or S.C. Regardless of the route, meperidine's effect lasts 2 to 4 hours.

The drug is dispersed throughout the body and readily crosses the placenta. It binds tightly to plasma proteins, with the highest concentrations occurring in the limbic system, thalamus, corpus striatum, hypothalamus, midbrain, and spinal cord. Metabolism occurs mainly in the microsomes of the hepatic endoplasmic reticulum, but it also takes place in the CNS, kidneys, lungs, and placenta. The drug's primary metabolite, normeperidine, is both active and toxic. Meperidine is excreted mainly in urine as metabolites, although small amounts appear in feces and breast milk. (See *Meperidine: Indications and dosages.*)

Contraindications and cautions

Don't give meperidine to patients with a known hypersensitivity to it or to patients with diarrhea from poisons, toxins, cephalosporins, or topical clindamycin until all toxic substances are cleared because the drug may slow GI motility. Also, don't give the drug to those with acute respiratory depression because it may worsen the condition.

Use extreme caution when giving the drug to patients with seizure disorders because it can trigger seizures. Give the drug carefully to patients with altered respiratory function because of the risk of respiratory depression, to those with head injury or increased intracranial pressure (especially from intracranial lesions) because it can mask changes in level of consciousness and elevate cerebrospinal fluid (CSF) pressure, and to those with prostatic hyperplasia, urethral stricture, or recent urinary tract surgery because it can cause urine retention.

Use meperidine cautiously in patients with atrial flutter or other supraventricular tachyarrhythmias because the drug's vagolytic action can increase ventricular response. Administer the drug with caution to patients with gallbladder disease because it may increase biliary contractions, to patients with abdominal disorders because it can alter the patient's perception of pain and obscure a diagnosis, and to patients with inflammatory bowel disease because of the risk of toxic megacolon. Because of meperidine's effect on GI motility, give it cautiously to those who've undergone GI surgery.

Meperidine increases the risk of prolonged CNS and respiratory depression in patients with hypothyroidism. Because of the potential for abuse, use caution when giving it to patients with a history of drug abuse, emotional instability, or suicidal tendencies.

Meperidine is a pregnancy risk category B drug (category D when given for prolonged periods or in high doses at term).

Preparation

Meperidine comes in preservative-free ampules and vials, as well as in syringes mixed with a preservative. Available strengths include 10, 25, 50, 75, and 100 mg/ml. Store vials and ampules at room temperature. Single doses in syringes are stable at room temperature for 24 hours.

For direct injection, dilute the drug with a compatible solution to a concentration of 10 mg/ml. For infusion, dilute it with a compatible solution to a concentration of 1 mg/ml.

Incompatibilities

Meperidine is incompatible with

DOSAGE FINDER

Meperidine: Indications and dosages

Control of moderate to severe pain

▶ For adults, give 50 to 150 mg I.M. or S.C. every 3 to 4 hours, 10 to 50 mg by direct injection every 2 to 4 hours, or 15 to 35 mg hourly by continuous infusion. The dosage depends on the severity of the patient's pain and his response to therapy.

▶ For children, administer 1.1 to 1.76 mg/kg (but less than 100 mg) I.M. or S.C. every 3 to 4 hours.

Adjunct to anesthesia

▶ For adults, administer a fractional dose of a 10 mg/ml solution by direct injection. Repeat this dose as needed. Or infuse 1 mg/ml concentration as needed.

▶ For children, administer 1 to 2.2 mg/kg I.M. or S.C. Don't exceed 100 mg.

aminophylline, amobarbital sodium, ephedrine sulfate, heparin, methicillin sodium, morphine sulfate, oxytetracycline hydrochloride, phenobarbital sodium, phenytoin sodium, sodium bicarbonate, sodium iodide, sulfadiazine, tetracycline, thiamylal sodium, and thiopental sodium.

Administration

- *Direct injection:* Give the diluted dose over a 3- to 5-minute period. Avoid a rapid injection.
- *Continuous infusion:* Using an infusion control device, administer the drug at 15 to 35 mg/hour. Avoid a rapid infusion.
- *I.M. injection:* Inject the ordered dose into any I.M. site.
- *S.C. injection:* Inject the ordered dose into any S.C. site. Use this route only if necessary because repeated injections can cause local tis-

MECHANISM OF ACTION

How meperidine controls pain

Meperidine inhibits pain transmission by mimicking the body's natural pain-control mechanisms, as explained in the following illustrations.

In the dorsal horn of the spinal cord, peripheral pain neurons meet central nervous system (CNS) neurons. At the synapse, the pain neuron releases substance P (a pain neurotransmitter). This agent helps transfer pain impulses to the CNS neurons that carry the impulses to the brain.

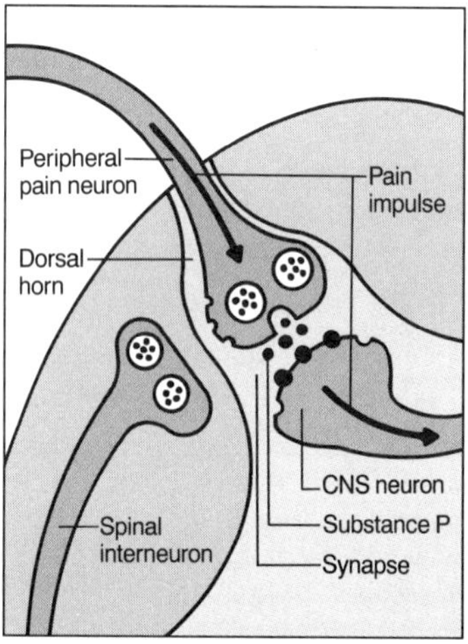

In theory, the spinal interneurons respond by releasing endogenous opiates. These opiates bind to the peripheral pain neuron to inhibit substance P's release and to retard the transmission of pain impulses.

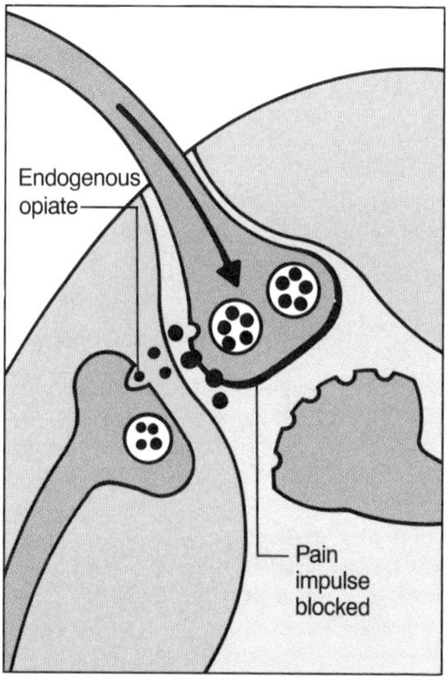

Meperidine supplements this pain-blocking effect by binding with free opiate receptors to inhibit the release of substance P. Meperidine also alters consciousness of pain, but how this mechanism works remains unknown.

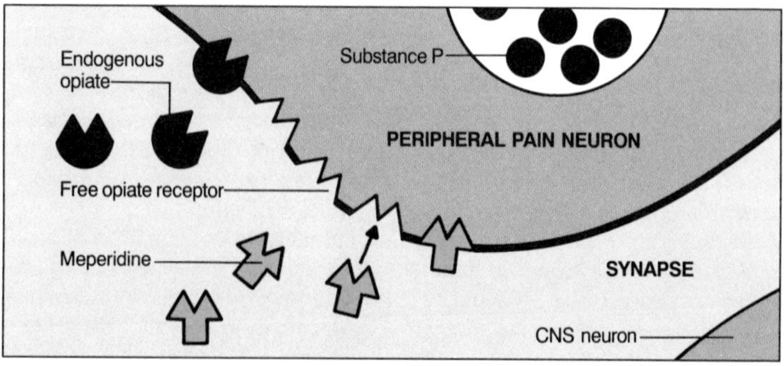

sue irritation and induration.

Adverse reactions

- *Life-threatening:* anaphylaxis, bradycardia, circulatory depression, severe respiratory depression, tachycardia.
- *Other:* abdominal pain, agitation, anorexia, ***clouded sensorium,*** coma, confusion, ***constipation,*** delirium, diaphoresis, dizziness, drowsiness, dry mouth, ***euphoria,*** facial flushing or redness, hallucinations, headache, ***hypotension,*** insomnia, malaise, mental dullness, ***nausea,*** nervousness, nightmares, oliguria, pain, palpitations, phlebitis at the injection site, pruritus, restlessness, ***sedation,*** seizures (with prolonged use), ***somnolence,*** syncope, tachycardia, tremor, unusual dreams, ***urine retention,*** urticaria, visual disturbances, ***vomiting,*** weakness.

Interactions

- *Anticoagulants:* increased anticoagulant effects.
- *Antidiarrheals:* increased risk of severe constipation.
- *Antihypertensives and diuretics:* potentiated hypotension.
- *Antimuscarinics:* increased risk of constipation or urine retention.
- *Estrogens and oral contraceptives:* inhibited meperidine metabolism.
- *Hydroxyzine:* enhanced analgesia and CNS depression.
- *Isoniazid:* aggravated adverse reactions to meperidine.
- *Magnesium sulfate:* potentiated CNS effects.
- *Metoclopramide:* decreased GI motility.
- *Monoamine oxidase (MAO) inhibitors:* severe respiratory depression, cyanosis, hypotension, coma, hyperexcitability, hypertension, hyperpyrexia, seizures, and tachycardia. Don't administer meperidine within 2 weeks of an MAO inhibitor.
- *Naloxone:* decreased CNS and respiratory depression and possible blocked analgesic effect.
- *Naltrexone:* blocked analgesic effect.
- *Neuromuscular blocking agents:* additive respiratory depression and severe constipation.
- *Other opioid analgesics and CNS depressants:* additive CNS effects, respiratory depression, and hypotension. Reduce the dose, as ordered.

Special considerations

Before administering the drug, have the patient lie down to minimize hypotension. Afterward, tell him to rise slowly to reduce dizziness.

For I.V. administration, make sure you're using a large enough vein to prevent infiltration. If you're giving the drug I.M., make sure you don't insert the needle around a nerve trunk, or the patient may experience transient sensorimotor paralysis.

To achieve better analgesia, give the drug before the pain becomes intense. You can help reduce the patient's anxiety about his pain by starting with a smaller dose given on a fixed schedule. Once the drug controls his pain, individualize the schedule and the effective dose. If your patient has renal or hepatic impairment, reduce his dosage.

Monitor the patient's respirations frequently during the I.V. infusion and every 15 minutes for an hour afterward. Keep resuscitation equipment and naloxone nearby. If his respirations drop below 8 breaths/minute, try to arouse him to stimulate his breathing. Notify the doctor, who may order naloxone or respiratory support. (See *Managing a meperidine overdose,* page 128.)

Because of the risk of toxicity, meperidine isn't recommended for chronic pain. After the patient stops

EMERGENCY INTERVENTION

Managing a meperidine overdose

An overdose of meperidine can cause bradycardia, bradypnea, cold and clammy skin, confusion, extreme nervousness and restlessness, extreme weakness, hypotension, pinpoint pupils, seizures, severe dizziness and drowsiness, and unconsciousness. If your patient develops such signs and symptoms, make sure he has a patent airway and provide respiratory support. Also, perform the following interventions, as ordered:

- To reverse respiratory depression, give 0.4 mg of naloxone by I.V. push. Keep monitoring the patient because meperidine has a longer duration of action than naloxone. The patient may need repeated doses or a continuous infusion of naloxone.
- To maintain blood pressure, administer I.V. fluids and vasopressors.
- Infuse ascorbic acid or ammonium chloride to acidify his urine and help him excrete the unchanged drug.

taking meperidine—especially after long-term use—assess him for signs of withdrawal. They may begin 3 to 4 hours after the last dose and usually peak within 8 to 12 hours. If a patient received meperidine regularly during pregnancy, monitor the neonate closely for signs of narcotic dependence.

Meperidine affects several laboratory tests. A lumbar puncture will reveal elevated CSF pressure caused by respiratory depression. The drug also prolongs the times of gastric emptying studies, delays visualization and causes a false image of a biliary tract obstruction during hepatobiliary imaging with technetium Tc 99m disofenin, and may increase serum amylase and lipase levels.

Metaproterenol sulfate

(Alupent, Metaprel)

Used to treat bronchial asthma and reversible bronchospasm, metaproterenol sulfate works by stimulating $beta_2$-adrenergic receptors. This action relaxes bronchial smooth muscle and the peripheral vasculature, resulting in bronchodilation. The drug, a sympathomimetic, has less effect on $beta_1$-adrenergic receptors and little or no effect on alpha-adrenergic receptors.

About 3% of an inhaled dose is absorbed intact through the lungs. The onset of action takes place within 1 minute of oral inhalation and 5 to 30 minutes of nebulization. Peak effects occur in about an hour. With oral inhalation, the duration of action lasts 1 to 4 hours for a single dose and 1 to 2½ hours after long-term use. With nebulization, the duration of action ranges from 2 to 6 hours for a single dose and 4 to 6 hours after long-term use.

Widely distributed throughout the body, metaproterenol is extensively metabolized on its first pass through the liver. It's excreted in urine, mainly as glucuronic acid conjugates. (See *Metaproterenol: Indications and dosages.*)

Contraindications and cautions

Don't administer metaproterenol to patients with preexisting cardiac arrhythmias associated with tachycardia because it stimulates the heart.

Use extreme caution when giving this drug to patients with hypertension, coronary artery disease, congestive heart failure, hyperthyroidism, or diabetes mellitus because it can worsen these conditions. Also give the drug carefully to patients who are sensitive to this drug or to other sympathomimetics.

Use caution if your patient has a seizure disorder or a sulfite sensitivity. Some preparations may contain sulfites.

The safety and efficacy of the inhalant form of this drug in children under age 12 haven't been established. Give this pregnancy risk category C drug carefully to pregnant women.

Preparation

Metaproterenol comes in a metered-dose inhaler that delivers 650 mcg in each metered spray. It also comes as a 0.4%, 0.6%, or 5% solution for administration undiluted with a hand-held nebulizer or diluted with an intermittent positive pressure breathing (IPPB) device.

Store the metered-dose inhaler below 120° F (49° C) and the solution below 104° F (40° C). Keep the solution in a tight container and protect it from light.

To prepare the drug for IPPB administration, dilute the 5% solution in about 2.5 ml of 0.9% sodium chloride solution or other diluent. The 0.4% unit-dose vial contains the equivalent of 0.2 ml of a 5% solution diluted to 2.5 ml with 0.9% sodium chloride solution. The 0.6% unit-dose vial contains the equivalent of 0.3 ml of a 5% solution diluted to 2.5 ml with 0.9% sodium chloride solution.

Incompatibilities

No incompatibilities have been reported.

Administration

• *Aerosol inhalation:* After shaking the container, have the patient close his lips around the inhaler's mouthpiece and exhale through his nose. Then give the drug while he inhales deeply through his mouth. Have him hold his breath for a few seconds and then exhale slowly. Let at least 2 minutes pass between inhalations.

• *Hand-held nebulizer:* Administer the drug full strength.

• *IPPB device:* Fill the chamber of the IPPB device with diluted solution. Tell the patient to put his lips around the mouthpiece and to breathe in and out through his mouth. (Young children may require a nose clip.) Continue the treatment until the mist is finished and the chamber is empty. You may need to shake the chamber midway through the treatment because the mist particles adhere to the chamber walls.

Adverse reactions

• *Life-threatening:* cardiac arrest (with excessive use).

• *Other:* bad taste in mouth, dizziness, drowsiness, headache, hypertension, muscle cramps, nausea, nervousness, palpitations, paradoxical bronchoconstriction (with exces-

DOSAGE FINDER

Metaproterenol: Indications and dosages

Bronchial asthma and reversible bronchospasm

▶ For adults and children age 12 and over, administer two or three inhalations with a metered-dose inhaler. Allow at least 2 minutes to pass between inhalations, and don't deliver more than 12 inhalations in 24 hours.

Alternatively, give 10 inhalations of an undiluted 5% solution with a hand-held nebulizer. Or give 0.2 to 0.3 ml of the 5% solution diluted with 0.9% sodium chloride solution, or 2.5 ml of a 0.6% solution using an intermittent positive pressure breathing device. Don't repeat a dose more often than every 4 hours for an acute attack.

EMERGENCY INTERVENTION

Managing a metaproterenol overdose

An overdose of metaproterenol may cause nausea and vomiting, cardiac arrhythmias, angina, hypertension, and seizures.

If these occur, monitor the patient's vital signs closely and take measures to support his cardiovascular status. If the doctor orders a cardioselective beta$_1$-adrenergic blocker such as acebutolol, atenolol, or metoprolol, administer it with extreme caution. These drugs can induce severe bronchospasm or an asthmatic attack.

sive use), tachycardia, tremor, vomiting, weakness.

Interactions

- *Antihypertensives and diuretics:* reduced effects of these drugs.
- *Beta-adrenergic blockers, especially propranolol:* antagonism of metaproterenol's bronchodilating effects.
- *Cardiac glycosides, general anesthetics (especially chloroform, cyclopropane, halothane, and trichlorethylene), levodopa, theophylline derivatives, and thyroid hormones:* increased risk of severe ventricular tachycardia, cardiac arrhythmias, and coronary insufficiency.
- *Cocaine, local:* increased central nervous system (CNS) and cardiovascular effects.
- *Maprotiline, monoamine oxidase inhibitors, and tricyclic antidepressants:* potentiated action of metaproterenol.
- *Nitrates:* reduced antianginal effects.
- *Other sympathomimetics:* additive effects and possible toxicity.
- *Ritodrine:* increased effects and potential adverse effects of both drugs.
- *Xanthines and other CNS stimulating drugs:* increased CNS stimulation.

Special considerations

During administration, monitor the patient for adverse reactions, which are dose-related and characteristic of sympathomimetics. High doses can cause CNS and cardiac stimulation, resulting in tachycardia, hypertension, or tremor. Adverse reactions may persist because of the drug's long duration of action. Observe elderly patients closely.

Signs and symptoms of a toxic reaction include nausea and vomiting, cardiac arrhythmias, and seizures. (See *Managing a metaproterenol overdose.*)

If necessary, you can administer aerosol treatments even though the patient is already taking metaproterenol tablets. But don't simultaneously administer the aerosol forms of metaproterenol and an adrenocorticoid. Let at least 5 minutes elapse between the administration of the two aerosols.

Metaproterenol has no reported effects on diagnostic tests.

Metaraminol bitartrate

(Aramine)

Used to relieve acute hypotension and severe shock (except hypovolemic shock), metaraminol bitartrate acts primarily on alpha-adrenergic receptors to increase blood pressure, which slows heart rate. It also produces a potent, indirect sympathomimetic effect by causing the release of norepinephrine. Prolonged use may deplete norepinephrine, decreasing the drug's pressor effects. (See *How metaraminol causes reflex bradycardia,* page 132.)

The drug's onset of action begins within 1 to 2 minutes of I.V. administration. The duration of action lasts about 20 minutes.

Metaraminol is probably distributed widely to body tissues, with the highest concentrations occurring in the kidneys, lungs, heart, and peripheral vasculature. The drug doesn't cross the blood-brain barrier. Whether it crosses the placenta isn't known. Metaraminol isn't metabolized. Thus, drug uptake into tissues – not metabolism – stops the drug's effects. Metaraminol is excreted in urine and feces, mostly as metabolites. Whether the drug passes into breast milk isn't known. (See *Metaraminol: Indications and dosages.*)

Contraindications and cautions

Metaraminol is contraindicated for patients with a known hypersensitivity to the drug or to sulfites, and for those with peripheral or mesenteric vascular thrombosis because it may worsen ischemia.

Give the drug carefully to patients with acidosis, hypercapnia, or hypoxia because these conditions decrease its effectiveness and may increase its adverse effects. Also give it cautiously to those with diabetes mellitus, Buerger's disease, peripheral vascular disease, hypertension, hyperthyroidism, hypercoagulability, or heart disease because its vasoconstrictive effects may aggravate symptoms or increase the risk of adverse reactions. Metaraminol may cause severe diuresis in patients with cirrhosis and a relapse in those who've had malaria.

A pregnancy risk category C drug, metaraminol should be given cautiously to pregnant patients.

DOSAGE FINDER

Metaraminol: Indications and dosages

Treatment of severe shock (except hypovolemic shock)

▶ For adults, administer 0.5 to 5 mg by direct injection. Then start a continuous infusion at a rate adjusted to maintain the desired blood pressure.

▶ For children, administer 0.01 mg/kg by direct injection.

Treatment of acute hypotension

▶ For adults, infuse 15 to 100 mg. Adjust the rate as necessary to maintain the desired blood pressure.

▶ For children, give 0.4 mg/kg by infusion. Adjust the rate as necessary to maintain the desired blood pressure.

Preparation

Metaraminol is available in a 10 mg/ml concentration that comes in a 10-ml vial. Store the drug at room temperature, and protect it from freezing and light.

Use the drug undiluted for direct injection. For infusion, add 15 to 100 mg of metaraminol – in some instances, up to 500 mg – to 500 ml of dextrose 5% in water, 0.9% sodium chloride solution, lactated Ringer's solution, or Ringer's injection. For pediatric administration, prepare a solution that has a concentration of 1 mg/25 ml. Use the diluted solution within 24 hours.

Incompatibilities

Metaraminol is incompatible with amphotericin B, barbiturates, dexamethasone sodium phosphate, erythromycin lactobionate, fibrinogen, hydrocortisone sodium succinate, methicillin sodium, methylprednisolone sodium succinate, penicillin G potassium, phenytoin sodium, prednisolone sodium phosphate, thiopen-

MECHANISM OF ACTION

How metaraminol causes reflex bradycardia

Metaraminol acts primarily on alpha-adrenergic receptors in vascular smooth muscle cells. This action causes vasoconstriction, which increases peripheral vascular resistance and raises or maintains blood pressure.

PERIPHERAL VASOCONSTRICTION

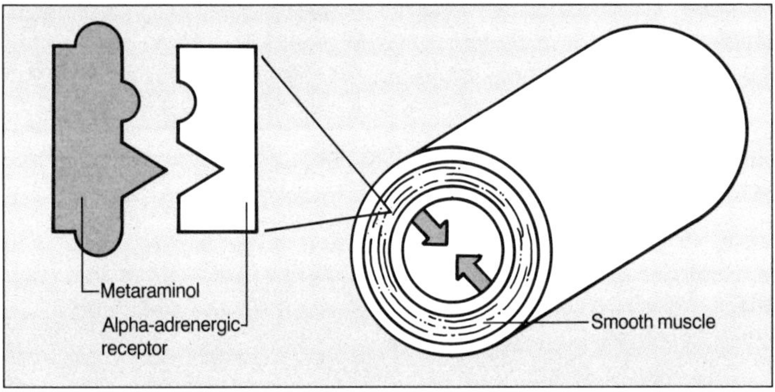

The resultant increase in arterial blood pressure stimulates pressoreceptors in the internal carotid artery and the aortic arch. These pressoreceptors then stimulate the compensatory reflex centers in the medulla. The result: increased vagal tone, which slows the heart rate and atrioventricular conduction.

INCREASED VAGAL TONE

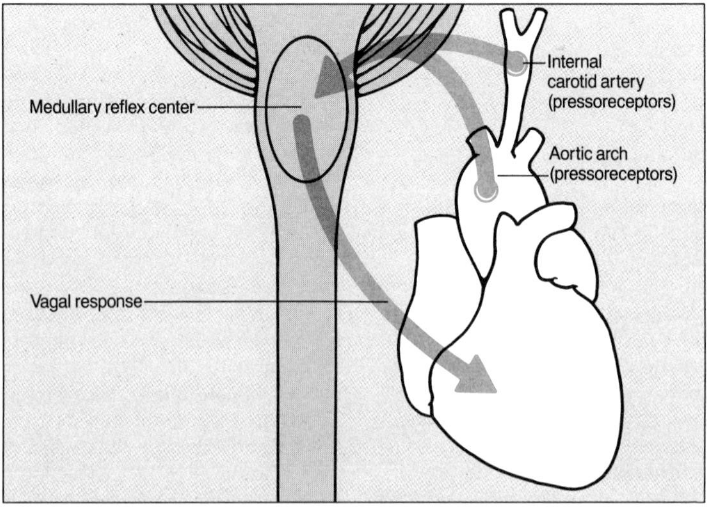

tal sodium, and warfarin sodium.

Administration

- *Direct injection:* Inject the drug slowly into a large vein. Don't use an ankle or a hand vein.
- *Intermittent infusion:* Using an infusion pump, piggyback the solution into a keep-vein-open line at a rate sufficient to maintain the desired blood pressure.
- *Continuous infusion:* Using an infusion pump, piggyback the drug into a free-flowing, compatible solution at a rate that maintains the desired blood pressure. Titrate the dosage based on the patient's response.

Adverse reactions

- *Life-threatening:* acute pulmonary edema, arrhythmias, cardiac arrest, cerebral hemorrhage, hypertension.
- *Other:* anxiety, apprehension, chest pain, decreased cardiac output (with prolonged use), faintness, flushing, hypotension, nausea, pallor, pruritus, rash, respiratory distress, restlessness, seizures, severe dizziness, severe headache, severe peripheral and visceral vasoconstriction, sweating, tissue sloughing at injection site, trembling, urticaria, weakness, wheezing.

Interactions

- *Alpha-adrenergic blockers:* decreased metaraminol pressor effects.
- *Antihypertensives and diuretics:* possible reduced antihypertensive effects.
- *Atropine sulfate:* blocked bradycardia and enhanced pressor effects of metaraminol.
- *Beta-adrenergic blockers:* possible diminished effects of both drugs.
- *Cardiac glycosides and levodopa:* increased risk of arrhythmias.
- *Diatrizoates and iothalamate:* heightened neurologic effects during aortography. Contrast material can be forced into the spine, causing paralysis.
- *Doxapram:* possible enhanced pressor effects of both drugs.
- *Ergonovine:* possible potentiated pressor effects, including severe hypertension and rupture of cerebral vessels.
- *Ergotamine:* risk of peripheral vascular ischemia and gangrene.
- *Guanadrel and guanethidine:* decreased antihypertensive effects of these drugs and possible potentiated pressor effects of metaraminol.
- *Hydrocarbon anesthetics, including halothane and methoxyflurane:* severe ventricular arrhythmias.
- *Maprotiline and tricyclic antidepressants:* potentiated cardiovascular effects of metaraminol, such as arrhythmias and tachycardia.
- *Mazindol:* possible potentiated metaraminol pressor effects.
- *Mecamylamine, methyldopa, and trimethaphan:* possible decreased hypotensive effects of these drugs and increased pressor effects of metaraminol.
- *Methylergonovine, methysergide, and oxytocin:* possible enhanced vasoconstriction.
- *Monoamine oxidase (MAO) inhibitors, especially furazolidone:* possible prolonged cardiac stimulation and vasopressor effects. Don't administer metaraminol within 2 weeks of an MAO inhibitor.
- *Nitrates:* possible diminished pressor effects of metaraminol and reduced antianginal effects of nitrates.
- *Rauwolfia alkaloids:* possible decreased hypotensive effect of these drugs.
- *Sympathomimetics:* possible enhanced cardiovascular effects.
- *Thyroid hormones:* possible enhanced coronary insufficiency.

Special considerations

First monitor the patient's central

EMERGENCY INTERVENTION

Managing a metaraminol overdose

A metaraminol overdose can cause nausea, vomiting, dizziness, severe chest pain, arrhythmias, hypertension, and excessive bradycardia.

If the patient develops these signs and symptoms, stop the infusion. Then take the following steps, as ordered:

- For arrhythmias, give propranolol.
- For severe hypertension, administer an alpha-adrenergic blocker, such as 5 to 10 mg of I.V. phentolamine. Repeat the dose, as necessary.
- For bradycardia, give atropine.
- To acidify the patient's urine and help him eliminate the drug, infuse ascorbic acid or ammonium chloride.

venous pressure to assess his circulating volume. This drug can't serve as a volume replacer, so if he has a fluid volume deficit, give fluids or volume expanders, as ordered.

Choose a large vein for an infusion. Don't use a vein in the ankle or the back of the hand, especially if the patient has peripheral vascular disease, diabetes mellitus, or hypercoagulability. A large vein helps prevent extravasation, which can cause tissue necrosis and sloughing. If extravasation does occur, stop the infusion at once and use a fine needle to infiltrate the area with 10 to 15 ml of 0.9% sodium chloride solution mixed with 5 to 10 mg of phentolamine. If administered within 12 hours, this should quickly reduce the effects of extravasation.

After you begin the infusion, let at least 10 minutes pass before increasing the dosage. A sharp rise in blood pressure may cause acute pulmonary edema and arrhythmias—even cardiac arrest. Keep emergency drugs on hand to reverse the effects of an overdose. (See *Managing a metaraminol overdose.*)

Monitor the patient's blood pressure every 5 minutes until it stabilizes, and then every 15 minutes. Also periodically check his pulse rate, breath sounds, the color and temperature of his extremities, and his urine output. Tell the doctor if the patient's urine output consistently declines. It may decrease initially but should rise as his blood pressure reaches a normal level.

Discontinue the drug slowly, and keep monitoring the patient's blood pressure, even after discontinuing the drug. An abrupt withdrawal could cause recurrent hypotension.

If the patient received metaraminol for an extended period, also monitor him for cumulative effects, including a continuing rise in blood pressure. Long-term use can also prevent the expansion of circulating volume and perpetuate shock.

Metaraminol may increase urine catecholamine levels.

Methoxamine hydrochloride

(Vasoxyl)

Methoxamine hydrochloride counteracts hypotension and paroxysmal supraventricular tachycardia by acting directly on alpha-adrenergic receptors of the peripheral vasculature, causing vasoconstriction. This action raises both systolic and diastolic blood pressure. The elevated blood pressure stimulates the carotid sinus reflex over the vagus nerve, stopping some paroxysmal supraventricular tachycardias.

With I.V. administration, the onset of action takes place immediately, peak action occurs in 30 seconds to 2 minutes, and pressor effects last 5 to 15 minutes. With I.M. administration, the drug starts working in 15 to 20 minutes, peak action occurs in 15 minutes, and pressor effects last 60 to 90 minutes.

The drug's distribution, metabolism, and excretion aren't known. (See *Methoxamine: Indications and dosages.*)

Contraindications and cautions

Don't give methoxamine to patients with a known hypersensitivity to the drug or to sulfites, or to patients with severe hypertension.

Give methoxamine cautiously to patients with bradycardia, partial heart block, or myocardial disease because it can exacerbate these conditions, and to patients with hyperthyroidism or pheochromocytoma because it can exacerbate the episodes of severe hypertension that these diseases cause. Also use the drug cautiously in those with vascular, peripheral, or mesenteric thrombosis because the area of ischemia and infarction may increase. And give the drug carefully to those with poor perfusion from severe arteriosclerosis because the decrease in cardiac output may be dangerous.

Use this pregnancy risk category C drug cautiously in pregnant women.

Preparation

Methoxamine comes in 1-ml ampules that contain 20 mg of the drug. Store ampules below 104° F (40° C), preferably between 59° and 86° F (15° and 30° C). Protect the drug from light and freezing.

To prepare the drug for infusion, dilute 30 to 40 mg in 250 ml of 5% dextrose in water.

DOSAGE FINDER

Methoxamine: Indications and dosages

Treatment of hypotension

▶ For adults, give a slow direct injection of 3 to 5 mg. Then give an I.M. injection of 10 to 15 mg, or infuse 30 to 40 mg in 250 ml of 5% dextrose in water, starting at a rate of 5 mcg/minute.

▶ For children, give a slow direct injection of 0.08 mg/kg or 2.5 mg/m^2. Then give an I.M. injection of 0.25 mg/kg or 7.5 mg/m^2.

Treatment of paroxysmal supraventricular tachycardia

▶ For adults, give 5 to 15 mg by direct injection over 3 to 5 minutes. The patient's systolic blood pressure shouldn't rise above 160 mm Hg.

Incompatibility

Methoxamine is incompatible with alkaline compounds.

Administration

- *Direct injection:* Slowly inject the ordered amount directly into a vein or an I.V. line containing a free-flowing, compatible solution.
- *Continuous infusion:* Administer the diluted drug at an infusion rate that maintains the desired blood pressure.
- *I.M. injection:* Inject the ordered dose of methoxamine into any I.M. injection site.

Adverse reactions

- *Life-threatening:* cerebral hemorrhage, respiratory distress.
- *Other:* anxiety, bradycardia, decreased cardiac output, decreased perfusion to vital organs, desire to void, dizziness, nausea and vomiting, nervousness, pallor, pilomotor response, precordial pain, seizures,

severe headaches, severe and prolonged hypertension, tremor, ventricular ectopic beats, weakness.

Interactions

- *Alpha-adrenergic blockers:* blocked pressor response to methoxamine, possibly causing severe hypotension.
- *Antihypertensives and diuretics:* reduced antihypertensive effects.
- *Atropine:* blocked reflex bradycardia and enhanced pressor effect of methoxamine.
- *Bretylium:* increased risk of arrhythmias.
- *Cardiac glycosides and levodopa:* possible cardiac arrhythmias.
- *Diatrizoates, iothalamate, and ioxaglate:* increased neurologic effects of these drugs.
- *Doxapram, guanadrel, guanethidine, mazindol, mecamylamine, methyldopa, methylphenidate, and trimethaphan:* increased pressor effects.
- *Ergot alkaloids and oxytocin:* increased vasoconstriction.
- *Halogenated hydrocarbon anesthetics:* increased risk of serious arrhythmias.
- *Nitrates:* reduced antianginal effects.
- *Rauwolfia alkaloids:* decreased hypotensive effects.
- *Sympathomimetics:* increased cardiovascular effects.
- *Thyroid hormones:* increased effects of both drugs.
- *Tricyclic antidepressants and maprotiline:* potentiated cardiovascular effects of methoxamine.

Special considerations

Before administering methoxamine to counteract hypotension, replace blood, plasma, fluids, and electrolytes as necessary.

Choose a large vein in the antecubital fossa to avoid extravasation, which can cause tissue necrosis and sloughing. If extravasation does occur, stop the infusion and use a fine needle to infiltrate the area with 10 to 15 ml of 0.9% sodium chloride solution mixed with 5 to 10 mg of phentolamine. This should counteract the effects of extravasation. Then restart the infusion.

During therapy, monitor the cardiac rhythm strip and blood pressure. Also watch for signs of an overdose. If excessive bradycardia develops, give atropine as ordered. For excessive hypertension, the patient will need an alpha-adrenergic blocker, such as phentolamine.

If the effects of methoxamine must be prolonged after an initial emergency I.V. dose, give supplemental doses by I.M. injection.

Methoxamine increases serum levels of plasma cortisol and corticotropin.

Methylergonovine maleate

(Methergine, Methylergabasine-Sandoz)

Methylergonovine maleate is indicated for severe postpartum and postabortion hemorrhage resulting from uterine atony or subinvolution. The drug controls bleeding by directly stimulating uterine and vascular smooth muscle, increasing the force and frequency of uterine contractions and constricting arterial vessels. The drug also increases cervical contraction. Large doses increase uterine tone and decrease periods of relaxation. (See *How methylergonovine increases uterine contractions,* page 138.)

After I.V. administration, the onset of action begins immediately, and the duration of action lasts up to 45 minutes. After an I.M. injection, the drug starts working in 2 to 5 minutes, and the duration of action lasts up to 3 hours. When given I.V., the drug's serum half-life has two phases, with the initial phase lasting 1 to 5 minutes, and the terminal phase, 30 minutes to 2 hours.

Methylergonovine is rapidly distributed into plasma, extracellular fluid, and tissues and probably metabolized in the liver. Although eliminated mainly in urine as metabolites, the drug is also excreted in feces; a negligible amount is excreted into breast milk. Neonates may take longer to eliminate the drug. (See *Methylergonovine: Indication and dosage.*)

DOSAGE FINDER

Methylergonovine: Indication and dosage

Emergency treatment of severe postpartum and postabortion hemorrhage caused by uterine atony or subinvolution

▶ Give adults 0.2 mg by I.V. or I.M. injection over at least 60 seconds. If necessary, repeat the dose every 2 to 4 hours up to a total of five doses.

Contraindications and cautions

Don't administer this pregnancy risk category C drug before placental expulsion, or it may cause captivation of the placenta. The drug is also contraindicated for inducing labor because it may cause uterine tetany or rupture, amniotic fluid embolism, or fetal trauma. Don't give this drug to patients with a hypersensitivity to ergot preparations.

Use methylergonovine cautiously in patients with hypertension or occlusive peripheral vascular disease because it can aggravate symptoms, and in patients with sepsis or hepatic or renal impairment because it can cause ergotism. Also use caution in patients with coronary artery disease because of the risk of angina or myocardial infarction.

Preparation

Methylergonovine comes in 1-ml ampules that contain 0.2 mg/ml. Store the drug below 46° F (8° C) in a light-resistant container, and protect it from freezing. Discard any solution that contains a precipitate or doesn't look clear and colorless.

You can dilute the drug with 5 ml of 0.9% sodium chloride solution to help ensure a slow injection.

Incompatibilities

No incompatibilities have been reported.

Administration

- *Direct injection:* Over a period of at least 60 seconds, inject the diluted or undiluted drug directly into a vein or an I.V. line with a free-flowing, compatible solution. Injecting the drug too rapidly may cause severe cardiovascular effects.
- *I.M. injection:* Inject the ordered dose into any I.M. injection site.

Adverse reactions

- *Life-threatening:* anaphylaxis, cerebrovascular accident, severe arrhythmias, shock.
- *Other:* blurred vision, chest pain, cool extremities, diaphoresis, dizziness, dyspnea, ergotism (agitation, confusion, dry mouth, hallucinations, muscle twitching, and palpitations), fever, headache, hypertension, joint pain, ***nausea,*** rash, seizures, sore throat, tachycardia, tinnitus, unusual bruising, ***vomiting,*** weakness.

MECHANISM OF ACTION

How methylergonovine increases uterine contractions

Methylergonovine produces vasoconstriction by stimulating vascular smooth muscle and increases the force and frequency of uterine contractions by directly stimulating the uterus. In larger doses, methylergonovine enhances uterine tone, causing briefer relaxation periods. Postpartum uterine contraction impedes uterine blood flow at the placental separation site.

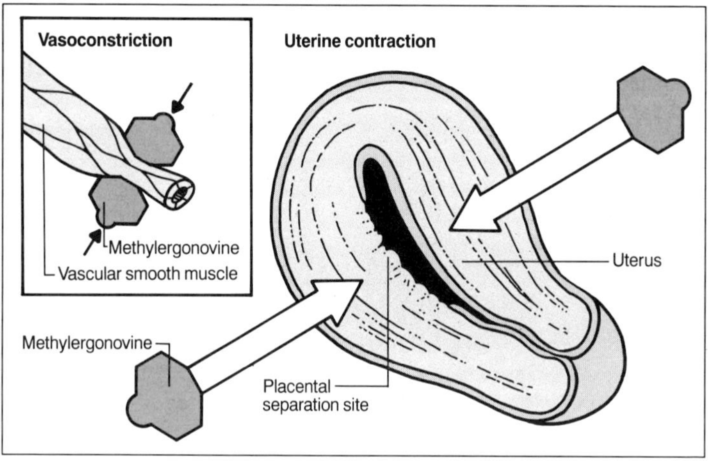

Interactions

- *Dopamine, I.V. oxytocin, and regional anesthetics:* increased vasoconstriction.
- *Other ergot alkaloids, vasoconstrictors, and vasopressors:* enhanced vasoconstriction.
- *Tobacco:* enhanced vasoconstriction (in heavy smokers).

Special considerations

Closely monitor the patient's blood pressure, pulse, and uterine response. Report frequent periods of uterine relaxation and any sudden changes in vital signs or the character or amount of vaginal bleeding. If the patient experiences severe uterine cramping, reduce the dosage as ordered.

An overdose may cause myocardial and peripheral ischemia, seizures, and severe hypertension. If an overdose occurs, provide symptomatic treatment, as ordered. Monitor the patient's cardiac rhythm strip for arrhythmias, as well as her vital signs and arterial blood gas and serum electrolyte levels. Administer nitroglycerin for myocardial ischemia, and diazepam or phenytoin for seizures. For peripheral ischemia, give the patient sodium nitroprusside, tolazoline, or phentolamine; for severe hypertension, sodium nitroprusside, chlorpromazine, or hydralazine.

Methylergonovine may decrease levels of serum prolactin, which may hinder lactation.

Methylprednisolone sodium succinate

(A-methaPred, Solu-Medrol)

Indicated for severe inflammation, shock, and lupus nephritis, this synthetic glucocorticoid suppresses pituitary release of corticotropin—thus preventing adrenal secretion of corticosteroids. As a result, methylprednisolone sodium succinate decreases inflammation, suppresses immune responses, stimulates bone marrow production, and alters protein, fat, and carbohydrate metabolism (see *How methylprednisolone works,* page 140).

The drug's onset of action is rapid. Peak effects occur in 1 to 3 hours, and the duration of action lasts 3 days to 3 weeks, depending on the dose. The serum half-life ranges from 2 to 3½ hours; the tissue half-life, up to 36 hours.

Methylprednisolone is distributed rapidly in the muscles, skin, liver, intestines, and kidneys. It binds with the protein transcortin and crosses the placenta. The drug is metabolized in the liver and in some tissues to form inactive compounds. These inactive metabolites—glucuronides and sulfates as well as some unconjugated products—are excreted by the kidneys. Small amounts of unmetabolized drug are eliminated in urine, and negligible amounts appear in bile. Methylprednisolone probably appears in breast milk, too. Excretion may be prolonged in hypothyroidism. (See *Methylprednisolone: Indications and dosages.*)

Contraindications and cautions

Methylprednisolone is contraindicated for patients with a known hypersensitivity to the drug, and for those with systemic fungal infection, sepsis syndrome, or septic shock because it may mask their symptoms or exacerbate their conditions. Except in life-threatening situations, the drug is also contraindicated for patients with viral or bacterial infections uncontrolled by antibiotics because the drug may mask symptoms. And, because the drug may exacerbate peptic ulcer disease, it's contraindicated for patients with this condition—except in life-threatening situations. Methylprednisolone contains benzyl alcohol, so avoid giving the drug to neonates.

Use methylprednisolone cautiously in patients with hyperthyroidism, hypothyroidism, or

DOSAGE FINDER

Methylprednisolone: Indications and dosages

Treatment of severe inflammation

▶ For adults, give 10 mg to 1.5 g I.V. or I.M. daily. The usual dosage is 10 to 250 mg every 4 hours.

Treatment of severe shock

▶ For adults, give 30 mg/kg I.V. initially, repeating the dose every 4 to 6 hours as needed. Or start with 100 to 250 mg, repeating the dose every 2 to 6 hours. As an alternative, the initial dose may be followed by an infusion of 30 mg/kg every 12 hours for 24 to 48 hours.

Treatment of severe lupus nephritis

▶ For adults, administer an intermittent infusion of 1 g for 3 days. Then give oral prednisolone or prednisone.

▶ For children, administer an intermittent infusion of 30 mg/kg I.V. on alternate days. Give a total of six doses, then give oral prednisolone or prednisone.

MECHANISM OF ACTION

How methylprednisolone works

Tissue trauma normally leads to tissue irritation, edema, inflammation, and scar tissue (shown in gray). But methylprednisolone counteracts the initial effects of tissue trauma, promoting healing (shown in color).

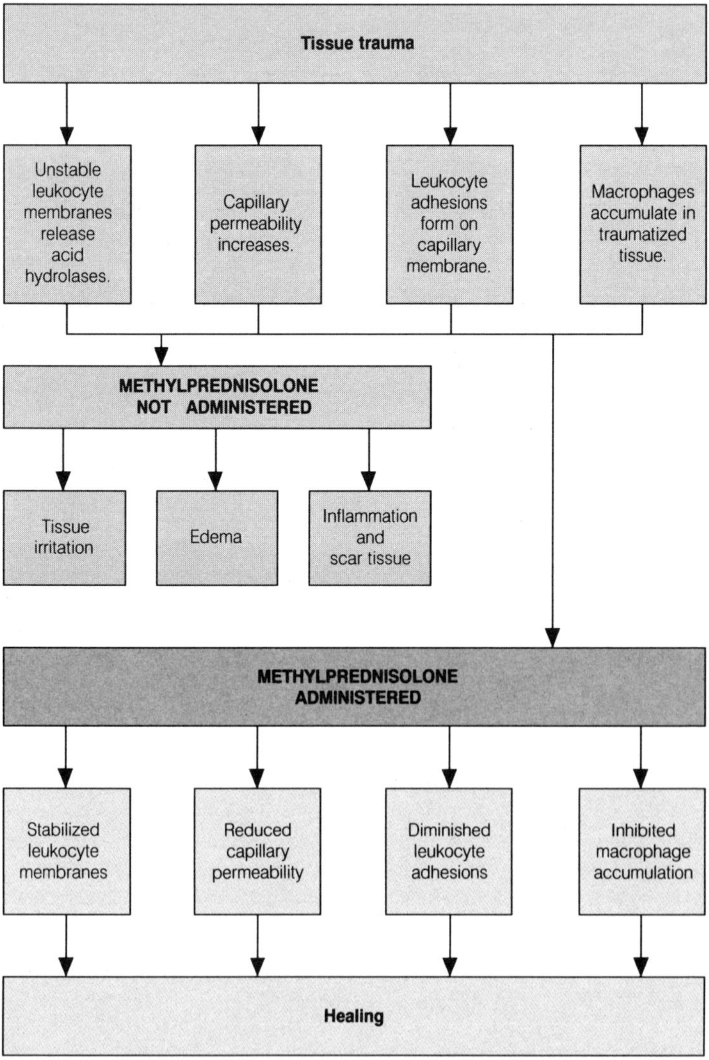

cirrhosis because the response may be exaggerated. Administer the drug cautiously to patients with psychoses because it may precipitate mental disturbances. Use caution with patients who have diverticulitis, nonspecific ulcerative colitis, or recent intestinal anastomosis because of the risk of perforation or abscess or other pyogenic infection.

To prevent an exacerbation of symptoms, give methylprednisolone carefully to patients with seizure disorders, renal insufficiency, diabetes mellitus, osteoporosis, or ocular herpes simplex infections. Also give the drug carefully to patients with a history of tuberculosis because of the risk of reactivation, to patients with renal dysfunction because of the risk of severe fluid retention, to patients with hepatic dysfunction or hypoalbuminemia because of the risk of toxicity, and to patients with open-angle glaucoma because of the risk of elevated intraocular pressure (IOP).

Use methylprednisolone cautiously in children because it may retard bone growth. It also may increase intracranial pressure, resulting in papilledema, oculomotor or abducens nerve paralysis, vision loss, and headache.

Because methylprednisolone is classified as a pregnancy risk category C drug, administer it cautiously to pregnant women.

Preparation

Methylprednisolone is available in vials containing the following amounts of drug and diluent: 40 mg/1 ml, 125 mg/2 ml, 500 mg/8.8 ml, 1 g/17.6 ml, and 2 g/30.6 ml. Reconstitute the drug with the diluent by depressing the vial's rubber stopper, then mixing. Store the reconstituted drug at room temperature and use within 48 hours (discard after 48 hours). Avoid freezing it. Never administer a cloudy solution and discard any unused portion after 48 hours. Dilute the solution for infusion with dextrose 5% in water, 0.9% sodium chloride solution, or dextrose 5% in 0.9% sodium chloride solution.

Incompatibilities

Methylprednisolone is incompatible with calcium gluconate, cephalothin sodium, cytarabine, glycopyrrolate, metaraminol bitartrate, nafcillin sodium, and penicillin G sodium.

Administration

- *Direct injection:* Over a period of at least 1 minute, administer the diluted drug into a vein or a free-flowing I.V. line with a compatible solution. In life-threatening situations, administer an initial massive dose over 3 to 15 minutes.
- *Intermittent infusion:* Administer the appropriate diluted dose, adjusting the flow rate based on the disorder and the patient's response.
- *Continuous infusion:* Infuse the appropriate diluted dose, adjusting the flow rate depending on the disorder and the patient's response.
- *I.M. injection:* Administer the ordered dose deep into the gluteal muscle. Never use the deltoid muscle, and don't use the same gluteal site repeatedly.

Adverse reactions

- *Life-threatening:* anaphylaxis.
- *Other:* bleeding, blurred vision, ***carbohydrate intolerance,*** depression, dyspnea, facial flushing, fever, ***fluid and electrolyte imbalance,*** hypertension, increased susceptibility to infection, ***insomnia,*** pain at injection site, palpitations, ***peptic ulcer,*** rash, rectal irritation, seizures, steroid withdrawal syndrome (an-

orexia, headache, hypotension, joint pain, lethargy, nausea, vomiting, weight loss), tachycardia.

Interactions

- *Anticholinesterase drugs:* severe weakness in patients with myasthenia gravis.
- *Asparaginase:* heightened risk of neuropathy and disturbances in erythropoiesis.
- *Barbiturates, phenytoin, rifampin:* risk of increased methylprednisolone metabolism.
- *Cardiac glycosides:* enhanced risk of arrhythmias or digitalis toxicity.
- *Estrogen:* risk of potentiated methylprednisolone effects.
- *Iodine 131 (^{131}I):* reduced thyroid uptake.
- *Indomethacin, nonsteroidal anti-inflammatory drugs, and other ulcerogenic drugs:* increased risk of ulcers.
- *Isoniazid:* risk of increased metabolism and excretion of isoniazid.
- *Mexiletine:* accelerated metabolism of mexiletine.
- *Oral anticoagulants:* possible increased blood coagulability.
- *Potassium-depleting diuretics and other potassium-depleting drugs:* enhanced potassium loss.
- *Salicylates:* decreased effects of salicylates.
- *Sodium-containing drugs and foods:* possible hypernatremia.
- *Streptozocin:* possible hyperglycemia.
- *Toxoids, live or inactivated vaccines:* diminished response to these agents.

Special considerations

Before starting methylprednisolone therapy, review test results, including the baseline electrocardiogram, blood pressure reading, and chest and spinal X-rays. You should also have results from a glucose tolerance test, hypothalamic-pituitary-adrenal axis function test, and an upper GI series (for patients predisposed to GI disorders).

During therapy, adjust the dosage as needed for a patient taking insulin, antithyroid drugs, or thyroid hormones. During long-term therapy, monitor the patient's weight, blood pressure, chest and spinal X-rays, hematopoietic test findings, electrolyte levels, glucose tolerance test results, and IOP.

Also, anticipate increasing the patient's protein intake because methylprednisolone promotes protein catabolism. Be aware that a patient's adrenal function should recover within 1 week after high-dose methylprednisolone therapy that lasts 1 to 5 days.

Methylprednisolone can interfere with the results of certain laboratory tests. The drug may cause decreased basophil, eosinophil, lymphocyte, and monocyte counts. Also, ^{131}I, serum protein-bound iodine, thyroxine, and serum calcium levels will be reduced. The drug may cause increased platelet and polymorphonuclear cell counts as well as increased serum lipid and urine glucose levels.

The nitroblue tetrazolium test for systemic bacterial infections may show false-negative results, and radionuclide brain imaging will reveal decreased contrast medium uptake. Because methylprednisolone suppresses the inflammatory response, the drug interferes with accurate skin testing.

Metoprolol tartrate

(Lopressor)

This $beta_1$-adrenergic blocker is used as an early treatment when an acute myocardial infarction is suspected or diagnosed. By lowering myocardial oxygen needs and possibly reducing arrhythmias, metoprolol tartrate diminishes the severity of myocardial ischemia, thereby decreasing the risks of reinfarction and death.

Metoprolol works by binding to postganglionic receptors in the myocardium and blocking the sympathetic neurotransmitter norepinephrine. In high doses, the drug also binds to $beta_2$-adrenergic receptors in bronchial and vascular smooth muscle.

The peak serum level occurs within 20 minutes after I.V. administration. The half-life of the drug in healthy or hypertensive patients ranges from 3 to 7 hours; in patients with poor hydroxylation, the half-life is 7½ hours.

The drug is widely distributed, with the highest concentrations found in the heart, liver, lungs, and saliva. About 12% is bound to serum albumin. Metoprolol crosses the placenta, producing almost equal fetal and maternal levels. It also crosses the blood-brain barrier, producing cerebrospinal fluid levels that are about 80% of plasma levels. Metabolism occurs mainly in the liver, producing three major, relatively inactive metabolites. Metoprolol is excreted in the urine via glomerular filtration and, to a lesser extent, through renal tubular secretion and reabsorption. About 10% of the drug is excreted unchanged; about 90%, as metabolites. The drug also appears in breast milk. (See *Metoprolol: Indication and dosage.*)

DOSAGE FINDER

Metoprolol: Indication and dosage

Early treatment of suspected or definitive acute myocardial infarction

▶ For adults, administer 5 mg by direct I.V. injection every 2 minutes for a total of three doses. Follow this with oral maintenance doses.

Contraindications and cautions

To avoid increasing the risk of myocardial depression, you shouldn't administer metoprolol to patients who have a known hypersensitivity to the drug, nor should you give it to patients who have first-, second-, or third-degree heart block, bradycardia (less than 45 beats/minute), a systolic pressure below 100 mm Hg, moderate to severe congestive heart failure (CHF), or cardiogenic shock.

Administer metoprolol cautiously to patients with CHF that's controlled by digitalis and diuretics because it may exacerbate the condition, to elderly patients or those with hepatic or renal disease because of the risk of drug toxicity and adverse effects, and to patients with bronchospastic disease because the drug may aggravate the symptoms. Also administer metoprolol cautiously to patients with myasthenia gravis because the drug may cause muscle weakness, to patients with diabetes mellitus or hyperthyroidism because the drug may mask symptoms, and to patients suffering from depression or psoriasis because the drug may exacerbate these conditions.

Because metoprolol is classified as a pregnancy risk category C drug, use it cautiously in pregnant women.

Preparation

Metoprolol is available in 5-ml ampules or prefilled syringes of 1 mg/ml. Store the drug at room

EMERGENCY INTERVENTION

Managing a metoprolol overdose

If you detect signs of a metoprolol overdose, discontinue the drug and notify the doctor immediately. Then perform the following interventions, as ordered:
- For bradycardia, give the patient atropine or prepare him for temporary pacemaker insertion.
- For premature ventricular contractions, administer lidocaine or phenytoin.
- For heart failure, administer oxygen, digitalis, and a diuretic.
- For hypotension, give the patient I.V. fluids and vasopressors, such as epinephrine.
- For bronchospasm, give a $beta_2$-agonist, such as isoproterenol.
- For seizures, administer diazepam or lorazepam.

temperature and protect it from light; avoid freezing it. Discard any solution that becomes discolored or forms a precipitate.

Incompatibilities
No incompatibilities have been reported.

Administration
- *Direct injection:* Rapidly inject the prescribed bolus dose into a free-flowing I.V. line.

Adverse reactions
- *Life-threatening:* respiratory distress with laryngospasm, severe bradycardia or hypotension.
- *Other:* abdominal pain, alopecia, CHF, cold extremities, confusion, depression, dizziness, dyspnea, fatigue, fever, first-degree heart block, hallucinations, intensified arrhythmias, nausea, palpitations, rash, Raynaud's syndrome, sleep disturbances, sore throat.

Interactions
- *Barbiturates, rifampin:* increased metabolism of metaprolol, causing decreased drug effectiveness.
- *Calcium channel blockers:* potentiated hypotensive effect.
- *Cardiac glycosides, catecholamine-depleting drugs (such as reserpine):* potentiation of hypotension or bradycardia.
- *Chlorpromazine, cimetidine:* increased beta blockade resulting from inhibited metoprolol metabolism.
- *Diazoxide:* prevention of tachycardia and enhanced hypotensive effect.
- *Estrogens, nonsteroidal anti-inflammatory drugs:* decreased antihypertensive effect.
- *Hydrocarbon inhalation anesthetics:* increased risk of myocardial depression and hypotension.
- *Insulin, oral antidiabetic agents:* amplified risk of hypoglycemia or hyperglycemia.
- *Lidocaine:* increased effect and risk of toxicity from reduced clearance of lidocaine.
- *Molindone:* enhanced metoprolol effects.
- *Monoamine oxidase inhibitors:* severe hypertension if metoprolol is given within 14 days of last dose.
- *Nondepolarizing neuromuscular blockers:* possible potentiated and prolonged action.
- *Other antihypertensive drugs:* potentiated hypotensive effect.
- *Phenothiazines:* possible increased plasma levels of both drugs.
- *Phenytoin (I.V.):* possible additive myocardial depression.
- *Ritodrine:* decreased ritodrine effects.
- *Sympathomimetics, xanthines:* possible antagonized beta blockade.

Special considerations
Administer metoprolol as soon as the patient's condition stabilizes. During administration, continuously monitor the patient's hemodynamic status, blood pressure, heart rate, and cardiac rhythm strip. If you note minor bradycardia or hypotension, notify the doctor, who may stop the injections or change to an oral form of the drug.

Report any signs of an overdose – severe hypotension, bradycardia, heart failure, bronchospasm, or seizures – and prepare to assist with emergency management. (See *Managing a metoprolol overdose.*)

Be aware that metoprolol can cause elevated blood urea nitrogen, serum lipoprotein, potassium, triglyceride, and uric acid levels.

DOSAGE FINDER

Morphine: Indications and dosages

Treatment of pain associated with myocardial infarction

▶ For adults, administer 8 to 15 mg I.V., followed by smaller doses every 3 to 4 hours as needed.

Treatment of severe, acute pain

▶ For adults, administer 5 to 20 mg I.M. or S.C. or 4 to 10 mg I.V. every 4 hours as needed.

▶ For children, give 100 to 200 mcg/kg I.M. or S.C. or 50 to 100 mcg/kg I.V. every 4 hours as needed. The maximum single dose is 10 mg.

Treatment of severe, chronic pain

▶ For adults, give 1 to 10 mg/hour by continuous infusion. The maintenance dosage is 20 to 150 mg/hour.

▶ For children, give 0.025 to 2.6 mg/kg/hour.

Morphine sulfate

(Astramorph, Astramorph PF, Duramorph PF)

Used to relieve severe pain, morphine sulfate binds with specific receptors (mainly the mu receptor) in the central nervous system (CNS) to alter the patient's perception of and emotional response to pain. A schedule II controlled substance, morphine is the drug of choice for pain associated with a myocardial infarction because it not only alleviates pain, but also reduces the myocardium's need for oxygen (see *How morphine reduces myocardial oxygen consumption*, page 146).

The drug's peak action occurs within 20 minutes of an I.V. dose; 10 to 30 minutes of an I.M. or S.C. dose. The effect lasts 4 to 5 hours, depending on the dose; the half-life ranges from 2 to 3 hours.

Morphine is rapidly distributed to the kidneys, spleen, lungs, and liver. Minimal protein binding occurs, and the drug readily crosses the placenta. Morphine is metabolized primarily in the liver and excreted in urine, mainly as metabolites. About 7% to 10% is excreted in feces. The drug also appears in breast milk. (See *Morphine: Indications and dosages.*)

Contraindications and cautions
Morphine is contraindicated for patients with a known hypersensitivity to the drug and for patients with acute respiratory depression because it may exacerbate this condition. What's more, morphine is contraindicated for those with diarrhea resulting from pseudomembranous colitis or poisoning because the drug may slow the elimination of toxins, and for those with pulmo-

MECHANISM OF ACTION

How morphine reduces myocardial oxygen consumption

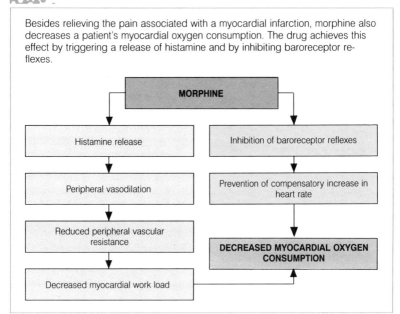

Besides relieving the pain associated with a myocardial infarction, morphine also decreases a patient's myocardial oxygen consumption. The drug achieves this effect by triggering a release of histamine and by inhibiting baroreceptor reflexes.

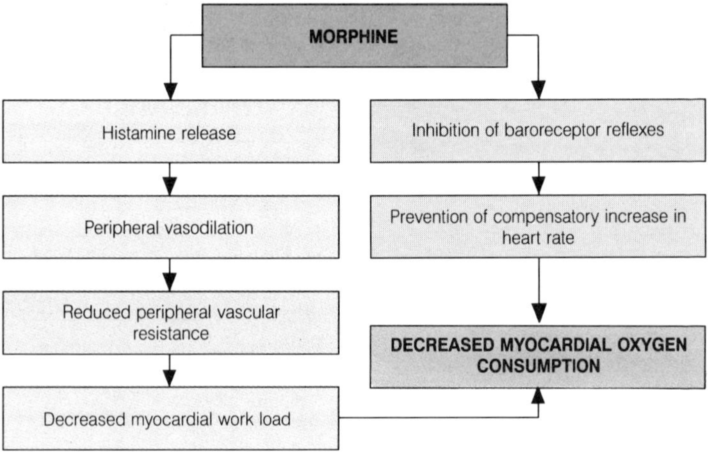

nary edema caused by a chemical respiratory irritant because the drug causes vasodilation and produces adverse hemodynamic effects.

Give morphine cautiously to patients with impaired respiratory function because of the risk of respiratory depression, to patients with hypothyroid conditions because of the risk of respiratory depression and prolonged CNS depression, to patients with arrhythmias because the drug can increase the vagal response through a vagolytic action, and to patients with seizure disorders because the drug may induce or exacerbate seizures.

Use morphine carefully in patients with acute abdominal conditions because the drug may mask symptoms, in those with gallbladder disease because the drug may increase biliary contractions, in those with inflammatory bowel disease because of the risk of toxic megacolon, and in those recovering from GI surgery because the drug may alter GI motility. Also give the drug cautiously to patients with hepatic or renal impairment because of the risk of toxicity. Patients with prostatic hyperplasia, urethral stricture, or recent urinary tract surgery who receive the drug may experience urine retention.

Give morphine cautiously to patients who've sustained a head injury and to those with increased intracranial pressure (from intracranial lesions) because morphine may mask clinical signs and elevate cerebrospinal fluid (CSF) pressure.

Because of the high potential for abuse, give morphine cautiously to patients with a history of drug dependency or emotional instability, including those with thoughts of suicide.

Give this pregnancy risk category C drug cautiously to pregnant patients.

Preparation

Morphine is available in concentrations of 0.5 mg/ml, 1 mg/ml, 2 mg/ml, 4 mg/ml, 5 mg/ml, 8 mg/ml, 10 mg/ml, and 15 mg/ml in 1-ml ampules, vials, and disposable units; in 2-ml disposable units; in 10-ml ampules; and in 20-ml vials. Store the drug at a temperature below 104° F (40° C). Protect it from light and freezing. For direct injection, dilute the drug with 4 or 5 ml of dextrose 5% in water. For slow infusion, dilute the drug with larger volumes. Morphine is compatible with most common I.V. solutions.

Incompatibilities

Morphine is incompatible with aminophylline, amobarbital sodium, chlorothiazide, heparin sodium, meperidine hydrochloride, methicillin sodium, minocycline hydrochloride, phenobarbital sodium, phenytoin sodium, promethazine hydrochloride, sodium bicarbonate, sodium iodide, soluble barbiturates, tetracyclines, and thiopental sodium.

Administration

- *Direct injection:* Over 4 to 5 minutes, inject the diluted drug into an I.V. line containing a free-flowing, compatible solution.
- *Continuous infusion:* Administer the diluted drug initially at a rate of 1 to 10 mg/hour. Then increase the rate until an effective dosage is achieved.
- *I.M. injection:* Inject the ordered dose of undiluted drug into any I.M. injection site.
- *S.C. injection:* Inject the ordered dose of undiluted drug into any S.C. injection site. Avoid repeated injections at the same site to help prevent local tissue irritation, pain, and induration.

Adverse reactions

- *Life-threatening:* anaphylaxis, bradycardia, circulatory collapse, respiratory depression, tachycardia.
- *Other:* agitation; coma; ***constipation; decreased mental acuity or depression;*** delirium; dizziness; dysphoria; euphoria; fainting; flushing; ***hypotension;*** insomnia; ***nausea;*** nervousness; oliguria; pain at infusion site; pruritus; restlessness; ***sedation;*** seizures; ***somnolence;*** sweating; ***urine retention;*** urticaria; visual disturbances; ***vomiting;*** warm face, neck, and upper trunk; and weakness.

Interactions

- *Antidiarrheals, antiperistaltics:* enhanced risk of constipation and CNS depression.
- *Antihypertensives, diuretics:* heightened risk of hypotension.
- *Antimuscarinics:* increased risk of constipation, paralytic ileus, and urine retention.
- *Buprenorphine:* risk of respiratory depression and reduced therapeutic morphine effect; risk of precipitating withdrawal symptoms in drug-dependent patients.
- *Hydroxyzine:* enhanced analgesia, CNS depression, and hypotension.
- *Metoclopramide:* antagonized effects on GI motility.
- *Monoamine oxidase inhibitors:* severe, unpredictable adverse reactions when given within 21 days of morphine. When given concomitantly, the morphine dose should be reduced.

EMERGENCY INTERVENTION

Managing a morphine overdose

When administering morphine, watch for signs and symptoms of an overdose including bradycardia, bradypnea, cold and clammy skin, dyspnea, hypotension, loss of consciousness, pinpoint pupils, seizures, severe dizziness and drowsiness, severe nervousness or restlessness, and severe weakness. If you detect an overdose, contact the doctor and take the following steps, as ordered:
• Establish and maintain an adequate airway and ventilation.
• Administer I.V. fluids and vasopressors.
• To reverse respiratory depression, administer 400 mcg to 2 mg of naloxone in a single I.V. dose. Monitor the patient's response, keeping in mind he may need another dose of naloxone because morphine's duration of action usually exceeds that of naloxone.

• *Naloxone:* antagonized analgesic, CNS, and respiratory depressant effects.
• *Naltrexone:* blocked therapeutic morphine effect and risk of precipitating withdrawal symptoms in drug-dependent patients.
• *Neuromuscular blockers:* deepened respiratory depression.
• *Opioid-agonist analgesics:* deepened CNS and respiratory depression, hypotension.
• *Other CNS depressants:* deepened CNS depression and risk of morphine tolerance and dependence.

Special considerations

Administer morphine with the patient supine to minimize hypotension. When he rises, have him move slowly to alleviate dizziness and faintness.

Keep emergency resuscitation equipment nearby if the patient is receiving I.V. morphine. During an infusion, monitor the patient's respirations frequently. Check him every 15 minutes for 1 hour following the infusion. Keep in mind that respiratory depression is more likely to occur in elderly and pediatric patients. If your patient's respirations fall below 8 breaths/minute, notify the doctor and arouse the patient to stimulate his breathing.

Watch for other signs of an overdose, as well. A rapid infusion can cause a life-threatening overdose because maximum CNS effects are delayed (see *Managing a morphine overdose*). Ambulatory patients and those without chronic pain have a higher incidence of adverse reactions than other patients.

Injected I.M. or S.C., morphine may be incompletely absorbed by a patient who is in shock and who has impaired blood volume and circulation. Repeating I.M. or S.C. injections in such a patient may result in an overdose when circulation and blood volume return and improve drug absorption.

Opioid agonists, such as morphine, stimulate vasopressin release. Thus, using morphine may increase the risk of water intoxication in postoperative patients.

Keep in mind that tolerance and dependence can develop from long-term morphine use. If a patient with severe chronic pain develops a tolerance to the drug, you may need to increase the dose. Withdrawal symptoms may appear within 24 hours of discontinuation and peak in 36 to 72 hours. Expect symptoms to disappear in 5 to 14 days.

Morphine can interfere with accurate results of various tests. For example, gastric emptying studies may show delayed emptying, and hepatobiliary imaging with technetium Tc 99m disofenin will show delayed visualization, falsely resembling common bile duct obstruction. Lumbar puncture will show elevated CSF pressure caused by respiratory depression, and serum amylase and lipase levels may appear increased.

Neostigmine methylsulfate

(Prostigmin)

An anticholinesterase agent, neostigmine methylsulfate blocks the effects of acetylcholinesterase at the neuromuscular junction. This action allows acetylcholine accumulation, resulting in a prolonged increase in skeletal muscle strength and intestinal muscle tone, bradycardia, ureteral constriction, bronchial and pupillary constriction, and salivary and sweat gland secretion.

You'll see the drug ordered as an antidote to nondepolarizing neuromuscular blocking agents and as a symptomatic treatment for myasthenia gravis. The drug also is used to reduce postoperative abdominal distention by stimulating GI motility and increasing gastric tone and to relieve nonobstructive urine retention by increasing detrusor muscle tone.

Following I.V. administration, the onset of action occurs in 5 minutes; the peak effect is reached between 20 and 30 minutes. Following an I.M. injection, the onset of action occurs in 20 to 30 minutes. With all routes, the duration of action is 2 to 4 hours, and the half-life is 47 to 60 minutes.

Neostigmine is distributed throughout most tissues, with the highest concentrations in the liver and heart; 15% to 25% of the drug is bound to serum albumin. Only after high doses does neostigmine cross the blood-brain barrier. It may cross the placenta. Neostigmine is hydrolyzed by cholinesterases at the neuromuscular junction and metabolized by hepatic microsomal enzymes. The drug is excreted in urine, via renal tubular secretion, as unchanged drug and inactive metabolites. Neostigmine doesn't appear in breast milk. (See *Neostigmine: Indications and dosages.*)

DOSAGE FINDER

Neostigmine: Indications and dosages

Antidote to nondepolarizing neuromuscular blocking agents

▶ For adults, slowly administer 0.5 to 2.5 mg I.V.; repeat the dose as needed, up to a total dose of 5 mg.

▶ For children, administer 0.04 mg/kg I.V. along with 20 mcg/kg of atropine.

Treatment of myasthenia gravis

▶ For adults, give 0.5 mg I.M. or S.C. Base subsequent doses on the patient's response.

▶ For children, give 10 to 40 mcg/kg I.M. or S.C. every 3 to 4 hours. You may give 10 mcg of atropine I.M. or S.C. with each dose or alternate doses to counteract any muscarinic effects.

Reduction of postoperative abdominal distention

▶ For adults, give 0.5 mg I.M. or S.C. as needed.

Treatment of urine retention

▶ For adults, administer 0.5 mg I.M. or S.C. Repeat the dose every 3 hours for five doses, or until the bladder empties.

Contraindications and cautions

Neostigmine is contraindicated for patients with a known or suspected hypersensitivity to the drug. Also, the drug shouldn't be given to patients with a mechanical obstruction of the intestinal or urinary tract because it increases intestinal and urinary muscle tone and activity.

Administer neostigmine cautiously to patients with asthma, bradycardia, arrhythmias, peptic ulcer, epilepsy, or hyperthyroidism because these conditions may be exacerbated. Also give the drug carefully to postoperative patients because respiratory difficulty may be aggravated by postoperative pain, sedation, secretions, or atelectasis.

A pregnancy risk category C drug, neostigmine should be used cautiously in pregnant patients.

Preparation

Neostigmine is available in 1-ml ampules of 1:2,000 (0.5 mg/ml) and 1:4,000 (0.25 mg/ml) and in multidose vials of 1:1,000 (1 mg/ml) and 1:2,000 (0.5 mg/ml). Protect the drug from light and from freezing temperatures. Neostigmine needs no further dilution.

Incompatibilities

No incompatibilities have been reported.

Administration

- *Direct injection:* Slowly inject the ordered dose into a free-flowing I.V. line of dextrose 5% in water, 0.9% sodium chloride solution, or another compatible I.V. solution.
- *I.M. injection:* Inject the ordered dose into any I.M. injection site.
- *S.C. injection:* Inject the ordered dose into any S.C. injection site.

Adverse reactions

- *Life-threatening:* anaphylaxis, aspiration of excessive oral secretions, respiratory paralysis, severe bradycardia, severe bronchospasm.
- *Other:* clumsiness; confusion; dyspnea; fasciculations; fatigue; irritability; ***muscarinic effects*** (**abdominal *cramps,*** blurred vision, diaphoresis, ***diarrhea,*** excessive salivation, increased bronchial secretions, lacrimation); muscle cramps; nausea; pupillary constriction; rash; thrombophlebitis; ***twitching or weakness; vomiting;*** wheezing.

Interactions

- *Aminoglycosides:* possible reversed neuromuscular blockade.
- *Antimuscarinic agents (especially atropine):* antagonized muscarinic effects of neostigmine.
- *Cholinesterase inhibitors:* risk of additive toxicity.
- *Depolarizing neuromuscular blocking agents (such as decamethonium and succinylcholine):* prolonged neuromuscular blockade.
- *Edrophonium:* increased risk of cholinergic crisis.
- *Guanadrel, guanethidine, mecamylamine, trimethaphan:* antagonized neostigmine effects.
- *Local ester-derivative anesthetics:* increased risk of toxicity from reduced metabolism of the anesthetic.
- *Magnesium:* risk of antagonized neostigmine effects.
- *Nondepolarizing neuromuscular blocking agents (such as gallamine, pancuronium, and tubocurarine):* antagonized effects of these blockers.
- *Procainamide, quinidine:* risk of antagonized neostigmine action.

Special considerations

Obtain a baseline respiratory rate and maintain a patent airway using suctioning, oxygen, and assisted ventilation, as needed. Also obtain a baseline heart rate and blood pressure. If the heart rate is below 80 beats/minute, give atropine before neostigmine, as ordered. (Some clinicians recommend giving adults 0.6 to 1.2 mg of atropine I.V. or 0.2 to 0.6 mg glycopyrrolate I.V. before or along with high neostigmine doses.)

When administering neostigmine I.V., keep a syringe of an anticholinergic, such as atropine, and emergency airway and resuscitation equipment on hand. Monitor the patient for signs of toxicity—especially increased muscarinic effects, such as severe bradycardia, excessive salivation, severe bronchospasm, and respiratory paralysis. If such signs occur, use the airway equipment, and administer the atropine or glycopyrrolate, as ordered.

If neostigmine is given to reverse the effects of a nondepolarizing neuromuscular blocker, keep the patient on assisted ventilation because the drug works best if the patient is hyperventilated to decrease his partial pressure of carbon dioxide level.

Periodically assess a myasthenic patient's vital capacity and muscle strength to monitor his response to neostigmine. Be alert for a cholinergic crisis marked by muscle weakness, adverse muscarinic effects, and fasciculations (resulting from excessive cholinergic stimulation). Cholinergic crisis usually occurs 1 hour after the last neostigmine dose.

Nitroglycerin

(Nitro-Bid, Nitrol, Nitrostat, Tridil)

Nitroglycerin is indicated as an adjunctive treatment of congestive heart failure and as a treatment of chest pain associated with myocardial infarction (MI) and acute angina pectoris. The drug also lowers blood pressure during surgery.

Nitroglycerin relaxes vascular smooth muscle, causing vasodilation and reducing myocardial oxygen demands. The subsequent improvement in myocardial blood flow to ischemic areas relieves angina, decreases peripheral venous stasis, and reduces venous ventricular volume and myocardial tension (preload). In high doses, nitroglycerin moderately decreases peripheral vascular resistance, reducing arterial pressure and ventricular outflow resistance (afterload).

The onset of action occurs immediately after an I.V. dose and 1 to 3 minutes after a sublingual or buccal dose. The peak effect is about 1 to 2 minutes after I.V. administration. The duration of action depends on the dose with I.V. administration but generally lasts several minutes; the duration for a sublingual dose is about 30 to 60 minutes. The elimination half-life is 1 to 4 minutes.

Nitroglycerin is widely distributed. Whether it crosses the placenta remains unknown. The drug is metabolized rapidly and almost completely in the liver, with the metabolites excreted in urine. Whether the drug appears in breast milk isn't known. (See *Nitroglycerin: Indications and dosages,* page 152.)

Contraindications and cautions

Nitroglycerin is contraindicated for patients with a history of hypersensitivity to this or other nitrates. The drug shouldn't be given to patients with increased intracranial pressure because it may raise cerebrospinal fluid pressure, to patients with hypotension or uncorrected hypovolemia because severe hypotension or shock may develop, to patients with constrictive pericarditis or pericardial tamponade because the drug may further impair coronary circula-

DOSAGE FINDER

Nitroglycerin: Indications and dosages

Adjunctive treatment of congestive heart failure, treatment of chest pain associated with myocardial infarction and acute angina pectoris, and reduction of elevated blood pressure during surgery

▶ For adults, initially administer 5 mcg/minute I.V. Increase this by 5 mcg/minute every 3 to 5 minutes until the desired response is achieved. If the response is inadequate at 20 mcg/minute, increase the dose by as much as 20 mcg/minute. Once a partial response is obtained, increase the interval between doses and reduce the dose. A safe maximum dosage hasn't been established.

Treatment of angina pectoris

▶ For adults, administer a 150- to 600-mcg sublingual or buccal tablet. Or administer one or two metered-dose sprays (400 or 800 mcg) onto or under the tongue. Give one dose every 5 minutes. If relief doesn't occur after the third dose, notify the doctor.

tion, or to those with hypertrophic cardiomyopathy because the drug may intensify angina.

Give nitroglycerin cautiously to patients with glaucoma because intraocular pressure may briefly increase. Use caution with patients who have hyperthyroidism because the resulting tachycardia may aggravate ischemia. Also exercise caution with patients who've recently sustained an MI because the drug may aggravate ischemia.

Administer the drug carefully to patients with severe hepatic impairment because of the increased risk of methemoglobinemia and to patients with severe renal impairment because excretion will be slow.

A pregnancy risk category C drug, nitroglycerin should be used cautiously in pregnant women.

Preparation

Several nitroglycerin preparations are available for I.V. use. Each comes with diluent and dosage instructions.

- Nitro-Bid comes in 1-, 5-, and 10-ml vials of 5 mg/ml. Dilute it with dextrose 5% in water (D_5W) or 0.9% sodium chloride solution. For a concentration of 50 mcg/ml, mix 1 ml of drug in 100 ml of solution; for 100 mcg/ml, mix 1 ml of drug in 50 ml of solution; for 200 mcg/ml, mix 2 ml of drug in 50 ml of solution.
- Nitrol is available in a 10-ml ampule containing 5 mg/ml. Dilute the drug by adding one 10-ml ampule (50 mg) to 500 ml of D_5W or 0.9% sodium chloride solution to yield 100 mcg/ml. For a maintenance infusion, dilute two ampules in 500 ml of solution for a concentration of 200 mcg/ml, or four ampules in 500 ml of solution to yield 400 mcg/ml.
- Nitrostat I.V. comes in a kit with a 10-ml ampule containing 0.8 mg/ml and a disposable I.V. infusion set. Mix the drug with 250 ml of D_5W or 0.9% sodium chloride solution for a concentration of 30 mcg/ml.
- Tridil I.V. is supplied in ampules of 5 mg/10 ml, 25 mg/5 ml, and 50 mg/10 ml. Mix a 25- or 50-mg ampule with 500 ml of D_5W or 0.9% sodium chloride solution for 50 or 100 mcg/ml concentrations, respectively. Diluting 5 mg of the drug in 100 ml of solution yields a concentration of 50 mcg/ml.

Mix and store each preparation in the glass bottle provided. Tubing is usually included, as well. Store preparations at room temperature and protect them from light and freezing. Although the reconstituted drug remains stable for 48 hours at room temperature, discard it after 24 hours to avoid contamination.

Keep in mind that the type of infusion set used affects the amount of drug delivered. Use only nonabsorbent tubing; polyvinylchloride (PVC) tubing may absorb up to 80% of the diluted drug from the solution. If you use PVC extension tubing for the infusion pump, you may negate the advantages of the non-PVC set supplied with the drug.

Sublingual nitroglycerin comes in 150-, 200-, 300-, 400-, and 600-mcg tablets. Store the tablets in the original container, which should be kept tightly closed to avoid exposure to air, heat, and moisture—conditions that speed the loss of potency.

A translingual spray containing 400 mcg per metered-dose is also available.

Incompatibilities
Avoid mixing I.V. nitroglycerin with any other drug because of the risk of incompatibility.

Administration
- *Continuous infusion:* Administer the diluted drug at the required rate (see *Drip rates for nitroglycerin infusions,* pages 154 and 155). Use a volume-control device and a microdrip regulator, and closely monitor the patient during the infusion.
- *Sublingual or buccal administration:* Have the patient wet the tablet with saliva and place it under the tongue or between the cheek and the gum, until the tablet is completely absorbed.
- *Translingual administration:* Spray the drug onto or under the tongue. Tell the patient to wait 10 seconds before swallowing.

Adverse reactions
- *Life-threatening:* reflex tachycardia, severe hypotension.
- *Other:* ***dizziness, flushing, headache,*** intoxication (alcohol in diluent), nausea, orthostatic hypotension, ***palpitations,*** syncope, vomiting, weakness.

Interactions
- *Acetylcholine, histamine, norepinephrine:* risk of decreased effects of these drugs.
- *Antihypertensives, ethanol, opioid analgesics, other vasodilators:* possible profound hypotension from additive vasodilation.
- *Beta blockers, calcium channel blockers, tricyclic antidepressants:* enhanced hypotension.
- *Ergot alkaloids:* risk of triggering angina and reversing nitroglycerin's antianginal effects.
- *Sympathomimetics:* reduced antianginal effects and increased hypotension.

Special considerations
During I.V. therapy, monitor the patient's blood pressure and heart rate and rhythm continuously. If the patient has a pulmonary artery catheter in place, monitor his pulmonary capillary wedge pressure.

Remember that responses to nitroglycerin vary greatly. If you detect severe hypotension, a sign of overdose, elevate the patient's legs and slow or temporarily stop the infusion. With sublingual or buccal administration, remove the tablet and wipe the administration site clean. If severe hypotension persists, administer an I.V. alpha-adrenergic agonist (methoxamine or phenylephrine), as ordered.

Monitor serum methemoglobin levels. If methemoglobinemia develops, administer high-flow oxygen and I.V. methylene blue, as ordered.

If the patient complains of a tingling sensation during sublingual use, have him place the tablet in the

Drip rates for nitroglycerin infusions

A doctor's order for nitroglycerin may be in micrograms per minute or micrograms per kilograms per minute. Using this chart, you can convert either to the drip rate you need for a standard concentration of 25 mg in 250 ml (100 mcg/ml).

For an order in micrograms per minute, use the first column of the chart. Find the number that's closest to the ordered number of micrograms per minute. Then look to the right to find the appropriate drip rate. For example, with an order of 65 mcg/minute, you'd find that the closest dosage is 66.667 mcg/minute. Looking to the right, you'd find that the corresponding drip rate is 40 microdrops/minute.

PRESCRIBED DOSAGE (mcg/minute)	DRIP RATE (microdrops/ minute)	PATIENT'S WEIGHT kg 35 / lb 77	kg 40 / lb 88	kg 45 / lb 99	kg 50 / lb 110	kg 55 / lb 121	kg 60 / lb 132	kg 65 / lb 143	kg 70 / lb 154
		PRESCRIBED DOSAGE (mcg/kg/minute)							
8.333	5	0.238	0.208	0.185	0.167	0.152	0.139	0.128	0.119
16.667	10	0.476	0.417	0.370	0.333	0.303	0.278	0.256	0.238
25.000	15	0.714	0.625	0.556	0.500	0.455	0.417	0.385	0.357
33.333	20	0.952	0.833	0.741	0.667	0.606	0.556	0.513	0.476
41.667	25	1.190	1.042	0.926	0.833	0.758	0.694	0.641	0.595
50.000	30	1.429	1.250	1.111	1.000	0.909	0.833	0.769	0.714
58.333	35	1.667	1.458	1.296	1.167	1.061	0.972	0.897	0.833
66.667	40	1.905	1.667	1.481	1.333	1.212	1.111	1.026	0.952
75.000	45	2.143	1.875	1.667	1.500	1.364	1.250	1.154	1.071
83.333	50	2.381	2.083	1.852	1.667	1.515	1.389	1.282	1.190
91.667	55	2.619	2.292	2.037	1.833	1.667	1.528	1.410	1.310
100.000	60	2.857	2.500	2.222	2.000	1.818	1.667	1.538	1.429
108.333	65	3.095	2.708	2.407	2.167	1.970	1.806	1.667	1.548
116.667	70	3.333	2.917	2.593	2.333	2.121	1.944	1.795	1.667
125.000	75	3.571	3.125	2.778	2.500	2.273	2.083	1.923	1.786
133.333	80	3.810	3.333	2.963	2.667	2.424	2.222	2.051	1.905
141.667	85	4.048	3.542	3.148	2.833	2.576	2.361	2.179	2.024
150.000	90	4.286	3.750	3.333	3.000	2.727	2.500	2.308	2.143
158.333	95	4.524	3.958	3.519	3.167	2.879	2.639	2.436	2.262
166.667	100	4.762	4.167	3.704	3.333	3.030	2.778	2.564	2.381

buccal pouch.

Following nitroglycerin administration, help the patient sit up and stand until he can tolerate orthostatic hypotension. If he has a headache, administer an analgesic, as indicated.

Nitroglycerin can interfere with the results of certain diagnostic tests. Serum cholesterol levels will appear decreased when measured by the Zlatkis-Zak color reaction method, and serum methemoglobin, urine catecholamine, and urine vanillylmandelic acid levels will be markedly increased.

Nitroprusside sodium

(Nipride, Nitropress)

Indicated for rapid blood pressure reduction in hypertensive emergencies and for controlled hypotension during anesthesia, nitroprusside sodium directly dilates vascular

For an order in micrograms per kilograms per minute, first find the number closest to the patient's weight (in kilograms or pounds). Follow that column down until you find the number closest to the prescribed dosage. Follow that line across to the drip rate column to find the appropriate rate. For example, if a doctor ordered 1 mcg/kg/minute for a 200-lb patient, you'd locate the column for 198 lb. Then you'd follow that column down to the line for 1.019 mcg/kg/minute. Finally, you'd follow this line across to the left and learn that you need a drip rate of 55 microdrops/minute.

DRIP RATE (microdrops/minute)	PATIENT'S WEIGHT							
kg	75	80	85	90	95	100	105	110
lb	165	176	187	198	209	220	231	242
	PRESCRIBED DOSAGE (mcg/kg/minute)							
5	0.111	0.104	0.098	0.093	0.088	0.083	0.079	0.076
10	0.222	0.208	0.196	0.185	0.175	0.167	0.159	0.152
15	0.333	0.313	0.294	0.278	0.263	0.250	0.238	0.227
20	0.444	0.417	0.392	0.370	0.351	0.333	0.317	0.303
25	0.556	0.521	0.490	0.463	0.439	0.417	0.397	0.379
30	0.667	0.625	0.588	0.556	0.526	0.500	0.476	0.455
35	0.778	0.729	0.686	0.648	0.614	0.583	0.556	0.530
40	0.889	0.833	0.784	0.741	0.702	0.667	0.635	0.606
45	1.000	0.938	0.882	0.833	0.789	0.750	0.714	0.682
50	1.111	1.042	0.980	0.926	0.877	0.833	0.794	0.758
55	1.222	1.146	1.078	1.019	0.965	0.917	0.873	0.833
60	1.333	1.250	1.176	1.111	1.053	1.000	0.952	0.909
65	1.444	1.354	1.275	1.204	1.140	1.083	1.032	0.985
70	1.556	1.458	1.373	1.296	1.228	1.167	1.111	1.061
75	1.667	1.563	1.471	1.389	1.316	1.250	1.190	1.136
80	1.778	1.667	1.569	1.481	1.404	1.333	1.270	1.212
85	1.889	1.771	1.667	1.574	1.491	1.417	1.349	1.288
90	2.000	1.875	1.765	1.667	1.579	1.500	1.429	1.364
95	2.111	1.979	1.863	1.759	1.667	1.583	1.508	1.439
100	2.222	2.083	1.961	1.852	1.754	1.667	1.587	1.515

smooth muscle, producing peripheral vasodilation and hypotensive action. The drug also decreases systemic resistance, reduces preload and afterload, and improves cardiac output in congestive heart failure and cardiogenic shock.

When used as an adjunctive treatment for myocardial infarction, nitroprusside reduces myocardial oxygen consumption and relieves persistent chest pain. However, the drug aggravates ischemia by redistributing blood away from the myocardium. As an adjunctive treatment for valvular regurgitation, nitroprusside reduces aortal and left ventricular impedance.

The onset of action is almost immediate after I.V. administration. Blood pressure returns to the pretreatment level 1 to 10 minutes after the completion of the infusion.

The distribution of nitroprusside isn't completely understood. After rapid conversion to cyanogen (a cyanide radical), probably via an interaction with sulfhydryl groups in

DOSAGE FINDER

Nitroprusside: Indications and dosages

Rapid reduction of blood pressure in hypertensive emergencies, induction of controlled hypotension during anesthesia, and reduction of preload and afterload in congestive heart failure or cardiogenic shock

▶ For adults not receiving other hypotensive drugs, give 0.5 to 10 mcg/kg/minute by continuous infusion. The average dose is 3 mcg/kg/minute. Discontinue the drug if 10 mcg/kg/minute for 10 minutes doesn't produce an adequate blood pressure reduction.

▶ For children not receiving other hypotensive drugs, give 1.4 mcg/kg/minute by continuous infusion. Adjust the rate slowly according to the response.

erythrocytes and tissues, the drug is converted to thiocyanate in the liver. The half-life of thiocyanate ranges from 3 to 7 days. Nitroprusside is excreted primarily in urine, entirely as metabolites. (See *Nitroprusside: Indications and dosages.*)

Contraindications and cautions

Nitroprusside is contraindicated in patients with a known hypersensitivity to the drug. It's also contraindicated for patients with inadequate cerebral circulation or coronary artery insufficiency (because of their reduced tolerance to hypotension) and for patients with compensatory hypertension (those with an atrioventricular shunt or coarctation of the aorta, for instance) because hypotension may be life-threatening. The drug shouldn't be used during emergency surgery for patients near death.

Give nitroprusside cautiously to patients considered poor surgical risks because hypotension may be life-threatening. Also, give the drug cautiously to patients with severe renal impairment because thiocyanate excretion will be decreased, to those with hepatic insufficiency because drug metabolism will be decreased, and to patients with hypothyroidism because thiocyanate inhibits iodine uptake and binding.

You should administer the drug carefully to patients with anemia or hypovolemia because it may decrease their tolerance to these conditions. Patients with Leber's optic atrophy or tobacco amblyopia must be given the drug carefully because they lack the enzyme needed to metabolize it. Also, administer nitroprusside cautiously to patients with pulmonary impairment because the drug may aggravate hypovolemia and to those with low serum vitamin B_{12} levels because the drug interferes with the metabolism and distribution of vitamin B_{12}. Use nitroprusside carefully with elderly patients, who commonly exhibit a heightened sensitivity to its antihypertensive effects.

Use this pregnancy risk category C drug cautiously in pregnant women.

Preparation

Nitroprusside is available as a powder in 50-mg vials. Reconstitute the drug with 2 to 3 ml of dextrose 5% in water (D_5W) or sterile water for injection without preservatives. Then dilute it in 250 to 1,000 ml of D_5W to the desired concentration. After reconstitution, cover the drug with aluminum foil or another opaque material. Store it at room temperature and protect it from light, heat, and moisture. The reconstituted solution is stable for 24 hours. Discard any discolored solution (blue, green, or dark red), which may indicate a reaction with another substance.

Incompatibilities
Nitroprusside is incompatible with bacteriostatic water for injection. Don't add any other drug or preservative to a nitroprusside solution.

Administration
• *Continuous infusion:* Using an infusion pump, piggyback the diluted solution into an I.V. line with a free-flowing, compatible solution. Infuse the nitroprusside at a rate that maintains the desired hypotensive effect. (See *Drip rates for nitroprusside infusions,* pages 158 and 159.)

Adverse reactions
When given at recommended dosages for short-term therapy, the drug seldom causes adverse effects.
• *Life-threatening:* cyanide toxicity (absent reflexes, coma, distant heart sounds, extremely shallow breathing, hypotension, imperceptible pulse, pink skin, widely dilated pupils); thiocyanate toxicity (anorexia, blurred vision, confusion, delirium, dizziness, dyspnea, excessive hypotension, fatigue, loss of consciousness, metabolic acidosis, rash, tinnitus, weakness).
• *Other:* ***abdominal pain,*** anxiety, apprehension, diaphoresis, ***dizziness, headache, muscle twitching,*** nasal stuffiness, ***nausea,*** palpitations, reflex tachycardia, restlessness, retrosternal discomfort, ***vomiting***.

Interactions
• *Dobutamine:* increased cardiac output and decreased pulmonary wedge pressure.
• *Estrogens, sympathomimetics:* diminished hypotensive effect.
• *Ganglionic blocking agents, general anesthetics (halothane), other antihypertensive drugs:* additive hypotensive effect.

Special considerations
Before administering nitroprusside, make sure the staff and equipment necessary for arterial blood pressure monitoring are available. The patient should be in an intensive care unit to ensure monitoring during therapy. Obtain his baseline vital signs.

EMERGENCY INTERVENTION

Managing a nitroprusside overdose

Toxic effects of nitroprusside result from excessive levels of the drug's metabolites—cyanide and thiocyanate. Signs of cyanide toxicity include absent reflexes, coma, distant heart sounds, hypotension, imperceptible pulse, pink skin, shallow breathing, and widely dilated pupils. Thiocyanate toxicity can produce blurred vision, confusion, delirium, dizziness, dyspnea, excessive hypotension, fatigue, loss of consciousness, rash, tinnitus, and weakness. If you detect any of these signs or symptoms, take the following steps, as ordered:
• Slow or stop the infusion. This usually decreases blood pressure within 10 minutes.
• Administer nitrates to prevent methemoglobin formation.
• For a massive overdose, administer amyl nitrite by inhalation every 15 to 30 seconds until a 3% sodium nitrite solution is available. Administer this solution at no more than 5 ml/minute, up to a total dose of 15 ml. Monitor the patient's blood pressure closely.
• Give I.V. sodium thiosulfate in a solution of 12.5 g/50 ml of dextrose 5% in water over 10 minutes. Monitor the patient; thiocyanate levels may rise rapidly in patients with renal impairment. Hemodialysis or peritoneal dialysis can remove excess thiocyanate.

Drip rates for nitroprusside infusions

A doctor's order for nitroprusside may be in micrograms per minute or micrograms per kilograms per minute. Using this chart, you can convert either to the drip rate you need for a standard concentration of 50 mg in 500 ml (100 mcg/ml).

For an order in micrograms per minute, use the first column of the chart. Find the number that's closest to the ordered number of micrograms per minute. Then look to the right to find the appropriate drip rate. For example, with an order of 60 mcg/minute, you'd find that the closest dosage is 58.333 mcg/minute. Looking to the right, you'd find that the corresponding drip rate is 35 microdrops/minute.

PRESCRIBED DOSAGE (mcg/minute)	DRIP RATE (microdrops/minute)	PATIENT'S WEIGHT							
		kg 35 / lb 77	kg 40 / lb 88	kg 45 / lb 99	kg 50 / lb 110	kg 55 / lb 121	kg 60 / lb 132	kg 65 / lb 143	kg 70 / lb 154
		PRESCRIBED DOSAGE (mcg/kg/minute)							
8.333	5	0.238	0.208	0.185	0.167	0.152	0.139	0.128	0.119
16.667	10	0.476	0.417	0.370	0.333	0.303	0.278	0.256	0.238
25.000	15	0.714	0.625	0.556	0.500	0.455	0.417	0.385	0.357
33.333	20	0.952	0.833	0.741	0.667	0.606	0.556	0.513	0.476
41.667	25	1.190	1.042	0.926	0.833	0.758	0.694	0.641	0.595
50.000	30	1.429	1.250	1.111	1.000	0.909	0.833	0.769	0.714
58.333	35	1.667	1.458	1.296	1.167	1.061	0.972	0.897	0.833
66.667	40	1.905	1.667	1.481	1.333	1.212	1.111	1.026	0.952
75.000	45	2.143	1.875	1.667	1.500	1.364	1.250	1.154	1.071
83.333	50	2.381	2.083	1.852	1.667	1.515	1.389	1.282	1.190
91.667	55	2.619	2.292	2.037	1.833	1.667	1.528	1.410	1.310
100.000	60	2.857	2.500	2.222	2.000	1.818	1.667	1.538	1.429
108.333	65	3.095	2.708	2.407	2.167	1.970	1.806	1.667	1.548
116.667	70	3.333	2.917	2.593	2.333	2.121	1.944	1.795	1.667
125.000	75	3.571	3.125	2.778	2.500	2.273	2.083	1.923	1.786
133.333	80	3.810	3.333	2.963	2.667	2.424	2.222	2.051	1.905
141.667	85	4.048	3.542	3.148	2.833	2.576	2.361	2.179	2.024
150.000	90	4.286	3.750	3.333	3.000	2.727	2.500	2.308	2.143
158.333	95	4.524	3.958	3.519	3.167	2.879	2.639	2.436	2.262
166.667	100	4.762	4.167	3.704	3.333	3.030	2.778	2.564	2.381

Monitor the patient's blood pressure every 5 minutes at the start of therapy and every 15 minutes thereafter. Observe him for adverse reactions, including signs and symptoms of toxicity (see *Managing a nitroprusside overdose*, page 157). Slowing the infusion rate or temporarily discontinuing the drug may alleviate adverse reactions.

Patients with low serum vitamin B_{12} levels or Leber's optic atrophy should receive hydroxocobalamin before and during nitroprusside administration as an antidote to cyanide. In patients with hepatic impairment, monitor plasma cyanogen concentrations daily after 1 or 2 days. If the patient develops metabolic acidosis, discontinue nitroprusside infusion and anticipate an alternate therapy.

Nitroprusside can influence the results of several laboratory tests. Plasma cyanide, cyanocobalamin, and thiocyanate levels may be elevated, as may serum lactate and creatinine levels. Serum bicarbonate

For an order in micrograms per kilograms per minute, first find the number closest to the patient's weight (in kilograms or pounds). Follow that column down until you find the number closest to the prescribed dosage. Follow that line across to the drip rate column to find the appropriate rate. For example, if a doctor ordered 2 mcg/kg/minute for a 120-lb patient, you'd locate the column for 121 lb. Then you'd follow that column down to the line for 1.970 mcg/kg/minute. Finally, you'd follow this line across to the left and learn that you need a drip rate of 65 microdrops/minute.

DRIP RATE (microdrops/ minute)		PATIENT'S WEIGHT							
	kg	75	80	85	90	95	100	105	110
	lb	165	176	187	198	209	220	231	242
		PRESCRIBED DOSAGE (mcg/kg/minute)							
5		0.111	0.104	0.098	0.093	0.088	0.083	0.079	0.076
10		0.222	0.208	0.196	0.185	0.175	0.167	0.159	0.152
15		0.333	0.313	0.294	0.278	0.263	0.250	0.238	0.227
20		0.444	0.417	0.392	0.370	0.351	0.333	0.317	0.303
25		0.556	0.521	0.490	0.463	0.439	0.417	0.397	0.379
30		0.667	0.625	0.588	0.556	0.526	0.500	0.476	0.455
35		0.778	0.729	0.686	0.648	0.614	0.583	0.556	0.530
40		0.889	0.833	0.784	0.741	0.702	0.667	0.635	0.606
45		1.000	0.938	0.882	0.833	0.789	0.750	0.714	0.682
50		1.111	1.042	0.980	0.926	0.877	0.833	0.794	0.758
55		1.222	1.146	1.078	1.019	0.965	0.917	0.873	0.833
60		1.333	1.250	1.176	1.111	1.053	1.000	0.952	0.909
65		1.444	1.354	1.275	1.204	1.140	1.083	1.032	0.985
70		1.556	1.458	1.373	1.296	1.228	1.167	1.111	1.061
75		1.667	1.563	1.471	1.389	1.316	1.250	1.190	1.136
80		1.778	1.667	1.569	1.481	1.404	1.333	1.270	1.212
85		1.889	1.771	1.667	1.574	1.491	1.417	1.349	1.288
90		2.000	1.875	1.765	1.667	1.579	1.500	1.429	1.364
95		2.111	1.979	1.863	1.759	1.667	1.583	1.508	1.439
100		2.222	2.083	1.961	1.852	1.754	1.667	1.587	1.515

and partial pressure of carbon dioxide levels may fall, and pH may be decreased.

Norepinephrine bitartrate
(Levophed)

This naturally occurring catecholamine stimulates alpha-adrenergic receptors to produce vasoconstriction, increasing coronary artery blood flow and blood pressure. The marked pressor effect primarily results from increased peripheral resistance. Norepinephrine bitartrate also stimulates beta$_1$-adrenergic receptors to stimulate the myocardium and increase cardiac output.

Norepinephrine is indicated to restore blood pressure in acute hypotension. However, when used to treat hypotension after a myocardial infarction, the drug may increase myocardial oxygen demand, counteracting its beneficial effects. The

DOSAGE FINDER

Norepinephrine: Indications and dosages

Treatment of acute hypotension and of severe hypotension during cardiac arrest

▶ For adults, give 8 to 12 mcg/minute initially. Then adjust the infusion rate (usually 2 to 4 mcg/minute) to maintain the patient's blood pressure in the desired range.

▶ For children, give 0.1 mcg/kg/minute initially. Then adjust the infusion rate (usually 2 mcg/minute) to maintain the patient's blood pressure in the desired range.

drug is also used as a temporary adjunct in advanced cardiac life support to restore blood pressure after an effective heartbeat and ventilation have been restored.

The drug's pressor effects begin almost immediately. They cease 1 to 2 minutes after the infusion stops.

Norepinephrine is distributed primarily to sympathetic nervous tissue. It crosses the placenta but not the blood-brain barrier. Metabolized in the liver and other tissues by the enzymes catechol-O-methyltransferase and monoamine oxidase, the drug is excreted in urine, primarily as metabolites, although 4% to 16% remains unchanged. Whether or not the drug appears in breast milk is unclear. (See *Norepinephrine: Indications and dosages.*)

Contraindications and cautions

Norepinephrine is contraindicated for patients with a known hypersensitivity to it, to other sympathomimetics, or to sulfites (which may be a component of a norepinephrine preparation). Don't give the drug to patients with hypotension from blood loss because of the risk of tissue hypoxia, lactic acidosis, low urine output, and severe vasoconstriction. Also don't administer the drug to patients with mesenteric or peripheral vascular thrombosis or other occlusive vascular disorders—such as arteriosclerosis, Buerger's disease, or diabetes mellitus—because norepinephrine may precipitate or aggravate ischemia. Avoid giving the drug to patients receiving cyclopropane or halothane anesthetics or to patients with hypoxia or hypercapnia because it can produce ventricular tachycardia or fibrillation. When treating shock, don't use the drug without replacing blood, plasma, fluids, or electrolytes.

Administer norepinephrine cautiously to patients with hyperthyroidism, hypertension, or severe cardiac disease and to all elderly patients. These patients have an increased risk of adverse reactions.

Give this pregnancy risk category D drug cautiously to pregnant women.

Preparation

Norepinephrine is available in 4-ml ampules containing 1 mg/ml. Store the ampules at room temperature. For infusion, mix one ampule of norepinephrine in 1,000 ml of dextrose 5% in water or dextrose 5% in 0.9% sodium chloride solution for a concentration of 4 mcg/ml. Adjust the concentration as necessary to reflect the patient's specific drug and fluid volume requirements. Discard any unused diluted solution after 24 hours and any solution that contains particulate matter or has become discolored (brown, pink, or yellow).

Incompatibilities

Drugs incompatible with norepinephrine include aminophylline, amobarbital sodium, cephalothin sodium, cephapirin sodium, chlorothiazide, chlorpheniramine maleate, lidocaine hydrochloride, pentobarbital sodium, phenobarbital sodium, secobarbital sodium, sodium bicarbonate, sodium iodide, streptomycin sulfate, and thiopental sodium. Also, don't combine the drug with whole blood or 0.9% sodium chloride solution alone.

Administration

• *Continuous infusion:* Administer the drug using a plastic I.V. catheter inserted deep into a large vein. Don't use leg veins in elderly patients or in patients with peripheral vascular disease. Use microdrip tubing and an infusion pump to carefully regulate the flow rate. Make sure the rate maintains blood pressure within the low-normal range—usually 80 to 100 mm Hg systolic or, for previously hypertensive patients, a maximum of 40 mm Hg below the baseline systolic pressure.

Adverse reactions

• *Life-threatening:* apnea, bradycardia, cerebral hemorrhage, hypertension (severe), increased peripheral vascular resistance, low cardiac output, seizures, ventricular tachycardia or fibrillation.
• *Other:* angina, anxiety, atrioventricular dissociation, bigeminy, dizziness, fever, ***headache,*** insomnia, junctional rhythm, ***low urine output,*** metabolic acidosis, pallor, precordial pain, restlessness, thyroid swelling, tissue necrosis and sloughing with extravasation, tremor, weakness.

Interactions

• *Amphetamines, doxapram, mazindol, methylphenidate:* enhanced central nervous system (CNS) stimulation and pressor effects.
• *Antihypertensives:* possible reduced pressor response.
• *Atropine:* increased pressor response.
• *Cardiac glycosides, levodopa:* increased risk of arrhythmias.
• *CNS stimulants:* potentiated stimulant effects.
• *Desmopressin, lypressin, vasopressin:* decreased antidiuretic effect.
• *Dihydroergotamine, ergonovine, methylergonovine, methysergide:* enhanced vasoconstriction.
• *Ergoloid mesylates, ergotamine:* risk of peripheral vascular ischemia and gangrene.
• *Ergonovine, ergotamine, methylergonovine, oxytocin:* potentiated pressor effect.
• *Guanadrel, guanethidine, mecamylamine, methyldopa:* diminished hypotensive effect of these drugs and enhanced pressor effect of norepinephrine.
• *Hydrocarbon inhalation anesthetics:* ventricular tachycardia or fibrillation.
• *Lithium:* decreased pressor response.
• *Maprotiline, tricyclic antidepressants:* potentiated cardiovascular effects.
• *Other sympathomimetics:* augmented CNS stimulation and cardiovascular effects.
• *Rauwolfia alkaloids:* decreased hypotensive effect of these drugs and prolonged action of norepinephrine.
• *Thyroid hormones:* increased hormone and norepinephrine effects.

Special considerations

During the infusion, check the patient's blood pressure every 2 minutes until he's stable, then every 5 to 15 minutes using intra-arterial monitoring. Monitor his cardiac rhythm strip continuously and report any arrhythmias. Also assess the patient's heart rate and rhythm every 5 to 15 minutes. As soon as possible, insert an indwelling urinary catheter and monitor the patient's urine output; if it drops below 30 ml/hour, notify the doctor.

Bradycardia, severe or persistent headache, severe hypertension, seizures, and vomiting may indicate an overdose. If these signs occur, notify the doctor and discontinue the infusion. As ordered, provide fluid and electrolytes, and administer an alpha-adrenergic blocker, such as 5 to 10 mg of phentolamine I.V.

Extravasation may cause local necrosis, so assess the infusion site for signs of this problem, such as blanching and coldness. If extravasation occurs, stop the infusion immediately and infiltrate the area with 5 to 10 mg of phentolamine in 5 to 10 ml of 0.9% sodium chloride solution. Use a 25G needle. Remove the I.V. line and protect the area from further trauma.

During a prolonged infusion, you can prevent blanching by rotating the I.V. sites. Including 5 to 10 mg of phentolamine in the infusion may prevent sloughing should extravasation occur. Also, including 10 mg of heparin in each 500 ml of norepinephrine may reduce the risk of venous thrombosis. If possible, avoid prolonged norepinephrine use to prevent ischemia of vital organs.

When therapy is completed, withdraw the drug slowly. Sudden cessation may cause severe hypotension. After the infusion, monitor the patient's vital signs hourly until he's stable. If his systolic pressure drops below 70 mm Hg, notify the doctor and restart the infusion, as ordered.

Norepinephrine can interfere with certain diagnostic tests. For example, the patient's electrocardiogram may show atrioventricular dissociation, bradycardia, bigeminy, junctional rhythm, tachycardia, or ventricular fibrillation. Also, serum glucose levels may be increased.

Phenobarbital sodium

(Luminal)

A schedule IV controlled substance, phenobarbital sodium appears to decrease nerve cell excitability in the cerebral cortex and reticular formation. The drug's anticonvulsant effects may stem from gamma-aminobutyric acid-like activity in the motor cortex, but the precise mechanism of action isn't understood.

Despite its slow onset, phenobarbital is indicated for status epilepticus and other acute seizure disorders not controlled by diazepam.

Following I.V. administration, the onset of action occurs in 5 minutes. The duration of action ranges from 4 to 6 hours, but the sedative effect may last up to 10 hours. The elimination half-life is 2 to 5 days.

Phenobarbital is widely distributed to all tissues, with the highest concentrations found in the brain, kidneys, and liver. The drug crosses the blood-brain barrier and the placenta. Metabolized in the liver, phenobarbital is excreted mainly in urine. Small amounts also appear in feces and breast milk. (See *Phenobarbital: Indication and dosages.*)

Contraindications and cautions

Don't give phenobarbital to patients who are hypersensitive to this or other barbiturates. Also, don't give the drug to patients with severe pulmonary disease because drug-induced respiratory depression further compromises ventilation, or to those with a history of acute intermittent or variegate porphyria because the drug worsens these disorders.

Give phenobarbital cautiously to patients with hepatic or renal impairment because its metabolism and excretion will be slowed. Also, give the drug carefully to patients with elevated serum ammonia levels because it impairs the liver's ability to metabolize ammonia and to those with cardiovascular disease or unstable blood pressure because of increased adverse cardiovascular effects. Patients with acute or chronic pain, elderly patients, and children may experience paradoxical central nervous system (CNS) excitement.

Use caution with patients who have diabetes mellitus, hyperthyroidism, or hypothyroidism because the drug may exacerbate their symptoms. Also use caution with patients who have a history of drug abuse, depression, or suicidal tendencies because of the drug's sedative effects and potential for abuse.

Use this pregnancy risk category D drug with extreme caution in pregnant women.

Preparation

Phenobarbital is available in single-dose vials, ampules, and prefilled syringes in concentrations of 30, 60, 65, 120, and 130 mg/ml. Discard any solution containing a precipitate. The drug is compatible with commonly used I.V. solutions.

Incompatibilities

Phenobarbital is incompatible with alcohol-dextrose solutions, cephalothin sodium, chlorpromazine hydrochloride, codeine phosphate, ephedrine hydrochloride, hydralazine hydrochloride, hydrocortisone sodium succinate, insulin (regular), levorphanol tartrate, meperidine hydrochloride, morphine sulfate, norepinephrine bitartrate, oxytetracycline hydrochloride, pentazocine lactate, prochlorperazine mesylate, promazine hydrochloride, promethazine hydrochloride, ranitidine hydrochloride, streptomycin sulfate, tetracycline hydrochloride, and vancomycin.

DOSAGE FINDER

Phenobarbital: Indication and dosages

Treatment of status epilepticus and other acute seizure disorders not controlled by diazepam

▶ For adults, slowly inject 200 to 600 mg at a rate not exceeding 60 mg/minute. Don't exceed a total dose of 20 mg/kg or 600 mg.

▶ For children, slowly inject 10 to 20 mg/kg over 10 to 15 minutes.

Administration

- *Direct injection:* Slowly inject the ordered dose into a vein or an I.V. line of a free-flowing, compatible solution. Don't exceed 60 mg/minute.

Adverse reactions

- *Life-threatening:* apnea, bronchospasm, hypotension, laryngospasm—all from rapid injection.
- *Other:* agranulocytosis, ataxia, bradycardia, coma, confusion, delirium, depression, diarrhea, ***drowsiness,*** epigastric pain, euphoria, fever, headache, hypoventilation, impaired judgment, joint or muscle pain, ***lethargy,*** megaloblastic anemia, nausea, nightmares, pain or thrombophlebitis at injection site, paradoxical excitement, rash, restlessness, rhinitis, severe subcutaneous necrosis, thrombocytopenic purpura, urticaria, vertigo.

Interactions

- *Ascorbic acid, chlorpromazine:* increased excretion of these agents.
- *Calcium channel blockers:* excessive hypotension.
- *Carbamazepine:* reduced serum levels and half-life of both drugs.

EMERGENCY INTERVENTION

Managing a phenobarbital overdose

If you detect signs of a phenobarbital overdose—clammy skin, cyanosis, hypotension, pupillary constriction, and eventually coma—take the following steps:

- Stop the drug infusion and notify the doctor.
- Maintain a patent airway and provide oxygen and assisted ventilation as necessary.
- Monitor the patient's vital signs and fluid balance. Keep him well hydrated with I.V. fluids and administer sodium bicarbonate to alkalinize urine and increase drug excretion.
- Administer a vasopressor for severe hypotension, as ordered.
- For a severe overdose, peritoneal dialysis and hemodialysis may be necessary.

- *Carbonic anhydrase inhibitors:* possible enhanced osteopenia.
- *Cardiac glycosides, corticosteroids, fenoprofen, levothyroxine, quinidine, tricyclic antidepressants, xanthines:* diminished effects, resulting from increased hepatic metabolism of these drugs.
- *CNS depressants:* deepened CNS depression.
- *Coumarin or indanedione-derivative anticoagulants:* decreased prothrombin time and diminished anticoagulant effects.
- *Cyclophosphamide:* increased leukopenia, resulting from reduced cyclophosphamide half-life.
- *Disopyramide, griseofulvin, mexiletine:* decreased serum concentrations of these drugs, reduced disopyramide efficacy.
- *Disulfiram, monoamine oxidase inhibitors:* reduced phenobarbital metabolism, prolonging its effect.
- *Divalproex sodium, valproic acid:* increased risk of CNS toxicity.
- *Doxycycline:* depressed antibiotic activity.
- *Estrogens:* reduced efficacy of estrogen.
- *Guanadrel, guanethidine, loop diuretics:* increased risk of orthostatic hypotension.
- *Halogenated inhalation anesthetics:* increased risk of hepatotoxicity or nephrotoxicity.
- *Haloperidol, loxapine, maprotiline, phenothiazines, primidone, thioxanthines:* risk of lowered seizure threshold.
- *Hydantoin anticonvulsants:* unpredictable metabolism of these agents.
- *Hypothermia-producing drugs:* increased risk of hypothermia.
- *Ketamine:* increased risk of hypotension and respiratory depression.
- *Leucovorin:* antagonized anticonvulsant effect.
- *Phenytoin:* possible increased or decreased phenytoin levels.
- *Vitamin D:* reduced vitamin efficacy.

Special considerations

Before giving the drug, make sure you have resuscitation equipment readily available. Obtain a baseline blood pressure and respiratory rate. During therapy, monitor the patient's blood pressure and respiratory rate. If his respiratory rate falls below 12 breaths/minute, notify the doctor; below 8 breaths/minute, arouse the patient and encourage him to breathe more deeply (at a rate of at least 12 breaths/minute). If you can't arouse the patient, manually ventilate him at 12 to 16 breaths/minute with a hand-held respirator. Have someone else notify the doctor immediately and prepare for intubation, as necessary.

Discontinue the drug immediately if a skin reaction occurs; it may signal a fatal reaction. Observe the injection site for signs of thrombophlebitis. If the patient reports local pain, stop the injection and check the placement of the cannula.

Watch for extravasation of this highly alkaline drug, which can cause tissue necrosis.

Monitor the patient for signs and symptoms of an overdose and intervene as necessary (see *Managing a phenobarbital overdose*).

In patients receiving anticoagulant therapy, closely monitor prothrombin time. Adjust the anticoagulant dosage as needed.

The drug may take up to 30 minutes to reach its peak effect after the initial dose. Maintain the serum level at 15 to 40 mcg/ml. Stop the injections when the seizures end or when you reach the total dosage.

Be aware that a tolerance may develop after about 2 weeks of therapy and that drug dependency and severe withdrawal symptoms may follow long-term therapy. To discontinue the drug, withdraw one dose each day for 5 to 6 days to prevent withdrawal symptoms and rebound rapid eye movement during sleep (which can cause nightmares).

Phenobarbital can interfere with some laboratory tests. It may impair the absorption of cyanocobalamin ^{57}Co and may cause a false-positive phentolamine test result. It can also reduce serum bilirubin levels, so don't give it within 24 hours of scheduled liver function tests.

Phentolamine mesylate

(Regitine, Rogitine)

This alpha-adrenergic blocker antagonizes the effects of epinephrine and norepinephrine, causing vasodilation and reducing peripheral vascular resistance. In patients with congestive heart failure (CHF), phentolamine mesylate reduces preload and pulmonary artery pressure, increases cardiac output, and exerts a positive inotropic effect.

The drug is indicated for left ventricular failure secondary to acute myocardial infarction (MI), for hypertensive crisis resulting from the interaction between a monoamine oxidase inhibitor and sympathomimetic amines, and for extravasation of norepinephrine.

The drug's onset of action occurs in 2 minutes. The duration of action lasts from 15 to 30 minutes.

The distribution of phentolamine isn't fully understood. Whether or not it crosses the blood-brain barrier or the placenta isn't known. Its metabolism is also unclear. Studies show about 10% of a dose is excreted unchanged in urine. What happens to the remainder isn't known. (See *Phentolamine: Indications and dosages,* page 166.)

Contraindications and cautions

Phentolamine is contraindicated for patients with a hypersensitivity to it or to related drugs. The drug may also be contraindicated for patients who've sustained an acute MI.

Use the drug cautiously in patients with coronary artery disease, angina, or a history of MI because reflex tachycardia may precipitate angina or CHF. Also use the drug cautiously in patients with gastritis or peptic ulcer to avoid exacerbating these disorders.

Give phentolamine, a pregnancy risk category C drug, cautiously to pregnant women.

Preparation

Phentolamine is supplied in 5-mg vials with 1-ml ampules of sterile

DOSAGE FINDER

Phentolamine: Indications and dosages

Treatment of left ventricular failure secondary to acute myocardial infarction
▶ For adults, give 0.17 to 0.4 mg/minute by continuous I.V. infusion.

Treatment of hypertensive crisis resulting from an interaction between a monoamine oxidase inhibitor and sympathomimetic amines
▶ For adults, administer 5 to 10 mg I.V. or I.M.

Treatment of norepinephrine extravasation
▶ For adults, inject 10 mg in 10 ml of 0.9% sodium chloride solution into the affected tissues within 12 hours of extravasation.

water for injection as the diluent. Keep the unreconstituted powder at room temperature. Reconstitute the powder with the diluent to a concentration of 5 mg/ml. The reconstituted solution remains stable for 48 hours at room temperature or for 7 days at 36° to 46° F (2.2° to 7.8° C). The manufacturer recommends using the solution immediately after reconstitution. For infusion, further dilute 5 to 10 mg of the drug in 500 ml of 0.9% sodium chloride solution.

Incompatibilities
No incompatibilities have been reported.

Administration
- *Direct injection:* Rapidly inject the dose into a vein or an I.V. line of a free-flowing, compatible solution.
- *Continuous infusion:* To prevent dermal necrosis and sloughing during concomitant infusion of norepinephrine, infuse the drug at the rate ordered for norepinephrine. Use an infusion pump to maintain the correct rate for left ventricular failure.
- *I.M. injection:* Inject the ordered dose into any I.M. injection site.

Adverse reactions
- *Life-threatening:* anaphylaxis, cerebrovascular spasm or occlusion, MI.
- *Other:* abdominal pain, ***acute and prolonged or orthostatic hypotension,*** angina, ***arrhythmias,*** confusion, ***diarrhea, dizziness,*** dyspnea, exacerbation of peptic ulcer, ***flushing,*** incoordination, ***nasal congestion, nausea,*** severe or sudden headache, slurred speech, ***tachycardia, vomiting, weakness.***

Interactions
- *Diazoxide:* diminished effects.
- *Dopamine:* antagonized peripheral vasoconstriction.
- *Ephedrine, metaraminol, phenylephrine:* decreased pressor response.
- *Epinephrine:* risk of severe hypotension and tachycardia.
- *Guanadrel, guanethidine:* increased incidence of bradycardia or orthostatic hypotension.
- *Methoxamine (preceded by phentolamine):* risk of blocked pressor response with severe hypotension.

Special considerations
During and after therapy, monitor the patient for severe hypotension, a sign of overdose. If this occurs, elevate his legs and replace fluids. If a vasopressor is needed, give him norepinephrine, as prescribed. (Epinephrine may cause a paradoxical drop in blood pressure.)

If shock occurs, also give norepinephrine. For arrhythmias, give a cardiac glycoside; don't use epinephrine.

When treating left ventricular failure, continuously monitor the cardiac rhythm strip and left ventricular function.

Results of a phentolamine test will be falsely positive when the drug is used in uremic patients or in patients receiving sedatives, opiates, or antihypertensive drugs.

Phenylephrine hydrochloride

(Neo-Synephrine injection)

Phenylephrine hydrochloride stimulates alpha-adrenergic receptors, causing vasoconstriction and increasing blood pressure. It has little, if any, effect on beta-adrenergic receptors. Indications for the drug include severe hypotension or shock, hypotensive emergencies during spinal anesthesia, and paroxysmal supraventricular tachycardia.

Phenylephrine's pressor effects begin almost at once after an I.V. dose and last for 15 to 20 minutes.

The drug is distributed in plasma and metabolized in the liver and intestines by the enzyme monoamine oxidase. Phenylephrine is excreted in urine. Studies don't indicate whether or not the drug appears in breast milk. (See *Phenylephrine: Indications and dosages.*)

DOSAGE FINDER

Phenylephrine: Indications and dosages

Treatment of severe hypotension or shock

▶ For adults, initially administer 0.1 to 0.18 mg/minute. After blood pressure stabilizes, give 0.04 to 0.06 mg/minute.

Treatment of hypotensive emergencies during spinal anesthesia

▶ For adults, initially administer 0.1 to 0.2 mg by slow I.V. injection. Subsequent doses should be less than 0.1 mg.

Treatment of paroxysmal supraventricular tachycardia

▶ For adults, initially administer 0.5 mg by slow I.V. injection; subsequent doses may be increased by increments of 0.1 to 0.2 mg. The maximum dose shouldn't exceed 1 mg.

Contraindications and cautions

Phenylephrine is contraindicated for patients with a history of hypersensitivity to it or to sulfites. Also, don't give the drug to patients with ventricular tachycardia because of its arrhythmogenic effects, to those with severe hypertension because the condition may be exacerbated, and to those with a myocardial infarction because of the risks of increased cardiac work load and aggravated ischemia. And don't give the drug to patients with mesenteric or peripheral vascular thrombosis, acute pancreatitis, or hepatitis; it may trigger or aggravate ischemia or infarction in the affected organs.

Give phenylephrine cautiously to patients with hyperthyroidism because of the increased risk of bradycardia, to those with incomplete heart block because the condition may worsen, to those with severe arteriosclerosis because of the risk of ischemia, and to those with myocardial disease because of the risks of increased cardiac work load and worsening heart failure. Use the drug cautiously in elderly patients because of their diminished cerebral and coronary circulation. Avoid the I.V. route in children if possible.

Phenylephrine is a pregnancy risk category C drug and should be used cautiously in pregnant women.

Preparation

Phenylephrine is available in 1-ml ampules and disposable cartridge units (10 mg/ml or 1% solution). Store the drug at room temperature and discard solutions that look brown or contain particulates.

For an infusion, dilute 10 mg in 500 ml of dextrose 5% in water or 0.9% sodium chloride solution. Discard diluted solutions after 48 hours. The drug is compatible with most I.V. solutions.

Incompatibilities

Phenylephrine is incompatible with alkaline solutions and iron salts.

Administration

- *Direct injection:* Give the drug over 1 minute for hypotensive crisis during spinal anesthesia. Inject the dose over 20 to 30 seconds for paroxysmal supraventricular tachycardia; rapid delivery may cause short paroxysms of ventricular tachycardia, ventricular extrasystoles, or a sensation of fullness in the head.
- *Continuous infusion:* Using microdrip tubing and an infusion pump, administer the diluted drug at a rate that maintains adequate blood pressure and tissue perfusion. To prevent extravasation, use a patent I.V. line inserted into a large vein in the antecubital fossa.

Adverse reactions

- *Life-threatening:* cerebral hemorrhage, decreased cardiac output, hypertension, respiratory distress, severe bradycardia, ventricular tachycardia.
- *Other:* angina, anxiety, blurred vision, decreased renal perfusion, decreased urine output, dizziness, ***headache, light-headedness,*** metabolic acidosis, necrosis or tissue sloughing (with extravasation), pallor, palpitations, paresthesia in extremity after injection, pilomotor response, restlessness, seizures, sweating, tremor, ventricular extrasystoles, vomiting, ***weakness.***

Interactions

- *Alpha-adrenergic blockers:* decreased phenylephrine duration of action and pressor effect.
- *Antihypertensives, diuretics:* risk of diminished pressor response.
- *Atropine sulfate, mazindol, methylphenidate, oxytocin:* potentiated pressor response, increasing risk of cerebral hemorrhage.
- *Beta-adrenergic blockers:* partial blockade of phenylephrine-induced myocardial stimulation. (May be used to block phenylephrine-induced ventricular arrhythmias.)
- *Diatrizoates, iothalamate, ioxaglate:* intensified neurologic effects.
- *Digitalis, hydrocarbon inhalation anesthetics, sympathomimetics:* risk of increased myocardial irritability and serious arrhythmias.
- *Dihydroergotamine, ergonovine, ergotamine, methylergonovine, methysergide:* enhanced vasoconstriction.
- *Doxapram, thyroid hormones:* increased pressor effects.
- *Guanadrel, guanethidine, monoamine oxidase inhibitors, maprotiline, tricyclic antidepressants:* risk of prolonged hypertension.
- *Levodopa:* increased risk of arrhythmias.
- *Mecamylamine, methyldopa, trimethaphan:* diminished hypotensive effects.
- *Nitrates:* reduced antianginal effect.
- *Rauwolfia alkaloids:* diminished hypotensive effects and risk of prolonged phenylephrine action.

Special considerations
Before or during therapy, correct hypovolemia because hypovolemic patients are more susceptible to the effects of severe vasoconstriction. Monitor central venous pressure or left ventricular filling pressure to detect hypovolemia. Keep in mind that the drug isn't a substitute for blood, plasma, fluid, or electrolytes, and that hypoxia and acidosis will reduce the drug's effectiveness.

During the infusion, check the patient's blood pressure every 2 minutes until he's stable, then every 5 to 15 minutes, using intra-arterial monitoring.

Continuously monitor the cardiac rhythm strip and assess the patient's heart rate every 5 to 15 minutes. Report any arrhythmias. But keep in mind that the rhythm strip may show bradycardia, ventricular tachycardia, or ventricular fibrillation because of the phenylephrine.

Insert an indwelling urinary catheter (before therapy begins, if possible), and monitor the patient's urine output. Inform the doctor if it falls below 30 ml/hour.

If you detect signs and symptoms of an overdose—such as a rapid, irregular, pounding heartbeat; hypertension; vomiting; a sensation of fullness in the head; or tingling in the hands or feet—stop the phenylephrine infusion and, as ordered, administer an alpha-adrenergic blocker, such as phentolamine.

Closely monitor the infusion site. If extravasation occurs, stop the infusion and restart it at another site. Infiltrate the area with 5 to 10 mg of phentolamine in 5 to 10 ml of 0.9% sodium chloride solution, using a fine needle. Start treatment within 12 hours if possible.

Discontinue the infusion slowly to avoid severe hypotension. Afterward, monitor the patient's vital signs hourly until he's stable. Watch for severe hypotension, and restart the infusion if the patient's systolic pressure drops below 70 mm Hg. Maintain his blood pressure slightly below his usual range.

Phenytoin sodium
(Dilantin)

A hydantoin derivative, phenytoin sodium is ordered to treat status epilepticus, ventricular tachycardia, paroxysmal atrial tachycardia, and arrhythmias caused by digitalis toxicity. How it achieves its anticonvulsant effect isn't fully understood. It appears to reduce the voltage and inhibit the spread of electrical stimulation within the motor cortex by stabilizing neuronal membranes and by either increasing the efflux or decreasing the influx of sodium ions across cell membranes. In patients with digitalis-induced arrhythmias, the drug exerts its antiarrhythmic effect by normalizing sodium influx to the Purkinje's fibers.

Phenytoin's onset of action is 3 to 5 minutes following I.V. administration; peak serum levels are reached in 1 to 2 hours. The drug's half-life averages 14 hours.

Phenytoin is distributed throughout the tissues, with the highest concentrations in the liver and adipose tissue. Between 70% and 95% of the drug is protein-bound (less in patients with renal or hepatic dysfunction). Serum levels are lower in patients with renal dysfunction. With small dosage increases, serum levels rise substantially. The drug crosses the placenta.

Phenytoin is metabolized in the liver, forming inactive metabolites. In children, the metabolism rate is

DOSAGE FINDER

Phenytoin: Indications and dosages

Treatment of status epilepticus

▶ For adults, administer 150 to 250 mg by direct injection. If necessary after 30 minutes, give 100 to 150 mg, or give 8 to 18 mg/kg at a rate not to exceed 50 mg/minute. The maximum daily dosage is 1.5 g.

▶ For children, give 10 to 15 mg/kg at a rate of 0.5 to 1.5 mg/kg/minute. The maximum daily dosage is 20 mg/kg.

Treatment of ventricular tachycardia, paroxysmal atrial tachycardia, or arrhythmias caused by digitalis toxicity

▶ For adults, inject 100 mg every 5 minutes until the arrhythmias disappear or 1 g has been given.

accelerated. The drug is excreted primarily in urine by glomerular filtration as glucuronides; 1% is excreted unchanged. Small amounts are excreted in feces, and the drug also appears in breast milk. Between 60% and 75% of a dose is excreted in 24 hours. Excretion may be enhanced by alkaline urine. (See *Phenytoin: Indications and dosages.*)

Contraindications and cautions

Don't give phenytoin to patients with a hypersensitivity to hydantoins. Because the drug delays conduction in the cardiac muscle, avoid using it in patients with sinus bradycardia, sinoatrial block, second- or third-degree atrioventricular (AV) block, or Stokes-Adams syndrome. Also, don't give it to patients whose seizures result from hypoglycemia.

Use phenytoin cautiously in patients with bradycardia, myocardial insufficiency, heart failure, or first-degree AV block because it depresses pacemaker action and reduces myocardial contractile force. Also give the drug cautiously to patients with respiratory depression because it may exacerbate symptoms, to those with hepatic impairment or renal disease because these conditions alter drug metabolism, and to those with diabetes mellitus or other hyperglycemic states because the drug may worsen hyperglycemia.

Give the drug carefully to patients with hypotension because of possible exacerbation, to those with impaired thyroid function because the drug decreases serum thyroxine (T_4), to those with blood dyscrasias because of the increased risk of serious infection, and to those with a fever lasting over 24 hours because drug levels may be decreased.

Phenytoin is classified as a pregnancy risk category D drug, so give it cautiously to pregnant women.

Preparation

Phenytoin is available in 100-mg and 250-mg ampules containing 50 mg/ml. Store the drug at room temperature; avoid freezing it.

Use only clear solutions. If a refrigerated solution has yellowed slightly, it should clear after warming slowly. If it doesn't, discard it.

An intermittent infusion isn't generally recommended because of the risk of an incompatibility. But you can use this method if phenytoin is mixed with 0.9% sodium chloride solution to a concentration of no more than 10 mg/ml. Mix the solution right before infusion and use an administration set with a 0.22-micron filter.

Incompatibilities

Phenytoin is incompatible with amikacin sulfate, aminophylline, bretylium tosylate, cephapirin sodium, clindamycin phosphate, codeine phosphate, dextrose 5% in water, dobutamine hydrochloride, fat emulsions, insulin (regular), lactated Ringer's, levorphanol tartrate, lidocaine hydrochloride, lincomycin hydrochloride, meperidine hydrochloride, metaraminol bitartrate, methadone hydrochloride, morphine sulfate, nitroglycerin, norepinephrine bitartrate, pentobarbital sodium, secobarbital sodium, 0.45% sodium chloride, 0.9% sodium chloride, and streptomycin sulfate.

Administration

- *Direct injection:* Inject the dose directly into a vein or into an I.V. line of a compatible solution that's infusing at a rate below 50 mg/minute. For elderly or debilitated patients, the rate should be 17 to 25 mg/minute. Before and after the injection, flush the I.V. tubing with 0.9% sodium chloride solution to remove the drug, reduce venous irritation, and prevent incompatibility with the primary solution. Don't inject the drug into the dorsal hand veins.
- *Intermittent infusion:* Infuse the drug within 1 hour at the prescribed rate. Don't exceed 50 mg/minute.

Adverse reactions

- *Life-threatening:* cardiovascular collapse, exfoliative dermatitis, severe central nervous system (CNS) depression, ventricular fibrillation.
- *Other:* anorexia, ***ataxia,*** blood dyscrasias, blurred vision, bullous or purpuric dermatitis, clumsiness, ***confusion,*** constipation, ***diplopia,*** dizziness, drowsiness, dysphagia, epigastric pain, fever, gingival hyperplasia, hypertrichosis, hypotension, insomnia, irritability, lupus erythematosus, lymphadenopathy, muscle weakness, ***nausea, nystagmus,*** osteomalacia, rash, seizures, ***slurred speech,*** taste abnormalities, toxic amblyopia, twitching, unusual excitement, ***vomiting.***

Interactions

- *Adrenocorticoids, carbamazepine, cardiac glycosides, corticotropin, cyclosporine, dacarbazine, disopyramide, doxycycline, estrogen-containing contraceptives, levodopa, quinidine:* decreased effects of these drugs from increased metabolism.
- *Alcohol (acute ingestion), amiodarone, anticoagulants, anticonvulsants, benzodiazepines, chloramphenicol, cimetidine, disulfiram, haloperidol, inhalation anesthetics:* enhanced phenytoin effects, resulting from increased serum levels.
- *Alcohol (chronic use), antacids, barbiturates, calcium sulfate, carbamazepine, CNS depressants, folic acid, primidone, rifampin, xanthines:* risk of decreased phenytoin levels.
- *Dopamine:* risk of potentiated hypotension.
- *Isoniazid, loxapine, maprotiline, monoamine oxidase inhibitors, phenothiazines, phenylbutazone, pimozide, sulfinpyrazone, sulfonamides, trazodone:* heightened phenytoin effects from increased serum levels.
- *Ketoconazole, miconazole:* altered metabolism and delayed peak serum levels of these agents.
- *Leucovorin:* antagonized anticonvulsant effects.
- *Levothyroxine:* reduced serum T_4 levels.
- *Lidocaine, propranolol:* additive myocardial depression.
- *Mexiletine:* risk of lowered mexiletine serum levels.
- *Nifedipine, verapamil:* risk of significantly altered serum levels.
- *Streptozocin:* risk of diminished therapeutic effects.
- *Valproic acid:* seizures resulting from interference with phenytoin protein binding.
- *Vitamin D:* risk of reduced efficacy.

Special considerations

During administration, monitor the patient's blood pressure and cardiac rhythm strip. Keep in mind that an infusion rate above 50 mg/minute can cause hypotension, cardiovascular collapse, and CNS depression.

Closely monitor the patient for seizure activity. Keep intubation and aspiration equipment readily available and pad the side rails, headboards, and footboards, as necessary. Because hydration affects the seizure threshold, monitor the patient's intake and output.

Also closely monitor the serum phenytoin level throughout therapy. The therapeutic serum level is 10 to 20 mcg/ml; the toxic level, above 20 mcg/ml; and the lethal level, 100 mcg/ml. If you note signs of toxicity—drowsiness, nausea, vomiting, nystagmus, ataxia, dysarthria, tremor, slurred speech, hypotension, respiratory collapse, and coma—immediately discontinue the drug infusion and notify the doctor.

Closely monitor the serum glucose levels of a diabetic patient. If you note an increase, adjust the insulin dosage as ordered. If a measles-like rash appears during the infusion, stop the infusion and notify the doctor. Assess the I.V. site frequently because phenytoin extravasation causes severe tissue damage.

Advise the patient that the drug may turn his urine pink, red, or a reddish brown color.

Phenytoin can interfere with certain laboratory test results. The drug may cause falsely lowered dexamethasone and metyrapone test results, reduced protein-bound iodine levels, and increased resin or red blood cell triiodothyronine uptake. Phenytoin also produces elevated serum alkaline phosphatase, gamma glutamyl transpeptidase, and glucose levels.

Physostigmine salicylate

(Antilirium)

Used to reverse the effects of anticholinergic drugs, physostigmine salicylate blocks the destruction of acetylcholine at both central and peripheral cholinergic neurotransmitter sites. The accumulated acetylcholine then counteracts the muscarinic effects of the anticholinergic overdose. (See *How physostigmine reverses anticholinergic drug effects*, page 174.)

Physostigmine also antagonizes the central nervous system depressant effects of benzodiazepines. But the drug isn't recommended for a benzodiazepine overdose because its action is nonspecific and the potential for physostigmine toxicity exists.

The onset of action occurs within 3 to 5 minutes. The drug's effects last 1 to 2 hours; the half-life is about 15 to 40 minutes.

Physostigmine is widely distributed throughout the body, easily crosses the blood-brain barrier, and probably crosses the placenta. The drug is hydrolyzed by cholinesterases at the neuromuscular junction. How physostigmine is excreted isn't fully understood. Small amounts appear in urine, and the drug may appear in breast milk. (See *Physostigmine: Indication and dosages.*)

Contraindications and cautions

Physostigmine is contraindicated for patients with a known hypersensitivity to the drug. It's also contraindicated for those with asthma, cardiovascular disease, diabetes mellitus, or gangrene because the drug may aggravate these conditions. And the drug shouldn't be given to patients with mechanical obstruction of the intestinal or urinary tract or with vagotonia because the increased muscle tone may worsen the obstruction.

Give physostigmine cautiously to patients with a history of seizures because of the increased risk of them and to patients with bradycardia or parkinsonian syndrome because their symptoms may worsen.

Classified as a pregnancy risk category C drug, physostigmine should be given cautiously to pregnant patients.

Preparation

Physostigmine is available in concentrations of 1 mg/ml in 2-ml ampules and 1-ml syringes. Solutions may appear slightly discolored (tinted red, blue, or brown). Discard any solution with marked discoloration. Store the drug in light-resistant containers at room temperature, and avoid freezing it.

Incompatibilities

No incompatibilities have been reported.

Administration

• *Direct injection:* Slowly administer the drug into a large vein or into I.V. tubing containing a free-flowing, compatible solution. Don't exceed 1 mg/minute for adults or 0.5 mg/minute for children. Rapid injection can cause bradycardia, breathing difficulty, excessive salivation, and seizures.

• *I.M. injection:* Inject the ordered dose into any I.M. site.

Adverse reactions

• *Life-threatening:* asystole, bronchospasm, cholinergic crisis, respiratory paralysis.

• *Other:* abdominal cramps, ***arrhythmias,*** blurred vision, bradycardia, ***diarrhea,*** dyspnea, ***excessive salivation, excitability,*** hallucinations, headache, hypotension, increased bronchial secretions, lacrimation, miosis, muscle cramps, nausea, palpitations, ***restlessness,*** seizures, ***sweating,*** thrombophlebitis, twitching, urinary frequency, vomiting, weakness.

Interactions

• *Acetylcholine, bethanechol, carbachol, methacholine:* enhanced effects of physostigmine.

• *Benzodiazepines:* risk of diminished effects of these drugs.

• *Procainamide, quinidine:* possibility of reversed cholinergic effects on muscle.

• *Succinylcholine:* additive depolarizing neuromuscular blockade.

DOSAGE FINDER

Physostigmine: Indication and dosages

Reversal of anticholinergic drug effects

▶ For adults who've received atropine or scopolamine, give twice the dose of the drug. For example, to reverse the effects of 0.5 mg I.V. of atropine, give 1 mg I.V. of physostigmine.

▶ For adults who've received another anticholinergic drug, initially give 0.5 to 2 mg I.V. or I.M. Repeat the dose every 20 minutes until the desired effect or adverse cholinergic effects occur. If life-threatening signs such as arrhythmias or coma recur, give 1 to 4 mg at 30- to 60-minute intervals, as needed.

▶ For children who've received another anticholinergic drug, initially give 0.02 mg/kg I.V., then repeat the dose at 5- to 10-minute intervals until the desired effect or adverse cholinergic effects occur. Don't exceed a total dose of 2 mg.

MECHANISM OF ACTION

How physostigmine reverses anticholinergic drug effects

Physostigmine acts at central and peripheral cholinergic sites of neurotransmission to prevent the destruction of acetylcholine. The first illustration shows the normal process of acetylcholine formation and breakdown. The second illustration shows how physostigmine blocks acetylcholine's breakdown, thus counteracting anticholinergic drug effects.

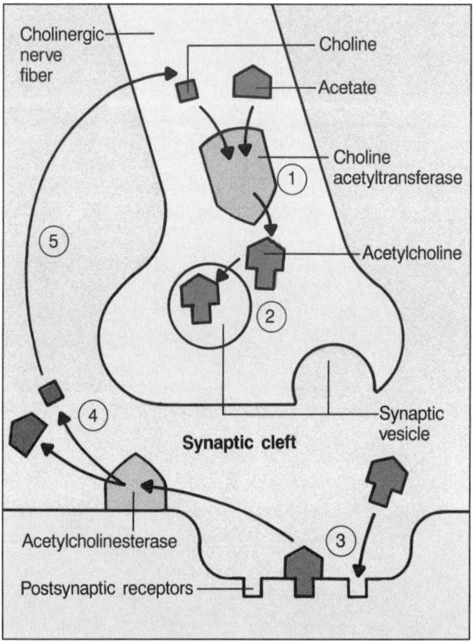

Acetylcholine is formed in the terminal endings of cholinergic nerve fibers when acetate and choline are combined by the action of choline acetyltransferase (1). Acetylcholine is then stored inside synaptic vesicles (2). When needed, it's released into the synaptic cleft. After activation of postsynaptic receptors (3), the enzyme acetylcholinesterase splits acetylcholine into acetate and choline (4). The choline is then transported back to the nerve ending for use again in acetylcholine synthesis (5).

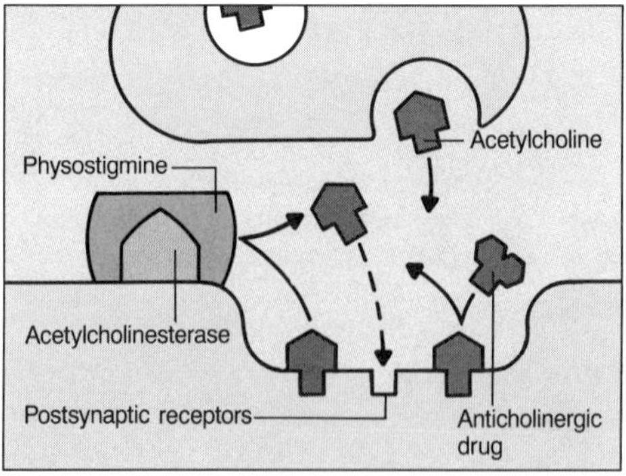

Physostigmine blocks the breakdown of acetylcholine by acetylcholinesterase. This increases the available acetylcholine, which prevents the anticholinergic drug from binding to postsynaptic receptors.

Special considerations

Before therapy, obtain baseline heart rate and blood pressure measurements. Make sure suction and cardiopulmonary resuscitation equipment and atropine sulfate are available.

During therapy, monitor the patient for arrhythmias, such as tachycardia or bradycardia, and hypotension. Immediately report significant changes. Monitor the patient for signs and symptoms of a cholinergic crisis, such as sweating and nausea. If you note them, reduce the dosage, as ordered.

Also watch for signs and symptoms of a physostigmine overdose—excessive salivation and urination, vomiting, and diarrhea. If you detect an overdose, discontinue the drug and notify the doctor. Then provide treatment as ordered. Administer 2 to 4 mg of atropine by I.V. injection at 3- to 10-minute intervals; for children, decrease the doses to 1 mg each. Give the patient 50 to 100 mg/minute of pralidoxime chloride to counteract ganglionic and skeletal muscle effects. Use mechanical ventilation, as needed, and suction the patient's secretions frequently.

Also, closely monitor the patient for changes in his level of consciousness. Because physostigmine's effects last only 1 to 2 hours, he may relapse into coma and require more physostigmine.

Procainamide hydrochloride

(Pronestyl)

A procaine derivative and a Class I antiarrhythmic, procainamide hydrochloride decreases myocardial automaticity and excitability, conduction velocity, and membrane responsiveness, prolonging the refractory period. The drug doesn't affect contractility or cardiac output unless myocardial damage has occurred.

Antiarrhythmic indications include paroxysmal atrial tachycardia, premature ventricular contractions, ventricular tachycardia and, in some cases, atrial fibrillation. Procainamide may also be ordered for malignant hyperthermia.

Peak serum levels occur immediately with I.V. infusion and 15 to 60 minutes after I.M. injection. The half-life of procainamide is 2½ to 5 hours; the half-life of its active metabolite, N-acetylprocainamide (NAPA), 7 hours. In patients with renal impairment or congestive heart failure (CHF), NAPA accumulation in serum reaches toxic levels while procainamide levels remain normal.

Procainamide is rapidly distributed to the liver, spleen, kidneys, lungs, heart, muscles, cerebrospinal fluid, and brain. About 14% to 23% is bound to plasma proteins, and the drug crosses the placenta.

Procainamide is metabolized in the liver, where about 25% is converted to NAPA; about 40% is converted in patients with rapid acetylation or renal impairment. The drug is excreted in urine by tubular secretion and glomerular filtration; 40% to 70% is excreted unchanged. Both procainamide and NAPA appear in breast milk. (See *Procainamide: Indications and dosages,* page 176.)

Contraindications and cautions

Procainamide is contraindicated for patients with a hypersensitivity to procaine or other local amide-type anesthetics. Also, don't give the

DOSAGE FINDER

Procainamide: Indications and dosages

Treatment of arrhythmias, including paroxysmal atrial tachycardia, premature ventricular contractions, ventricular tachycardia, and atrial fibrillation

▶ For adults, slowly give an initial dose of 100 mg by direct I.V. injection or infusion. (Don't exceed 50 mg/minute.) Repeat the dose as needed to control arrhythmias. The maximum dosage is 1 g by direct injection or 500 to 600 mg by infusion over 25 to 30 minutes at 2 to 6 mg/minute. To keep arrhythmias under control, administer a titrated maintenance dose of 1 to 6 mg/minute, or give 500 mg to 1 g I.M. every 4 to 6 hours.

▶ For children, the dosage hasn't been established. Recommendations include giving 3 to 6 mg/kg I.V. (without exceeding 100 mg), then repeating this dose as necessary at 10- to 30-minute intervals (without exceeding 30 mg/kg in 24 hours), and giving 3 to 6 mg/kg I.V. over 5 minutes, followed by a maintenance infusion of 0.02 to 0.08 mg/kg/minute.

▶ For infants, give 1 mg/kg by direct I.V. injection, repeated every 5 minutes up to a total of 15 mg/kg. Follow this with a maintenance infusion of 20 to 50 mcg/kg/minute.

Treatment of malignant hyperthermia

▶ For adults, give 200 to 900 mg by direct I.V. injection. Then give a maintenance infusion of 0.02 to 0.08 mg/kg/minute.

drug to patients with second- or third-degree atrioventricular (AV) heart block because of the risk of further myocardial depression or to patients with atypical ventricular tachycardia (torsades de pointes) because the drug may exacerbate the condition.

Give the drug cautiously to patients with digitalis toxicity, severe first-degree AV block, or bundle-branch block because of the risk of enhanced myocardial depression, ventricular tachycardia, or asystole. Also use caution with patients who have CHF or hepatic or renal impairment because of the risk of toxicity and with patients who have bronchial asthma because of the risk of hypersensitivity.

Give the drug cautiously to patients with myasthenia gravis because it may worsen symptoms. Similarly, use caution with patients who have systemic lupus erythematosus (SLE) because the drug may exacerbate the condition.

A pregnancy risk category C drug, procainamide should be given cautiously to pregnant patients.

Preparation

Available in 10-ml (100 mg/ml) and 2-ml (500 mg/ml) vials, procainamide should be stored at room temperature and protected from light and freezing. Don't use the drug if it appears markedly discolored or if a precipitate has formed.

For an injection or a loading infusion, dilute 1 g of the drug with 50 ml of dextrose 5% in water (D_5W) to yield 20 mg/ml. For a continuous infusion, dilute 1 g of the drug with 500 ml of D_5W to yield 2 mg/ml. In patients with fluid restrictions, dilute 1 g of the drug with 250 ml of D_5W to yield 4 mg/ml. Keep in mind that procainamide may form a complex with dextrose, causing a gradual loss of potency.

Incompatibilities

Procainamide is incompatible with bretylium tosylate, ethacrynate sodium, and phenytoin sodium.

Administration

- *Direct injection:* Administer the

dose over 2 minutes or longer directly into the vein or into I.V. tubing containing a free-flowing, compatible solution.

- *Intermittent infusion:* Give the loading infusion at 1 ml/minute for 25 to 30 minutes. Therapeutic effects usually occur after an infusion of 100 to 200 mg. If you don't see any effect after 500 mg, wait at least 10 minutes for drug distribution and then continue.
- *Continuous infusion:* Using an infusion pump, administer the diluted solution at the ordered rate, usually from 2 to 6 mg/minute. (See *Drip rates for procainamide infusions.*)
- *I.M. injection:* Inject the dose into any I.M. site. Use this route only when an I.V. route can't be used.

Drip rates for procainamide infusions

This chart provides the drip rates you'll need to achieve common infusion rates for a standard concentration of 1 g in 500 ml (2 mg/ml).

PRESCRIBED DOSAGE (mg/minute)	DRIP RATE (microdrops/minute)
1	30
2	60
3	90
4	120
5	150
6	180

Adverse reactions

- *Life-threatening:* severe hypotension, tachycardia (sympathetic response to hypotension), ventricular asystole or fibrillation (from rapid administration).
- *Other:* agranulocytosis, ***anorexia, bitter taste,*** bleeding or bruising, chills, confusion, depression, ***diarrhea,*** dizziness, drowsiness, fatigue, ***fever,*** flushing, hallucinations, joint swelling or pain, light-headedness, ***maculopapular rash,*** nausea, pruritus, rash (SLE-like syndrome), ***vomiting,*** weakness.

Interactions

- *Antiarrhythmics:* risk of additive or antagonized effects.
- *Antidyskinetics, antihistamines, antimuscarinics (especially atropine and related drugs):* risk of intensified atropine-like effects.
- *Antihypertensives:* risk of additive hypotension.
- *Antimyasthenics:* risk of decreased effects of these drugs.
- *Bethanechol:* antagonized cholinergic effects.
- *Bone marrow depressants:* increased leukopenia and thrombocytopenia.
- *Bretylium:* diminished inotropic effects and potentiated hypotension.
- *Cimetidine:* elevated serum procainamide levels.
- *Lidocaine:* additive central nervous system effects.
- *Neuromuscular blockers:* prolonged or enhanced effects of these drugs.
- *Pimozide:* risk of arrhythmias.

Special considerations

Before administering the drug, make sure you have phenylephrine or norepinephrine available to treat severe hypotension. Find out if the patient is sensitive to benzyl alcohol or sulfites; if so, inform the doctor because procainamide may contain these additives. Be aware that patients with CHF or renal impairment may require lower doses.

During therapy, monitor the patient's response to the drug and ad-

EMERGENCY INTERVENTION

Managing a procainamide overdose

The signs and symptoms of a procainamide overdose include confusion, dizziness or fainting, drowsiness, nausea and vomiting, oliguria, severe hypotension, and an unusually rapid or irregular heartbeat. If your patient develops such signs and symptoms, discontinue the drug immediately. Then take these measures:

- Maintain a patent airway and ventilate the patient as necessary.
- Administer replacement fluids.
- Give the patient norepinephrine or phenylephrine, as ordered.
- Infuse ⅙ M sodium lactate injection to reverse procainamide's cardiotoxic effects, as ordered.

Hemodialysis may be ordered to reduce the serum half-life of procainamide and N-acetylprocainamide.

just the dosage, as ordered. Continuously monitor his blood pressure, cardiac rhythm strip, and other indicators of cardiac function. Discontinue administration if the patient develops excessive hypotension, widened QRS complexes, or signs of impending myocardial infarction. Also discontinue therapy if the patient develops signs of SLE or hemolytic anemia. For a patient with ventricular tachycardia, discontinue the infusion if the ventricular rate declines significantly without the return of regular AV conduction. (See *Managing a procainamide overdose.*)

Procainamide can affect the results of some tests. The Coombs' test may show a false-positive result. An electrocardiogram will show a widened QRS complex, prolonged PR and QT intervals, and reduced QRS and T-wave voltage. White blood cell and platelet tests will show decreased counts, while serum alkaline phosphatase, bilirubin, lactate dehydrogenase, and alanine aminotransferase (ALT), formerly SGPT, tests may show increased levels.

Propranolol hydrochloride

(Inderal)

Indicated for life-threatening arrhythmias, propranolol hydrochloride competitively blocks beta-adrenergic receptors in the myocardium and in bronchial and vascular smooth muscle. By these actions, the drug reduces heart rate, decreases myocardial contractility and cardiac output, and increases systolic ejection time and cardiac volume. Propranolol also reduces conduction velocity and myocardial automaticity.

The drug lowers blood pressure not only by blocking peripheral adrenergic receptors, but also by decreasing sympathetic outflow from the central nervous system and suppressing renin release.

The onset of action is immediate; the duration of action lasts from 3½ to 6 hours. The half-life of the drug ranges from 10 minutes to 6 hours.

Propranolol is widely distributed throughout the tissues, including the lungs, liver, kidneys, and heart. More than 90% is bound to plasma proteins. The drug crosses the blood-brain barrier and placenta. Metabolized in the liver, propranolol is excreted primarily in urine, with between 1% and 4% removed in feces. Fecal excretion rises in patients who have severe renal impairment. Small amounts of propranolol appear in breast milk. (See *Propran-*

olol: Indication and dosages.)

DOSAGE FINDER

Propranolol: Indication and dosages

Treatment of life-threatening arrhythmias

▶ For adults, give 1 to 3 mg by direct I.V. injection. Repeat the dose after 2 minutes and again after 4 hours, if necessary.

▶ For children, initially give 10 to 100 mcg/kg by slow I.V. injection over 10 minutes. Repeat the dose as needed every 6 to 8 hours.

Contraindications and cautions

Propranolol is contraindicated for patients with a known hypersensitivity to the drug. It's also contraindicated for patients with Raynaud's syndrome or malignant hypertension because of the risk of peripheral arterial insufficiency and for patients with bronchial asthma because beta-adrenergic blockade may lead to increased airway resistance and bronchospasm. Other contraindications include sinus bradycardia, heart block greater than first degree, myocardial infarction with a systolic pressure below 100 mm Hg, congestive heart failure (CHF) unless it results from tachyarrhythmia treatable with propranolol, and usually cardiogenic shock. Further myocardial depression can occur with these conditions. Avoid giving propranolol to patients with myasthenia gravis because it may exacerbate symptoms.

Give propranolol cautiously to patients with cardiac impairment because the drug may precipitate CHF, to patients with hyperthyroidism because the drug may mask tachycardia, to patients with nonallergic bronchospastic disease because the drug may increase airway resistance and bronchospasm, and to patients with hepatic or renal impairment because of an increased risk of adverse reactions. In patients with diabetes mellitus who are taking oral hypoglycemic drugs, propranolol may trigger hyperglycemic reactions or hypoglycemia, possibly inhibiting pancreatic insulin release.

Administer propranolol cautiously to children because the drug's pediatric safety and efficacy haven't been established. Because propranolol is classified as a pregnancy risk category C drug, administer it cautiously to pregnant patients.

Preparation

Propranolol comes in 1-ml ampules containing 1 mg/ml. Store it at room temperature, and protect it from light and freezing. The drug is compatible with 0.9% sodium chloride solution and dextrose 5% in water.

Incompatibilities

No incompatibilities have been reported.

Administration

• *Direct injection:* Administer the drug at a maximum rate of 1 mg/minute through an I.V. line containing a free-flowing, compatible solution.

Adverse reactions

• *Life-threatening:* atrioventricular (AV) dissociation, cardiac arrest, CHF, complete heart block, intensified AV block, pulmonary edema, ventricular fibrillation.

• *Other:* alopecia (reversible), ***bradycardia,*** confusion, constipation, ***diarrhea, dizziness,*** dry mouth, eosinophilia (transient), ***fatigue,*** flatulence, fluid retention, hallucinations, ***hypotension, increased airway resistance, insomnia,*** irritability,

EMERGENCY INTERVENTION

Managing a propranolol overdose

Treat the complications of a propranolol overdose using these interventions, as ordered:
- For hypotension with severe bradycardia, give I.V. atropine and, if necessary, isoproterenol, dobutamine, or epinephrine. Glucagon may also be ordered.
- For premature ventricular contractions, administer I.V. lidocaine or phenytoin.
- For cardiac failure, administer oxygen, a diuretic, and digitalis. A transvenous pacemaker may be used if drug therapy is unsuccessful.
- For hypotension, place the patient in the Trendelenburg position and administer I.V. fluids (unless he has pulmonary edema) and an I.V. vasopressor.
- For seizures, administer I.V. diazepam (or, if necessary, phenytoin).
- For bronchospasm, give isoproterenol or a theophylline derivative.

laryngospasm, ***lethargy,*** light-headedness, lupuslike reactions, ***mental depression,*** migraine, ***nausea,*** partial heart block, peripheral arterial insufficiency, peripheral neuropathy, pharyngitis, respiratory distress, rhinitis, ***vomiting.***

Interactions
- *Antiarrhythmic drugs (such as lidocaine, phenytoin, procainamide, or quinidine):* risk of additive or antagonistic cardiac effects and magnified toxic effects of these drugs.
- *Atropine, other antimuscarinics:* risk of reversing propranolol-induced bradycardia.
- *Cimetidine:* reduced propranolol clearance, resulting from inhibited hepatic metabolism.
- *Diuretics, other antihypertensives:* potentiated hypotension.
- *Levodopa:* antagonized hypotensive and positive inotropic effects.
- *Neuromuscular blockers:* risk of potentiated effects.
- *Phenothiazines:* enhanced hypotensive effects, especially with high phenothiazine doses.
- *Sympathomimetics (such as isoproterenol and epinephrine):* antagonized beta-adrenergic effects.
- *Tricyclic antidepressants:* antagonized cardiac effects.

Special considerations
During therapy, carefully monitor the patient's cardiac rhythm strip, blood pressure, and central venous pressure. Note any signs or symptoms of a propranolol overdose, and provide treatment, as ordered. (See *Managing a propranolol overdose.*)

For elderly patients, adjust the dosage as ordered to reflect their response. Give lower doses to patients with hepatic impairment.

After prolonged atrial fibrillation, restoration of a normal atrial rhythm may dislodge thrombi from the atrial wall, resulting in thromboembolism. Thus, an anticoagulant may be given before the normal atrial rhythm is restored.

As soon possible, switch to an oral form of propranolol.

The drug may alter some laboratory test results. Antinuclear antibody titers may show dose-related increases. Blood urea nitrogen; serum creatinine; alkaline phosphatase; lactate dehydrogenase; aspartate aminotransferase (AST), formerly SGOT; alanine aminotransferase (ALT), formerly SGPT; lipoprotein; triglyceride; potassium; and uric acid levels may also show increases. Intraocular pressure will be reduced, and a radionuclide cardiac scan may show decreased myocardial uptake of thallous chloride.

Pyridostigmine bromide

(Mestinon, Regonol)

A cholinesterase inhibitor, pyridostigmine bromide is used as an antidote to nondepolarizing neuromuscular blockers, such as tubocurarine, metocurine, gallamine, and pancuronium. Pyridostigmine is also indicated for the treatment of myasthenia gravis.

By blocking the effects of acetylcholinesterase at the neuromuscular junction, pyridostigmine allows acetylcholine to accumulate. This results in prolonged and enhanced effects, including miosis, bradycardia, increased intestinal and skeletal muscle tone, constriction of bronchi and ureters, and increased salivary and sweat gland secretion. Accumulations at receptor sites reverse muscle paralysis induced by nondepolarizing neuromuscular blockers. Accumulations at the motor end plate increase muscle strength and response to repetitive nerve stimulation.

Pyridostigmine's onset of action occurs within 2 to 5 minutes of I.V. administration and less than 15 minutes after I.M. administration. Its duration of action ranges from 2 to 3 hours; its half-life is about 90 minutes.

Widely distributed throughout the body, pyridostigmine crosses the placenta. In high doses, the drug also crosses the blood-brain barrier. Hydrolyzed by cholinesterases and metabolized by liver enzymes, pyridostigmine is excreted in urine. The drug also appears in breast milk. (See *Pyridostigmine: Indications and dosages.*)

DOSAGE FINDER

Pyridostigmine: Indications and dosages

Antidote to nondepolarizing neuromuscular blockers, such as tubocurarine, metocurine, gallamine, and pancuronium

▶ For adults, give 10 to 20 mg or 0.1 to 0.25 mg/kg of pyridostigmine I.V. with or shortly after giving 0.6 to 1.2 mg of atropine I.V. or 0.2 to 0.6 mg of glycopyrrolate I.V. (about 0.2 mg of glycopyrrolate for each 5 mg of pyridostigmine).

Treatment of myasthenia gravis

▶ For adults, give 2 mg I.V. or I.M. every 2 to 3 hours, or give about $1/30$ of the patient's oral maintenance dose.

▶ For neonates of mothers with myasthenia gravis, give 50 to 150 mcg/kg I.M. every 4 to 6 hours.

Contraindications and cautions

Pyridostigmine is contraindicated for patients with a hypersensitivity to this or other anticholinesterase drugs or bromides. Also avoid giving the drug to patients with a mechanical obstruction of the intestinal or urinary tract because of increased smooth muscle tone and activity.

Give pyridostigmine cautiously to patients with asthma, pneumonia, postoperative atelectasis, urinary tract infections, and arrhythmias (especially bradycardia and atrioventricular block), and recent coronary occlusion because the drug may exacerbate these conditions. Use caution with patients who have epilepsy, hyperthyroidism, peptic ulcer, and vagotonia; the drug may mask signs of these conditions. And because the drug may exacerbate breathing difficulty caused by pain, sedation, or secretions, give it cau-

EMERGENCY INTERVENTION

Managing a pyridostigmine overdose

When administering pyridostigmine, assess the patient for muscarinic effects, which indicate a drug overdose. These effects include abdominal cramps, diaphoresis, diarrhea, excessive bronchial and salivary secretions, lacrimation, nausea, and vomiting. If you note these effects, take the following actions, as ordered:
• Promptly discontinue pyridostigmine.
• Maintain a patent airway, using suctioning, oxygen, and assisted ventilation, as necessary.
• Give the patient 1 to 4 mg atropine I.V., then additional doses every 5 to 30 minutes, as needed.

tiously after surgery.

Classified as a pregnancy risk category C drug, pyridostigmine should be given carefully to pregnant patients.

Preparation
Pyridostigmine is available in a concentration of 5 mg/ml in 2-ml ampules and 5-ml vials. Store the drug at room temperature, and protect it from light and freezing.

Incompatibilities
Pyridostigmine is unstable in alkaline solutions.

Administration
• *Direct injection:* Slowly administer the undiluted drug into an I.V. line containing a free-flowing, compatible solution. Watch for thrombophlebitis at the I.V. site.
• *I.M. injection:* Inject the ordered dose into any I.M. injection site.

Adverse reactions
• *Life-threatening:* bradycardia, bronchospasm, excessive salivation (leading to aspiration), hypotension, respiratory paralysis.
• *Other:* ***abdominal cramps,*** acne, agitation, anxiety, blurred vision, clumsiness, confusion, ***diaphoresis, diarrhea (severe),*** fasciculations, headache, increased bronchial secretions, increased weakness (especially in arms, neck, shoulders, and tongue), irritability, lacrimation, ***nausea,*** pupillary constriction, restlessness, seizures, slurred speech, thrombophlebitis at injection site, twitching, unsteadiness, ***vomiting.***

Interactions
• *Aminoglycosides, capreomycin, hydrocarbon inhalation anesthetics (such as halothane), lincomycin, polymyxins, quinine:* risk of antagonized antimyasthenic effects.
• *Antimuscarinic agents (especially atropine):* antagonized muscarinic effects of pyridostigmine and reduced GI motility.
• *Depolarizing neuromuscular blockers (such as succinylcholine):* prolonged neuromuscular blockade.
• *Edrophonium:* risk of cholinergic crisis (pyridostigmine overdose) with increased muscle weakness and worsening of patient's condition.
• *Guanadrel, guanethidine, mecamylamine, procainamide, quinidine, trimethaphan:* risk of antagonized antimyasthenic effects.
• *Local ester-derivative anesthetics:* increased risk of anesthesia toxicity.
• *Nondepolarizing neuromuscular blockers:* antagonized effects.
• *Other cholinesterase inhibitors (such as demecarium, echothiophate, and possibly topical malathion):* risk of additive toxicity.
• *Parenteral local anesthetics:* antagonized antimyasthenic effects.

Special considerations
Determine the patient's baseline re-

spiratory rate, heart rate, and blood pressure. If his heart rate is below 80 beats/minute, administer atropine before pyridostigmine. Also, when giving high doses of pyridostigmine, administer 0.6 to 1.2 mg of atropine or 0.2 to 0.6 mg of glycopyrrolate, as ordered. These drugs block the muscarinic effects of pyridostigmine. Keep a separate syringe of atropine on hand during therapy in case of overdose.

When giving the drug to reverse the effects of nondepolarizing neuromuscular blockers, keep the patient on a ventilator and wait 15 to 30 minutes for the full effects. Monitor the patient for signs and symptoms of a recurring respiratory depression. Delayed recovery is associated with hypokalemia, debilitation, carcinomatosis, aminoglycoside antibiotic therapy, and the use of anesthetics (such as ether).

Monitor the patient for signs and symptoms of an overdose (see *Managing a pyridostigmine overdose*). Be alert too for signs of a cholinergic crisis, which can occur with a pyridostigmine overdose. In a cholinergic crisis, muscle weakness usually occurs 1 hour after the last pyridostigmine dose and is accompanied by adverse muscarinic effects and fasciculations. Weakness that occurs 3 or more hours after the last pyridostigmine dose may indicate myasthenic crisis and the need for more drug. An edrophonium chloride (Tensilon) test may be used to differentiate a cholinergic crisis from a myasthenic crisis.

Severe myasthenia gravis is associated with accelerated pyridostigmine metabolism and excretion. Thus, the drug's effects are diminished in patients with this disorder. Also, in myasthenia gravis, muscle groups may respond differently to the drug. One muscle group may have no response, while another develops increased strength.

Quinidine gluconate

A Class I antiarrhythmic, quinidine gluconate exerts direct and indirect antimuscarinic effects on cardiac tissue. The drug reduces myocardial automaticity, conduction velocity, and membrane responsiveness—possibly by inhibiting the movement of potassium ions across cell membranes. The drug also reduces vagal tone and prolongs the effective refractory period. All these effects contribute to the drug's ability to block reentrant arrhythmias. (See *How quinidine corrects arrhythmias,* pages 184 and 185.) Its alpha-adrenergic blocking action also increases beta-adrenergic effects, including peripheral vasodilation.

Quinidine is indicated for atrial fibrillation or flutter, paroxysmal atrial or junctional tachycardia, premature atrial or ventricular contrac-

DOSAGE FINDER

Quinidine: Indications and dosages

Treatment of arrhythmias, including atrial fibrillation or flutter, paroxysmal atrial or junctional tachycardia, premature atrial or ventricular contractions, and ventricular tachycardia

▶ For adults, initially infuse 16 mg/minute (1 ml/minute). Then adjust the dosage as necessary to control arrhythmias. The usual dose needed to control ventricular arrhythmias is 300 mg or less. The maximum daily dose is 4 g.

▶ For children, infuse 30 mg/kg or 900 mg/m^2 daily in five divided doses.

MECHANISM OF ACTION

How quinidine corrects arrhythmias

When a reentrant arrhythmia develops in an area of myocardial damage, quinidine can help reestablish normal conduction.

Normally, an impulse travels down a conduction pathway, splits in two directions, and enters a common pathway. As shown, myocardial damage produces a one-way block, preventing normal tissue activation. The unblocked impulse travels up through the damaged area, which slows conduction. After the impulse passes through the damaged area, it reactivates the myocardial tissue, triggering a reentrant arrhythmia.

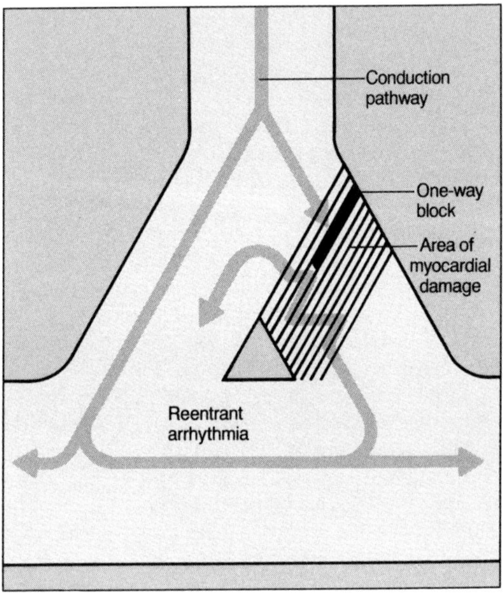

tions, and ventricular tachycardia.

A peak plasma level occurs in 3 to 4 hours. The plasma half-life is normally 6 to 8 hours but may range from 3 to 16 hours or longer.

Quinidine is distributed to all tissues except the brain, with 80% to 90% bound to plasma proteins (primarily albumin). The highest concentrations appear in the heart, liver, kidneys, and skeletal muscles. The drug also is distributed to the red blood cells and binds to hemoglobin. Quinidine crosses the placenta. Metabolized in the liver, quinidine is thought to be excreted by glomerular filtration, with 10% to 20% excreted unchanged in urine within 24 hours. Excretion increases in acidic urine and decreases in alkaline urine. Less than 5% is eliminated in feces; small amounts are found in breast milk. (See *Quinidine: Indications and dosages,* page 183.)

Contraindications and cautions

Quinidine is contraindicated for patients with a hypersensitivity to the drug or to other cinchona derivatives. Also, avoid giving the drug to patients with myasthenia gravis because it may increase weakness. Because quinidine causes additive cardiac depression, it's contraindicated for patients with digitalis-

Quinidine produces a two-way block in the pathway that stops the returning impulse. This prevents the development of a reentrant arrhythmia and helps reestablish normal conduction.

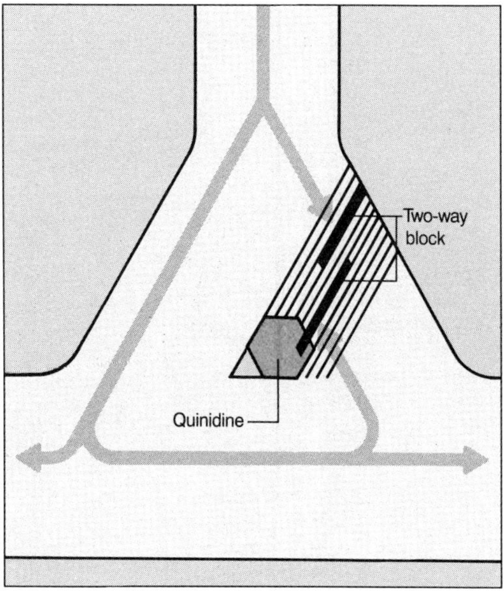

induced atrioventricular (AV) conduction disorders, complete AV block, severe intraventricular conduction defects associated with a widened QRS complex, or escape junctional or ventricular rhythms.

Give quinidine cautiously to patients with incomplete AV block because of the potential for complete block. Also use caution with patients who have congestive heart failure (CHF) or hypotension because quinidine may decrease myocardial contractility or blood pressure, aggravating these conditions.

Administer the drug cautiously to patients with asthma, emphysema, weakness, or febrile infection because their symptoms can mask those of quinidine hypersensitivity. Also, give the drug cautiously to patients with digitalis toxicity because quinidine may intensify cardiac depression and inhibit intracardial conduction, to patients with hypokalemia because of possible reduced drug effects, and to patients with psoriasis or a history of thrombocytopenia because the drug may worsen these disorders.

Give quinidine carefully to elderly patients and those who have hepatic or renal impairment because of decreased quinidine metabolism and the risk of toxicity. Administer the drug carefully to children because

EMERGENCY INTERVENTION

Managing a quinidine overdose

Signs and symptoms of a quinidine overdose include an absent P wave, anuria, apnea, ataxia, extrasystole, hallucinations, hypotension, irritability, lethargy, respiratory distress, seizures, thrashing, twitching, and a widening QRS complex, PR interval, or QT interval. If you note these signs or symptoms, take the following steps, as ordered:

- Give supplemental oxygen and ventilatory support.
- Assist with cardiac pacing and administer hypertensives, urine acidifiers, and I.V. fluids.
- Replace fluids, then give metaraminol or norepinephrine to treat hypotension.
- Infuse $1/6$ M sodium lactate to reduce quinidine's cardiotoxic effects.

pediatric safety and efficacy haven't been determined. And because quinidine is classified as a pregnancy risk category C drug, give it cautiously to pregnant patients.

Preparation

Quinidine is available in 10-ml vials (80 mg/ml). Store the drug at room temperature, and protect it from light and freezing. For an intermittent infusion, dilute the drug with dextrose 5% in water (D_5W) to the ordered concentration. For a continuous infusion, dilute 800 mg (one vial) of quinidine in 40 ml of D_5W to yield 16 mg/ml. Don't use any solutions that have turned brown, and discard all diluted solutions after 24 hours.

Incompatibilities

Quinidine is incompatible with alkaline solutions, amiodarone hydrochloride, and iodide salts.

Administration

- *Intermittent infusion:* Administer the solution through an I.V. line over the prescribed period.
- *Continuous infusion:* Start the infusion at 1 ml/minute. Then adjust the infusion rate to control arrhythmias.

Adverse reactions

- *Life-threatening:* aggravated CHF, agranulocytosis, anaphylaxis, hemolytic anemia, hemorrhage, hepatotoxicity, hypoglycemia (severe), respiratory arrest, thrombocytopenia, torsades de pointes (usually self-limiting polymorphic ventricular tachycardia), ventricular fibrillation.
- *Other:* angioedema, bleeding or bruising, blurred vision or other vision changes, ***cinchonism,*** confusion, ***diarrhea,*** dyspnea, electrocardiogram (ECG) changes, fainting, fatigue, ***fever,*** jaundice, ***lightheadedness,*** nausea, pallor, photosensitivity, pleuritic chest pain, polyarthritis, premature ventricular contractions, pruritus, rash, ***severe headache,*** tachycardia, ***tinnitus,*** vertigo, ***vomiting,*** weakness, wheezing.

Interactions

- *Antiarrhythmics (lidocaine, phenytoin, procainamide, propranolol):* risk of additive cardiac effects.
- *Anticholinergic drugs:* potentiated effects.
- *Antihypertensives:* risk of potentiated hypotension because quinidine may lower blood pressure.
- *Antimuscarinic drugs:* risk of intensified atropine-like effects.
- *Bethanechol:* risk of antagonized cholinergic effects.
- *Bretylium:* risk of diminished inotropic effects and potentiated hypotension.
- *Cardiac glycosides:* risk of in-

creased serum levels of these drugs.
- *Cholinergic drugs:* reduced effectiveness in terminating paroxysmal atrial tachycardia.
- *Cimetidine and drugs that alkalinize urine (acetazolamide, sodium bicarbonate, some antacids, thiazide diuretics):* increased serum levels of quinidine, resulting from decreased metabolism.
- *Hepatic enzyme inducers:* risk of reduced serum levels of quinidine from enhanced hepatic metabolism.
- *Neuromuscular blockers (gallamine, metocurine, pancuronium, succinylcholine, tubocurarine):* potentiated effects.
- *Nifedipine:* risk of decreased quinidine levels; risk of increased levels when nifedipine is discontinued.
- *Pimozide:* risk of arrhythmias (prolonged QT interval).
- *Potassium-containing drugs:* heightened quinidine effects.
- *Quinine:* increased risk of cinchonism.
- *Verapamil:* risk of hypotension in patients with hypertrophic cardiomyopathy.
- *Warfarin:* heightened warfarin effects.

Special considerations

During the infusion, continuously monitor the patient's blood pressure and cardiac function. A rapid infusion of as little as 200 mg of quinidine may cause blood pressure to drop by 40 to 50 mm Hg. Also monitor the patient's serum quinidine and potassium levels; quinidine levels above 8 mcg/ml are toxic.

Stop the infusion immediately if the patient develops signs and symptoms of an overdose. (See *Managing a quinidine overdose.*) Also, discontinue the drug if the cardiac rhythm strip reveals excessive widening of the QRS complex (25% greater than before infusion), excessive prolongation of the PR and QT intervals, or an absent P wave. And discontinue the drug when a rapid heart rate declines to 120 beats/minute, or when the normal sinus rhythm is restored.

Quinidine can alter the results of some diagnostic tests. The patient's ECG will show a widened QRS complex, prolonged QT interval, and T-wave flattening. Serum alkaline phosphatase; aspartate aminotransferase (AST), formerly SGOT; and alanine aminotransferase (ALT), formerly SGPT, levels may be elevated, while serum glucose levels may be decreased.

Sodium bicarbonate

Indicated for cardiac arrest and metabolic acidosis, sodium bicarbonate works as a systemic alkalinizing agent. The drug increases plasma bicarbonate and buffers excess hydrogen ion concentration, thereby reversing acidosis.

The onset of action is immediate. The drug's duration of action isn't known.

Sodium bicarbonate is distributed throughout extracellular fluid and probably crosses the placenta. The drug is metabolized by dissociation in water to form sodium and bicarbonate ions. The bicarbonate anions are converted to carbonic acid, then to carbon dioxide (CO_2), which is excreted by the lungs. Usually less than 1% of the drug is excreted in urine by glomerular filtration. The drug probably appears in breast milk. (See *Sodium bicarbonate: Indications and dosages,* page 188.)

Contraindications and cautions

Sodium bicarbonate is contraindi-

DOSAGE FINDER

Sodium bicarbonate: Indications and dosages

Dosages will vary based on the severity of the acidosis, pertinent test results, and the patient's age, weight, and condition.

Treatment of cardiac arrest

▶ For adults and children age 2 and over, give a direct I.V. injection of 1 mEq/kg. Then give 0.5 mEq/kg every 10 minutes, depending on arterial blood gas (ABG) measurements.

▶ For children under age 2, give a direct I.V. injection of 1 mEq/kg over 1 to 2 minutes. Then give additional doses every 10 minutes. If ABG and pH levels are available, determine these doses by multiplying body weight (in kilograms) by 0.3. Then, multiply this figure by the base deficit (mEq/liter). If ABG and pH levels aren't available, give additional doses of 1 mEq/kg during the cardiac arrest, to a maximum of 8 mEq/kg daily.

Treatment of metabolic acidosis associated with chronic renal failure

▶ For adults and older children, infuse 2 to 5 mEq/kg over 4 to 8 hours. Base subsequent doses on the patient's response to the drug, and carbon dioxide and blood pH test results.

cated for patients with metabolic or respiratory alkalosis because the drug may exacerbate these conditions, for patients with chloride loss from vomiting or continuous GI suctioning because of the increased risk of severe alkalosis, for patients with hypocalcemia because of the heightened risk of alkalosis resulting in tetany, and for patients at risk for developing diuretic-induced hypochloremic alkalosis.

Give the drug cautiously to patients with renal insufficiency, edematous sodium-retaining conditions – such as cirrhosis of the liver, congestive heart failure, or toxemia of pregnancy – and hypertension. The drug's sodium content may exacerbate these conditions.

Give this pregnancy risk category C drug cautiously to pregnant women.

Preparation

Sodium bicarbonate is available in 5-ml (2.4 mEq) flip-top and pin-top vials containing 4% solution (6.48 mEq/ml); 10-ml (5 mEq) disposable syringes containing 4.2% solution (0.5 mEq/ml); 500-ml (297.5 mEq) containers of 5% solution (0.595 mEq/ml); 10-ml (8.9 mEq) ampules and 50-ml (44.6 mEq) ampules and disposable syringes containing 7.5% solution (0.892 mEq/ml); and 10-ml (10 mEq) disposable syringes and 50-ml (50 mEq) vials and disposable syringes containing 8.4% solution (1 mEq/ml).

Store the drug at room temperature, but below 104° F (40° C). Protect it from freezing and heat. Don't use the solution if it looks cloudy or contains a precipitate.

To increase stability, refrigerate the sodium bicarbonate and syringe ahead of time and rinse the syringe twice with refrigerated sterile water for injection. Minimize air contact by expelling air from the syringe and taping the plunger in place to reduce movement caused by escaping CO_2. The 7.5% solution in the polypropylene syringe remains stable up to 100 days if refrigerated or up to 45 days at room temperature.

To dilute sodium bicarbonate for infusion, follow the manufacturer's instructions, using sterile water for injection or a standard electrolyte solution. For neonates and children under age 2, use a 4.2% sodium bicarbonate solution or dilute a 7.5%

or 8.4% solution with dextrose 5% in water at a 1:1 ratio.

Incompatibilities

Sodium bicarbonate is incompatible with the following drugs, compounds, and solutions: alcohol 5% in dextrose 5%; amino acids; ascorbic acid injection; calcium salts; carmustine; cisplatin; codeine phosphate; corticotropin; dextrose 5% in lactated Ringer's injection; dobutamine hydrochloride; dopamine hydrochloride; epinephrine hydrochloride; fat emulsion 10%; glycopyrrolate; hydromorphone hydrochloride; insulin (regular); Ionosol B, D, or G with invert sugar 10%; isoproterenol hydrochloride; labetalol hydrochloride; levorphanol tartrate; magnesium sulfate; meperidine hydrochloride; methadone hydrochloride; methicillin sodium; methylprednisolone sodium succinate; metoclopramide hydrochloride; morphine sulfate; norepinephrine bitartrate; oxytetracycline hydrochloride; penicillin G potassium; pentazocine lactate; pentobarbital sodium; phenobarbital sodium; procaine hydrochloride; promazine hydrochloride; Ringer's injection and lactated Ringer's injection; secobarbital sodium; ⅙ M sodium lactate; streptomycin sulfate; succinylcholine chloride; tetracycline hydrochloride; thiopental sodium; tubocurarine chloride; vancomycin hydrochloride; and vitamin B complex with vitamin C.

Administration

- *Direct injection:* Flush the I.V. line before and after giving the drug. With adults and children age 2 and over, inject it rapidly into a patent primary I.V. line. With children under age 2, inject the drug into a patent primary I.V. line over 1 to 2 minutes. A rapid injection in children (10 ml/minute) can cause hypernatremia, decreased cerebrospinal fluid pressure, intracranial hemorrhage, and alkalosis accompanied by hyperirritability or tetany.
- *Continuous infusion:* Flush the I.V. line before and after giving the drug. Infuse the diluted drug into a patent I.V. line over 4 to 8 hours.

Adverse reactions

- *Life-threatening:* intracranial hemorrhage in children under age 2 (with rapid administration), metabolic alkalosis.
- *Other:* bradypnea; fatigue; increased thirst; irregular heartbeat; mental changes; muscle cramps, pain, or twitching; necrosis, sloughing, or ulceration (with extravasation); nervousness; restlessness; swollen feet or lower legs; unpleasant taste in the mouth; weakness.

Interactions

- *Amphetamines, quinidine:* risk of toxicity resulting from inhibited urine excretion of these drugs.
- *Anabolic steroids, androgens:* heightened risk of edema.
- *Antidyskinetics:* reduced therapeutic effects of these drugs.
- *Antimuscarinics, especially atropine-related compounds:* reduced effectiveness, delayed excretion, and increased adverse effects of these drugs.
- *Corticosteroids:* increased risk of hypernatremia with frequent or high-dose administration of sodium bicarbonate.
- *Ephedrine:* lengthened half-life and prolonged action of ephedrine, especially if alkaline urine persists for several days.
- *Lithium:* enhanced excretion and risk of decreased effectiveness of lithium.
- *Mecamylamine:* delayed excretion and prolonged effects of mecamylamine.

- *Methenamine:* reduced methenamine effectiveness.
- *Mexiletine:* delayed mexiletine excretion.
- *Potassium-sparing diuretics, potassium supplements:* altered serum potassium levels of these drugs.
- *Potassium-wasting diuretics:* enhanced risk of hypochloremic alkalosis.
- *Salicylates:* increased excretion of these drugs.
- *Warfarin, indanedione-derived anticoagulants:* reduced effectiveness of these drugs resulting from decreased absorption.

Special considerations

Keep in mind that the American Heart Association no longer recommends the routine use of sodium bicarbonate during the initial stages of advanced cardiac life support.

Before giving the drug, obtain baseline electrolyte values. Before and during therapy, correct any electrolyte imbalances, especially hypokalemia and hypocalcemia. Monitor the patient's arterial blood gases, pH, and serum bicarbonate levels, as well as his renal function.

Before administering sodium bicarbonate to a patient in cardiac arrest, lower his level of partial pressure of carbon dioxide in arterial blood with manual or mechanical hyperventilation. Then give him the drug.

Repeatedly administer small doses of the drug to avoid an overdose and metabolic alkalosis. Excessive doses may induce hypokalemia and predispose the patient to arrhythmias. If alkalosis occurs, have the patient rebreathe expired air from a mask or paper bag. Treat severe alkalosis with calcium gluconate I.V., as ordered.

Don't attempt to fully correct a sodium bicarbonate deficit during the first 24 hours of therapy; this may produce metabolic alkalosis resulting from delayed compensatory mechanisms.

Sodium bicarbonate use can affect some laboratory test results. Blood and urine pH and serum potassium levels may rise. Also, a gastric acid secretion test will show an antagonized response to pentagastrin.

Streptokinase

(Kabikinase, Streptase)

Streptokinase promotes thrombolysis by converting plasminogen to plasmin (fibrinolysin), which degrades fibrin clots, fibrinogen, and precoagulant factors V and VII. The drug also decreases blood and plasma viscosity and reduces the tendency of red blood cells (RBCs) to form aggregates, thereby increasing the perfusion of collateral blood vessels. Streptokinase is strongly antigenic, with the antibodies diminishing the drug's effect.

The drug is indicated for pulmonary embolism, deep vein thrombosis, arterial embolism or thrombosis, and acute, obstructing coronary artery thrombi associated with evolving, acute myocardial infarction. Streptokinase also is used to treat arteriovenous cannula occlusion.

The onset of action is rapid. The duration of action lasts a few hours after therapy stops. The drug's initial half-life is about 18 minutes (because of antibody action against streptokinase); subsequent half-life is about 83 minutes (in the absence of antibodies).

Streptokinase is distributed in the plasma, and minimal amounts may cross the placenta. The drug isn't metabolized. Instead, it's rapidly cleared from the circulation by antibodies and the reticuloendothelial system. Reperfusion of the myocardium usually occurs 20 minutes to 2 hours after the start of therapy; the average time is 45 minutes. The drug may appear in breast milk. (See *Streptokinase: Indications and dosages.*)

DOSAGE FINDER

Streptokinase: Indications and dosages

Treatment of pulmonary embolism, deep vein thrombosis, and arterial embolism or thrombosis

▶ For adults, infuse a loading dose of 250,000 IU over 30 minutes. Set the rate at 30 ml/hour (for a 750,000 IU vial) or 90 ml/hour (for a 250,000 IU vial). Follow this with a maintenance dose of 100,000 IU/hour, administered by continuous infusion. Continue the infusion for 24 hours to treat pulmonary embolism, for 24 to 72 hours to treat arterial embolism or thrombosis, and for 72 hours to treat deep vein thrombosis.

Treatment of acute, obstructing coronary artery thrombi associated with evolving, acute myocardial infarction

▶ For adults, give 1.5 million IU over 1 hour by continuous infusion. No maintenance dose is required. Or give an initial dose of 20,000 IU through a coronary artery catheter placed using the Judkins or Somes technique; follow this with 200 IU/minute for 60 minutes.

Treatment of arteriovenous cannula occlusion

▶ For adults, give 100,000 to 250,000 IU in 2 ml of I.V. solution by direct injection into the obstructed catheter.

Contraindications and cautions

Because thrombolytic therapy increases the risk of bleeding, streptokinase is contraindicated for patients with active internal bleeding, intracranial neoplasm, or severe uncontrolled hypertension, as well as patients who've suffered a cerebrovascular accident or undergone intracranial or intraspinal surgery in the past 2 months. Streptokinase also is contraindicated for patients with previous severe allergic reactions to the drug.

Give streptokinase cautiously to patients with conditions that carry an associated risk of bleeding. These include a dissecting aneurysm, cerebrovascular disease within the past 2 months, childbirth, invasive procedures or surgery within the past 10 days, uncontrolled coagulation defects or other hemostatic defects (including those secondary to severe hepatic or renal disease), subacute bacterial endocarditis, diabetic hemorrhagic retinopathy, severe GI bleeding within the past 10 days, GI lesion or ulcer, moderate hypertension, recent trauma (minor or severe, including possible internal injury caused by cardiopulmonary resuscitation), and active tuberculosis with a recent onset of cavitation.

Use caution with patients who have mitral stenosis and atrial fibrillation or other indications of a thrombus in the left side of the heart. Also, give the drug carefully to patients whose condition increases the risk of cerebral embolism.

Because of the risk of systemic infection, give streptokinase cautiously to patients with sepsis at or near a thrombus site, an obstructed I.V. catheter, or an occluded arteriovenous cannula. Administer the drug carefully to patients with a recent streptococcal infection as well as to those who have received streptokinase or anistreplase therapy within the last 5 days to 6 months because the elevated streptokinase antibody levels may cause resistance to therapy and increase the risk of an allergic reaction.

Because streptokinase is a pregnancy risk category C drug, give it cautiously to pregnant patients.

Preparation

Streptokinase comes in powder form in 5-ml vials containing 250,000, 600,000, or 750,000 IU; in 6.5-ml vials containing 250,000, 750,000, or 1.5 million IU; and in 50-ml infusion bottles of 1.5 million IU. Store unopened vials at room temperature.

Just before an infusion, reconstitute streptokinase with 0.9% sodium chloride injection or dextrose 5% injection. Further dilute the drug, generally to a volume of 45 ml (for a loading dose infusion) or to a multiple of 45 ml with a maximum of 500 ml (for a continuous maintenance infusion), using the same solution used for reconstitution. Use a 0.22- or 0.45-micron filter. Also, use a volumetric or syringe pump because the reconstituted streptokinase solution may alter the drop size, influencing the accuracy of drop-counting infusion devices.

For arteriovenous cannula clearance, reconstitute the drug using 2 ml of 0.9% sodium chloride injection or dextrose 5% injection for each 250,000 IU of streptokinase. Add the diluent slowly, directing it at the side of the vial, rather than onto the powder. Roll and tilt the vial gently; avoid shaking it, which may cause foaming and increased flocculation. Slight flocculation doesn't interfere with safe use; however, solutions containing many particles should be discarded.

Store reconstituted solutions at 36° to 39° F (2.2° to 3.9° C) and discard them after 24 hours. Don't add any other drugs to the solution.

Incompatibilities

Streptokinase is incompatible with dextran. Further, the manufacturer recommends that no other medication be added to the streptokinase solution container and that streptokinase not be administered through the same I.V. line as other medications.

Administration

Streptokinase should be administered only by a person who's trained to manage thrombotic disease and who works in an institution equipped to monitor thrombin time and perform other necessary laboratory tests.

- *Direct injection:* Slowly deliver the drug into the occluded arteriovenous cannula. Then, clamp the cannula for 2 hours and closely observe the patient for adverse reactions. After 2 hours, aspirate the contents of the cannula and flush with 0.9% sodium chloride solution. Reconnect the cannula.
- *Continuous infusion:* Administer the diluted drug through a peripheral I.V. line using an infusion pump.
- *Intra-arterial administration:* Give the ordered dose through a coronary artery catheter placed using the Judkins or Somes technique.

Adverse reactions

- *Life-threatening:* anaphylaxis, severe hemorrhage.
- *Other:* abdominal pain or swelling; backache; bleeding or oozing from cuts or wounds; bloody or black, tarry stools; constipation (paralytic ileus or intestinal obstruction caused by hemorrhage); dizziness; dyspnea; epistaxis; fast, slow, or irregular heartbeat; ***fever;*** hematemesis; he-

maturia; hemoptysis; mild or severe headache; muscle pain or stiffness; nausea; phlebitis at infusion site; pruritus; rash; sudden or severe hypotension; swelling of eyes, face, lips, or tongue; unexpected or unusually heavy vaginal bleeding; urticaria; wheezing.

Interactions

- *Antifibrinolytic drugs (aminocaproic acid):* reversal of streptokinase effects.
- *Aspirin, azlocillin, carbenicillin (parenteral), indomethacin, mezlocillin, piperacillin, ticarcillin:* increased risk of bleeding because of altered platelet function.
- *Cefamandole, cefoperazone, moxalactam, plicamycin:* increased risk of severe hemorrhage.
- *Corticosteroids, corticotropin, ethacrynic acid, nonacetylated salicylates:* heightened risk of severe hemorrhage.
- *Dextran, dipyridamole, divalproex, phenylbutazone, sulfinpyrazone, valproic acid:* increased risk of bleeding because of altered platelet function.
- *Heparin, oral anticoagulants:* increased risk of hemorrhage.

Special considerations

Before therapy, obtain a blood sample for thrombin time, activated partial thromboplastin time, prothrombin time, hematocrit, fibrin/fibrinogen degradation product titer, fibrinogen concentration, and platelet count tests. This is especially important for patients who are receiving heparin. Although pretreatment with heparin or drugs affecting platelets increases the risk of bleeding, it also may improve the long-term results.

Keep corticosteroids on hand to treat allergic reactions and aminocaproic acid on hand to control bleeding. Also, have emergency resuscitation equipment available.

Because exposure to streptococci (the source of streptokinase) is common, a loading dose is used to neutralize the antibodies present in many patients. To help establish the dose, determine the patient's resistance to streptokinase. Don't administer a loading dose larger than 1 million IU.

Before and during therapy, invasive arterial procedures should be avoided. If such a procedure is necessary, use a puncture site in the arm and apply pressure to the site for 15 minutes afterward.

During therapy, perform venipunctures carefully and as infrequently as possible. Avoid I.M. injections and unnecessary handling of the patient.

Check the patient's pulses and the color and sensation of his limbs every hour. Monitor him for excessive bleeding every 15 minutes for the first hour, every 30 minutes for the second through eighth hours, then once a shift. Check percutaneous puncture sites and cuts for oozing because streptokinase may lyse fibrin deposits at these sites.

If you note bleeding, discontinue therapy. If necessary, administer whole blood, packed RBCs, and cryoprecipitate or fresh frozen plasma. Don't administer dextran. Administer aminocaproic acid, as ordered.

If reperfusion arrhythmias occur, administer lidocaine or procainamide, as ordered. Defibrillation may be needed for ventricular fibrillation or tachycardia.

If sudden hypotension occurs during high-dose therapy, reduce the infusion rate. If necessary, place the patient in the Trendelenburg position. If a fever persists during therapy, administer acetaminophen.

To avoid dislodging deep venous

thrombi, don't take blood pressure readings of the patient's legs.

Soon after streptokinase therapy, administer heparin, if ordered, to minimize the risk of recurrent thrombosis and pulmonary emboli.

Streptokinase may alter the results of some laboratory tests. The erythrocyte sedimentation rate may increase or temporarily decrease. Fibrinogen, other plasma protein, hematocrit, and hemoglobin levels may fall. Fibrin split product levels may increase. Alanine aminotransferase (ALT), formerly SGPT, and aspartate aminotransferase (AST), formerly SGOT, will show transient elevations during or shortly after an infusion. And thrombin time will be two to five times greater than the control value.

DOSAGE FINDER

Verapamil: Indications and dosages

Treatment of supraventricular tachyarrhythmias, vasospastic angina, and reentrant paroxysmal atrial tachycardia unresponsive to vagal stimulation

▶ For adults, give 5 to 10 mg by direct I.V. injection over 2 minutes (3 minutes in elderly patients). If the response is inadequate, give 10 mg 30 minutes later. In patients with renal or hepatic impairment, try to avoid giving a second dose. If a second dose is necessary, reduce the amount and administer it 60 to 90 minutes after the initial dose.

▶ For children ages 1 to 15, administer 0.1 to 0.3 mg/kg by direct I.V. injection; don't exceed 5 mg. If necessary, repeat the dose in 30 minutes, but don't exceed 10 mg as a single dose.

▶ For children under age 1, administer 0.1 to 0.2 mg/kg by direct I.V. injection.

Verapamil hydrochloride

(Calan, Isoptin)

An antiarrhythmic, verapamil hydrochloride dilates the coronary arteries, increasing myocardial oxygen supply, and slows sinoatrial (SA) and atrioventricular (AV) node conduction, reducing the heart rate. Although the drug decreases myocardial activity and cardiac output, a corresponding drop in afterload counters these effects. The drug is used to treat supraventricular tachyarrhythmias and vasospastic angina, and to convert reentrant paroxysmal atrial tachycardia unresponsive to vagal stimulation. (See *How verapamil works.*)

The onset of action occurs in 1 to 5 minutes. The drug's antiarrhythmic effect lasts about 2 hours; its hemodynamic effect, about 10 to 20 minutes. Verapamil's half-life is biphasic—4 minutes for the first phase, 2 to 5 hours for the second.

About 90% of verapamil is bound to plasma proteins. The drug is distributed to cerebrospinal fluid and crosses the placenta. Rapidly and completely metabolized in the liver to demethylated metabolites, verapamil is excreted in urine and feces; 16% is excreted within 5 days. The drug appears in breast milk. (See *Verapamil: Indications and dosages.*)

Contraindications and cautions

Verapamil is contraindicated for second- or third-degree AV block because of the risk of excessive bradycardia; for patients with severe hypotension, cardiogenic shock, or pulmonary artery wedge pressure greater than 20 mm Hg because the drug may exacerbate these conditions; and for patients with Wolff-

MECHANISM OF ACTION

How verapamil works

Verapamil hydrochloride increases the myocardial oxygen supply and slows the heart rate. Apparently, the drug produces these effects by blocking the slow calcium channel as shown in the illustration below. This action inhibits the influx of extracellular calcium ions across both myocardial and vascular smooth muscle cell membranes. Verapamil achieves this blockade without changing serum calcium concentrations.

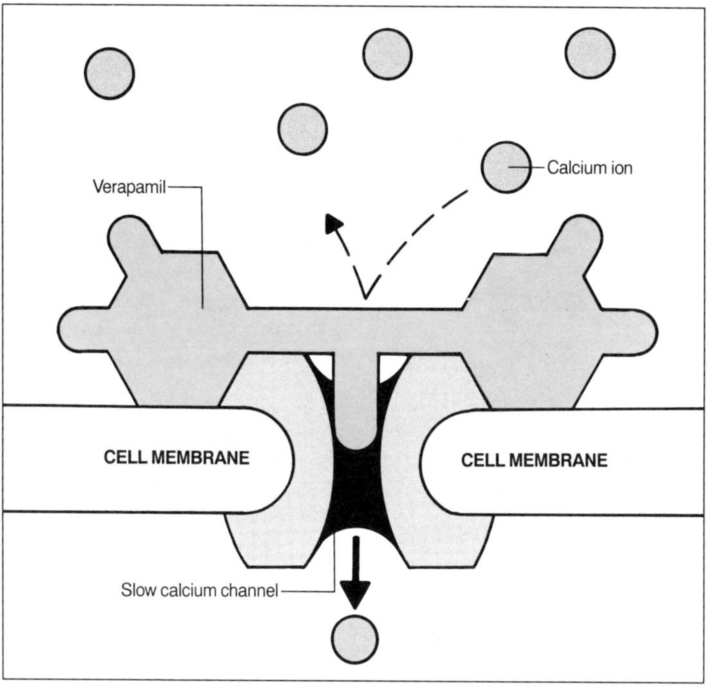

This calcium blockade causes the coronary arteries (and, to a lesser extent, the peripheral arteries and arterioles) to dilate, decreasing afterload and increasing the myocardial oxygen supply. The blockade also slows sinoatrial and atrioventricular node conduction, slightly reducing the heart rate.

Parkinson-White syndrome because the drug may precipitate severe arrhythmias.

Use caution when giving verapamil to patients with a known hypersensitivity to the drug. Also use caution when giving the drug to patients with Duchenne-type muscular dystrophy because of the risk of respiratory paralysis and to patients with extreme bradycardia or heart failure because of the reduction in SA and AV node activity. Give the drug cautiously to patients with hy-

EMERGENCY INTERVENTION

Managing a verapamil overdose

Signs of a verapamil overdose include hypotension, a rapid ventricular rate caused by antegrade conduction, and bradycardia with second- or third-degree atrioventricular (AV) block progressing to asystole. If you detect such signs, take these measures, as ordered:

- To treat hypotension, administer I.V. fluids and place the patient in the Trendelenburg position. If necessary, give him dobutamine, dopamine, calcium chloride, isoproterenol, metaraminol, or norepinephrine.
- To treat a rapid ventricular rate caused by antegrade conduction (such as that seen in patients with atrial flutter or fibrillation, or Wolff-Parkinson-White or Lown-Ganong-Levine syndrome), use direct current cardioversion or give lidocaine or procainamide.
- To treat bradycardia with second- or third-degree AV block progressing to asystole, give atropine, calcium chloride, isoproterenol, or norepinephrine. Or the patient may require a temporary pacemaker.

pertrophic cardiomyopathy, moderate ventricular dysfunction, and sick sinus syndrome because their symptoms may worsen, to patients with mild to moderate hypotension because the drug may exacerbate the condition, and to patients with renal or hepatic impairment because of the increased risk of toxicity.

Administer verapamil cautiously to children (particularly neonates) because its efficacy in children hasn't been established. Finally, give verapamil cautiously to pregnant patients because it's classified as a pregnancy risk category C drug.

Preparation

Verapamil is supplied as a solution of 2.5 mg/ml. Store the solution at room temperature, protecting it from light and freezing. The drug remains stable in most infusion solutions for 24 hours at 77° F (25° C) when protected from light. Verapamil is compatible with dextrose 5% in water, 0.9% sodium chloride solution, and lactated Ringer's solution.

Incompatibilities

Verapamil is incompatible with albumin, amphotericin B, co-trimoxazole (sulfamethoxazole and trimethoprim), dobutamine hydrochloride, hydralazine hydrochloride, nafcillin sodium, and sodium bicarbonate. Precipitation will occur in any solution with a pH above 6.0.

Administration

- *Direct injection:* Administer the undiluted drug at a rate of 5 to 10 mg over at least 2 minutes. Inject it directly into a vein or an I.V. line containing a free-flowing, compatible solution. With elderly patients, give the drug over at least 3 minutes to minimize adverse effects.

Adverse reactions

- *Life-threatening:* asystole, severe pulmonary edema, ventricular fibrillation.
- *Other:* alopecia, atrial fibrillation, blurred vision, bradycardia, ***congestive heart failure (CHF), constipation,*** depression, diaphoresis, dizziness, drowsiness, dry mouth, dyspnea, ecchymosis, first-degree AV block, headache, ***hypotension,*** muscle fatigue, nausea, peripheral edema, purpura, vertigo.

Interactions

- *Anticoagulants (oral), hydantoins, salicylates, sulfonamides, sulfonylureas:* decreased effectiveness be-

cause of possible displacement from binding sites.
- *Antihypertensives:* risk of additive effects.
- *Beta-adrenergic blockers:* increased risk of CHF and AV block.
- *Carbamazepine, cyclosporine, prazosin, theophylline, valproate:* elevated serum levels of these drugs and increased risk of toxicity.
- *Cimetidine:* risk of decreased verapamil clearance.
- *Dantrolene (I.V.):* risk of cardiovascular collapse.
- *Digoxin:* increased serum levels of digoxin.
- *Disopyramide:* additive effects and possibly fatal impairment of left ventricular function.
- *Estrogens, nonsteroidal anti-inflammatory drugs, sympathomimetics:* risk of reduced antihypertensive effects of verapamil.
- *Lithium:* decreased serum levels of lithium.
- *Metoprolol:* increased bioavailability of metoprolol.
- *Quinidine:* heightened hypotensive effects.

Special considerations

During therapy, continuously monitor the patient's cardiac rhythm strip. Keep emergency resuscitation equipment on hand. (See *Managing a verapamil overdose.*)

Expect to give a lower dose to patients with severe cardiac impairment and to those receiving beta blockers. Monitor these patients closely for adverse effects. If you note signs of CHF, such as dependent edema or dyspnea, notify the doctor.

Verapamil can alter some test results. An electrocardiogram may show a prolonged PR interval, and levels of alanine aminotransferase (ALT), formerly SGPT, and aspartate aminotransferase (AST), formerly SGOT, may temporarily increase.

Suggested readings

Drug Information for the Health Care Professional, 2 vols., 11th ed. Rockville, Md.: United States Pharmacopeial Convention, Inc., 1991.

Drug Information 91—American Hospital Formulary Service. Bethesda, Md: American Society of Hospital Pharmacists, 1991.

Facts and Comparisons. St. Louis, Mo.: Facts and Comparisons, Inc. Updated monthly.

Nursing92 Drug Handbook. Springhouse, Pa: Springhouse Corp., 1992.

Physician's Desk Reference, 45th ed. Oradell, N.J.: Medical Economics Company Inc., 1991.

Trissel, L.A. *Handbook on Injectable Drugs,* 5th ed. Bethesda, Md.: American Society of Hospital Pharmacists, 1988.

SELF-TEST

Test your knowledge and skills at your own pace by answering the multiple-choice questions on pages 199 to 201. Answers appear on page 201.

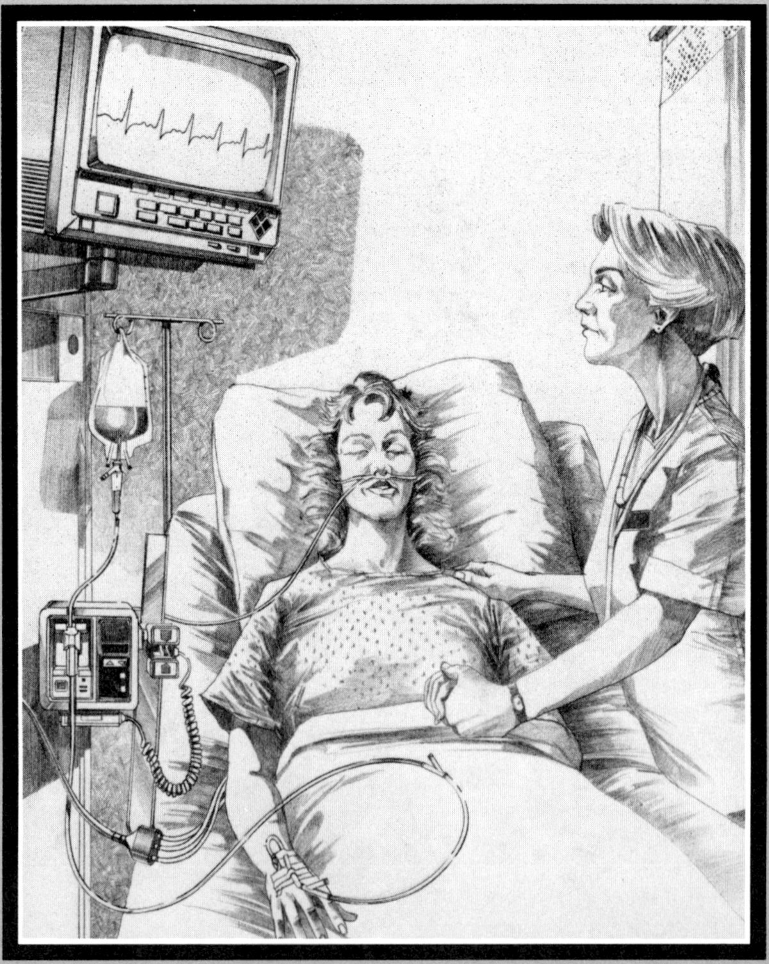

QUESTIONS

1. *Which of the following would you inject locally to treat dopamine extravasation?*
a. 0.9% sodium chloride solution
b. sterile water
c. phentolamine
d. phenylephrine

2. *When administering dobutamine, you should monitor the patient's blood pressure, heart rate, and:*
a. urine output.
b. daily weight.
c. cardiac rhythm.
d. capillary refill time.

3. *Morphine is the analgesic of choice for treating:*
a. myocardial infarction.
b. end-stage renal disease.
c. severe liver impairment.
d. head injury.

4. *When given after a myocardial infarction, metoprolol:*
a. prevents bradycardia.
b. reduces the severity of myocardial ischemia.
c. increases blood pressure.
d. prevents heart block.

5. *Dantrolene serves as an adjunct in the treatment of:*
a. ventricular fibrillation.
b. severe hypotension.
c. active peptic ulcer.
d. malignant hyperthermia crisis.

6. *You should monitor a patient who is receiving epinephrine and chlorpromazine for:*
a. severe hypotension and bradycardia.
b. severe hypotension and tachycardia.
c. severe hypertension and bradycardia.
d. severe hypertension and tachycardia.

7. *Chlorpheniramine serves as an adjunct in the treatment of:*
a. cardiac arrhythmias.
b. acetaminophen toxicity.
c. severe hypertension.
d. anaphylaxis.

8. *The usual dose of I.V. calcium chloride for a hypocalcemic adult ranges from:*
a. 2 to 4 mEq.
b. 7 to 14 mEq.
c. 15 to 20 mEq.
d. 20 to 25 mEq.

9. *How long after giving bretylium for ventricular fibrillation should you see signs that the drug is working?*
a. 20 to 60 minutes
b. 15 to 20 minutes
c. 1 to 5 minutes
d. 5 to 10 minutes

10. *If a hypoglycemic patient doesn't respond to glucagon, he probably:*
a. has insufficient hepatic stores of glycogen.
b. received too small a dose.
c. received too large a dose.
d. received the drug too slowly.

11. *During advanced cardiac life support (ACLS), you'd administer atropine to:*
a. decrease heart rate and increase blood pressure.
b. increase heart rate and blood pressure.
c. decrease heart rate and blood pressure.
d. increase heart rate and decrease blood pressure.

12. *In a patient with central nervous system trauma, atropine can cause:*
a. pupil dilation.
b. pupil constriction.
c. increased reflexes.
d. decreased reflexes.

13. *The drug of choice for treating anaphylaxis is:*
a. esmolol.
b. ephedrine.
c. epinephrine.
d. norepinephrine.

14. *Ergonovine is an:*
a. antidepressant.
b. oxytocic.
c. antispasmodic.
d. antihistamine.

15. *The drug of choice for treating status epilepticus is:*
a. phenytoin.
b. diazepam.
c. phenobarbital.
d. magnesium sulfate.

16. *Monitor a pulmonary edema patient who is receiving I.V. furosemide for:*
a. extravasation.
b. muscle weakness and cramps.
c. bradycardia.
d. complete heart block.

17. *What type of insulin should a patient with diabetic ketoacidosis receive?*
a. NPH
b. lente
c. regular
d. PZI

18. *Which of these reverses magnesium sulfate toxicity?*
a. epinephrine
b. dextrose in water
c. naloxone
d. calcium gluconate

19. *Neostigmine serves as an antidote to an overdose of:*
a. succinylcholine.
b. pancuronium.
c. biperiden.
d. promethazine.

20. *For an adult with severe hypertension, the nitroprusside infusion rate shouldn't exceed:*
a. 5 mcg/kg/minute.
b. 10 mcg/kg/minute.
c. 20 mcg/kg/minute.
d. 25 mcg/kg/minute.

21. *You would give verapamil to treat:*
a. ventricular arrhythmias.
b. heart block.
c. atrial arrhythmias.
d. hypotension.

22. *Isoproterenol does all of the following* except:
a. increase myocardial contractility.
b. increase diastolic pressure.
c. increase cardiac output.
d. relieve bronchospasm.

23. *The recommended method for administering anistreplase is:*
a. I.M. injection.
b. intermittent infusion.
c. direct injection.
d. continuous infusion.

24. *During ACLS, lidocaine may be given by any of these routes* except:
a. intracardiac.
b. endotracheal.
c. direct I.V. injection.
d. I.M. injection.

25. *Metaraminol increases blood pressure by:*
a. indirectly causing the release of norepinephrine.
b. pulling interstitial fluid into the intravascular space.
c. causing the kidneys to conserve fluid.
d. increasing the heart rate.

26. *When administering phenytoin in an emergency, which of the following is* not *an important consideration?*
a. checking the patient's serum phenytoin levels before administration
b. giving the drug at a rate of 50 mg/minute or less
c. frequently checking for extravasation
d. diluting the drug with 0.9% sodium chloride solution to a concentration of 10 mg/ml

27. *Which statement about aminophylline is* not *correct?*
a. Smoking accelerates plasma clearance of aminophylline.
b. Combining aminophylline with ephedrine causes excessive stimulation.
c. Aminophylline and theophylline are interchangeable.
d. A patient with cardiac, renal, or hepatic dysfunction requires a reduced dosage.

28. *You should administer digoxin immune FAB cautiously to patients who are sensitive to:*
a. beef.
b. lamb.
c. poultry.
d. pork.

29. *Amyl nitrate can help counteract what type of poisoning?*
a. cyanide
b. lead
c. digoxin
d. organophosphate

30. *If you note crystals in a mannitol solution, you should:*
a. add EGTA to the solution.
b. discard the solution.
c. place the container in warm water until the crystals dissolve.
d. add 0.9% sodium chloride solution.

31. *You can safely give metaproterenol to a patient with:*
a. hypertension.
b. bradycardia.
c. a seizure disorder.
d. tachycardia.

32. *All of the following are loop diuretics* except:
a. furosemide.
b. ethacrynate sodium.
c. bumetanide.
d. nitroprusside.

33. *During ACLS, a patient should receive sodium bicarbonate:*
a. every 10 minutes.
b. every 5 minutes.
c. based on clinical findings.
d. after successful resuscitation.

34. *For an adult with severe agitation, the usual initial dose of promazine ranges from:*
a. 25 to 50 mg.
b. 50 to 150 mg.
c. 150 to 200 mg.
d. 200 to 300 mg.

35. *Heparin does all of the following* except:
a. inhibit the action of Factors IX, X, XI, and XII.
b. dissolve clots through its fibrinolytic action.
c. potentiate the effects of antithrombin.
d. activate fibrin-stabilizing factor to prevent clots.

36. *Which of the following does* not *signal a pyridostigmine overdose?*
a. dry, parched skin
b. abdominal cramps
c. diarrhea
d. excessive bronchial secretions

37. *Which of the following can cause respiratory depression that naloxone can't reverse?*
a. diazepam
b. morphine
c. meperidine
d. oxymorphone

38. *When administering digoxin in an emergency, you must do all of the following* except:
a. check the patient's apical pulse for a full minute.
b. obtain a digoxin level.
c. divide the loading dose over 24 hours.
d. obtain the patient's ideal body weight.

39. *Nitroglycerin does all of the following* except:
a. reduce myocardial oxygen consumption.
b. reduce preload.
c. reduce afterload.
d. increase blood pressure.

ANSWERS

1. c	**9.** d	**17.** c	**25.** a	**33.** c
2. c	**10.** a	**18.** d	**26.** d	**34.** b
3. a	**11.** b	**19.** b	**27.** c	**35.** b
4. b	**12.** a	**20.** b	**28.** b	**36.** a
5. d	**13.** c	**21.** c	**29.** a	**37.** a
6. b	**14.** b	**22.** b	**30.** c	**38.** c
7. d	**15.** b	**23.** c	**31.** b	**39.** d
8. b	**16.** b	**24.** a	**32.** d	

APPENDIX AND INDEX

ANTIDOTES TO DRUG OVERDOSES AND POISONS

ANTIDOTE AND INDICATIONS	DOSAGE AND ADMINISTRATION	NURSING CONSIDERATIONS
acetylcysteine (Airbron, Mucomyst, Mucosol, Parvolex) • Acetaminophen toxicity	• *Adults and children:* 140 mg/kg P.O., followed by 70 mg/kg q 4 h for 17 doses (total of 1,330 mg/kg).	• Use cautiously in elderly or debilitated patients and in those with asthma or severe respiratory insufficiency. • Don't use with activated charcoal because charcoal limits acetylcysteine's effectiveness. • Don't combine with oxytetracycline, tetracycline, erythromycin lactobionate, amphotericin B, ampicillin, iodized oil, chymotrypsin, trypsin, or hydrogen peroxide. Give separately.
activated charcoal (Actidose-Aqua, Charcoaide, Charcocaps, Liqui-Char, Superchar) • Overdose of amphetamines, aspirin, atropine, barbiturates, cocaine, cardiac glycosides, glutethimide, ipecac syrup, opiates, phenothiazines, quinine, sulfonamides, tricyclic antidepressants, and poisoning with antimony, arsenic, camphor, malathion, oxalic acid, parathion, phenol, poisonous mushrooms, strychnine	• *Adults:* initially, 1 g/kg (30 to 100 g) P.O., or 5 to 10 times the amount of poison ingested as a suspension in 180 to 240 ml of water. • *Children ages 1 to 12:* 20 to 50 g P.O. as single dose. • *Children under age 1:* 1 g/kg P.O. as single dose.	• Don't give to semiconscious or unconscious patients. • If possible, administer within 30 minutes of poisoning. Administer larger dose if patient has food in his stomach. • Don't administer with ipecac syrup because charcoal inactivates ipecac. If patient needs ipecac syrup, give charcoal after patient has finished vomiting. • Don't give in ice cream, milk, or sherbet because they reduce adsorptive capacities of charcoal. • Powder form is most effective. Mix with tap water to form thick syrup. A small amount of fruit juice or flavoring may be added to make charcoal more palatable. • Dose may need to be repeated if patient vomits shortly after administration.
aminocaproic acid (Amicar) • Alteplase, streptokinase, urokinase toxicity	• *Adults:* initially, 5 g P.O. or as slow I.V. infusion, followed by 1 to 1.25 g hourly until bleeding is controlled. Don't exceed 30 g daily.	• Use cautiously with oral contraceptives and estrogens because they may increase risk of hypercoagulability. • For infusion, dilute solution with sterile water for injection, 0.9% sodium chloride solution, D_5W, or Ringer's solution. • Monitor coagulation studies, heart rhythm, and blood pressure.
amyl nitrite • Cyanide poisoning	• *Adults:* 0.2 or 0.3 ml by inhalation for 30 to 60 seconds q 5 minutes until patient regains consciousness.	• To administer, wrap ampule in cloth and crush. Hold near patient's nose and mouth so he can inhale vapor. • Monitor patient for orthostatic hypotension. • Patient may experience headache after administration.

(continued)

ANTIDOTES TO DRUG OVERDOSES AND POISONS *(continued)*

ANTIDOTE AND INDICATIONS	DOSAGE AND ADMINISTRATION	NURSING CONSIDERATIONS
atropine sulfate • Cholinesterase toxicity	• *Adults:* initially, 1 to 2 mg by direct I.V. injection, then 2 mg q 5 to 60 minutes until symptoms subside. In severe cases, initial dose may be as much as 6 mg; then give q 5 to 60 minutes. Administer over 1 to 2 minutes.	• Contraindicated for patients with glaucoma, myasthenia gravis, obstructive uropathy, or unstable cardiovascular status. • Monitor intake and output to assess for urine retention.
botulism antitoxin, bivalent equine • Botulism	• *Adults and children:* 1 vial I.V. initially and q 4 h p.r.n., until patient's condition improves. Dilute antitoxin 1:10 in D_5W, $D_{10}W$, or 0.9% sodium chloride solution before administration. Give first 10 ml of dilution over 5 minutes; after 15 minutes, you may increase rate.	• Test for sensitivity before administration. • Keep epinephrine 1:1,000 available in case of adverse reaction. • Bivalent antitoxin contains antibodies against types A and B *Clostridium botulinum.* Antitoxins against all other types are available only from Centers for Disease Control in Atlanta: Monday to Friday, 8 a.m. to 4:30 p.m. (E.S.T.), (404) 329-3670; nights, weekends, and holidays (emergencies only), (404) 329-2888. • Obtain accurate patient history of allergies, especially to horses, and reactions to immunizations. • Administer antitoxin as soon as possible for best results.
crotaline antivenin, polyvalent • Crotalid (rattlesnake) bites	• *Adults and children:* initially, 10 to 50 ml or more I.M. or S.C., depending on severity of bite and patient's response. Smaller patients should receive larger initial dose than larger patients. If patient received large amount of venom, inject 70 to 100 ml I.V. directly into superficial vein. Base subsequent doses on patient's response; may give 10 ml q ½ to 2 h p.r.n.	• Don't use with antihistamines because of enhanced toxicity of crotalid venom. • Immobilize patient immediately and splint the affected limb. • Test patient for sensitivity before administration. Give 0.02 to 0.03 ml of a 1:10 dilution in 0.9% sodium chloride solution intradermally. Read results after 5 to 10 minutes. • If patient was bitten in limb, inject part of initial dose at various sites around limb above swelling; don't inject in finger or toe. • Keep epinephrine 1:1,000 available in case of adverse reaction. • Obtain accurate patient history of allergies, especially to horses, and reactions to immunizations. • Type and crossmatch as soon as possible because hemolysis from venom prevents accurate crossmatching. • Watch patient carefully for delayed allergic reaction or relapse. • Children, who have less resistance and less body fluid to dilute venom, may need twice the adult dose. • Discard unused reconstituted drug.

ANTIDOTES TO DRUG OVERDOSES AND POISONS *(continued)*

ANTIDOTE AND INDICATIONS	DOSAGE AND ADMINISTRATION	NURSING CONSIDERATIONS
deferoxamine mesylate (Desferal) • Acute iron intoxication (adjunctive treatment)	• *Adults and children:* 1 g I.M. or I.V. followed by 500 mg I.M. or I.V. for two doses q 4 h; then 500 mg I.M. or I.V. q 4 to 12 h. Don't infuse more than 15 mg/kg hourly. Don't administer more than 6 g in 24 hours.	• Contraindicated for patients with severe renal disease or anuria. Use cautiously in patients with impaired renal function. • Keep epinephrine 1:1,000 available in case of allergic reaction. • Use I.M. route if possible. Use I.V. route only when patient has cardiovascular collapse or is in shock. • If giving I.V., switch to I.M. as soon as possible. • To reconstitute, add 2 ml of sterile water for injection to each ampule. Make sure drug dissolves completely. To reconstitute for I.V. administration, dissolve as for I.M. use but in 0.9% sodium chloride solution, D_5W, or lactated Ringer's solution. • Monitor intake and output carefully. • Warn patient that his urine may turn red. • Reconstituted solution can be stored for up to 1 week at room temperature. Protect from light.
digoxin immune FAB (ovine) (Digibind) • Potentially life-threatening digoxin or digitoxin intoxication	• *Adults and children:* I.V. infusion over 30 minutes or as a bolus if cardiac arrest is imminent. Dosage varies according to amount of overdose; average dose is 10 vials (400 mg), but if toxicity resulted from acute digoxin ingestion and neither serum digoxin level nor estimated ingestion amount is known, increase to 20 vials (800 mg).	• Use cautiously in patients allergic to ovine proteins because drug is derived from digoxin-specific antibody fragments obtained from immunized sheep. Perform skin test before administration in these patients. • Use only in patients in shock or cardiac arrest; with ventricular arrhythmias, such as ventricular tachycardia or fibrillation; with progressive bradycardia, such as severe sinus bradycardia; or with second- or third-degree atrioventricular block not responsive to atropine. • Monitor potassium levels closely. • Infuse through a 0.22-micron membrane filter, if possible. Administer as a bolus injection only if cardiac arrest is imminent. • Refrigerate powder for reconstitution. If possible, use reconstituted drug immediately, although you may refrigerate it for up to 4 hours. • In most patients, signs of digitalis toxicity disappear within a few hours of receiving dose. • Drug interferes with digitalis immunoassay measurements, resulting in misleading standard serum digoxin levels until drug is cleared from body (about 2 days). • Total serum digoxin levels may rise after administration of this drug, reflecting FAB-bound (inactive) digoxin.

(continued)

ANTIDOTES TO DRUG OVERDOSES AND POISONS *(continued)*

ANTIDOTE AND INDICATIONS	DOSAGE AND ADMINISTRATION	NURSING CONSIDERATIONS
edetate calcium disodium (Calcium Disodium Versenate, Calcium EDTA) • Lead poisoning	***For blood levels > 50 mcg/dl*** • *Adults and children:* 1 g/m² I.M. or I.V. daily for 3 to 5 days. For I.V. infusion, dilute in D_5W or 0.9% sodium chloride solution and administer over 1 to 2 hours. ***For blood levels > 100 mcg/dl*** • *Adults and children:* 1.5 g/m² I.M. or I.V. daily for 3 to 5 days, usually in conjunction with dimercaprol. For I.V. infusion, dilute in D_5W or 0.9% sodium chloride solution and administer over 1 to 2 hours. If necessary, administer a second course no sooner than 4 days later; preferably, 2 to 3 weeks should elapse between courses.	• Contraindicated for patients with severe renal disease or anuria. • Avoid rapid I.V. infusion; I.M. route is preferred, especially for children. • Don't use I.V. route in patients with lead encephalopathy because intracranial pressure may increase; use I.M. route instead. • With large dose, administer dimercaprol to avoid toxicity. • Force fluids to facilitate lead excretion, except in patients with lead encephalopathy. • Before administration, obtain baseline lead levels. Also, obtain urinalysis, blood urea nitrogen, and serum alkaline phosphatase, calcium, creatinine, and phosphorus measurements. Then monitor on first, third, and fifth days of treatment. Monitor electrocardiogram (ECG) periodically. • If procaine hydrochloride has been added to I.M. solution to minimize pain, watch for local reaction.
edetate disodium (Disodium EDTA, Disotate, Endrate) • Hypercalcemic crisis	• *Adults:* 50 mg/kg in 500 ml of D_5W or 0.9% sodium chloride solution by slow I.V. infusion. Don't exceed 3 g/day. • *Children:* 40 to 70 mg/kg diluted in D_5W or 0.9% sodium chloride solution to maximum concentration of 30 mg/ml by slow I.V. infusion. Don't exceed 70 mg/kg/day.	• Contraindicated for patients with anuria, known or suspected hypocalcemia, significant renal disease, active or healed tubercular lesions, history of seizures or intracranial lesions, or generalized arteriosclerosis associated with aging. • Use cautiously in patients with limited cardiac reserve, congestive heart failure, hypokalemia, or diabetes. • Avoid rapid I.V. infusion because profound hypocalcemia may occur, leading to tetany, seizures, cardiac arrhythmias, and respiratory arrest. • Monitor blood pressure and ECG, and test renal function frequently. • Obtain serum calcium levels after each dose. Keep I.V. calcium available in case serum calcium levels drop precipitously. • Keep patient in bed for 15 minutes after infu-

ANTIDOTES TO DRUG OVERDOSES AND POISONS *(continued)*

ANTIDOTE AND INDICATIONS	DOSAGE AND ADMINISTRATION	NURSING CONSIDERATIONS
edetate disodium *(continued)*		sion to avoid postural hypotension. • Don't confuse drug with edetate calcium disodium, which is used to treat lead toxicity. • Record I.V. site used, and try to avoid using same site repeatedly to decrease risk of thrombophlebitis. • Monitor patient for fever, chills, back pain, emesis, muscle cramps, and urinary urgency, which may occur 4 to 8 hours after administration. Report such reactions to doctor, who'll usually order supportive treatment. Symptoms usually subside within 12 hours. • Not currently drug of choice for hypercalcemia because other safer and more effective treatments exist.
ipecac syrup • To induce vomiting in poisoning	• *Adults:* 15 ml P.O., followed by 200 to 300 ml of water. • *Children age 1 and over:* 15 ml P.O., followed by about 200 ml of water or milk. • *Children under age 1:* 5 to 10 ml P.O., followed by 100 to 200 ml of water or milk. Repeat dose once after 20 minutes, if necessary.	• Contraindicated for semicomatose, unconscious, or severely inebriated patients and for those with seizures, shock, or absent gag reflex. • Don't give after ingestion of petroleum distillates (such as kerosene or gasoline) or volatile oils; retching and vomiting may cause aspiration and lead to bronchospasm, pulmonary edema, or aspiration pneumonitis. Instead, administer vegetable oil to delay absorption of these substances. • Don't give after ingestion of caustic substances such as lye; further injury to esophagus and mediastinum can occur during emesis. • If two doses don't induce vomiting, tell doctor, who'll probably order gastric lavage. • For antiemetic toxicity, administer within 1 hour. • If patient also needs activated charcoal, administer charcoal after patient has vomited or charcoal will neutralize emetic effect. • Suggest to parents of children over age 1 that they keep 1 oz (30 ml) of ipecac syrup available for immediate use in case of emergency. • Drug induces vomiting within 30 minutes in more than 90% of patients; average time is usually less than 20 minutes. • Patient's stomach usually empties completely; vomitus may contain some intestinal material as well. • No systemic toxicity occurs with doses of 30 ml or less.

(continued)

ANTIDOTES TO DRUG OVERDOSES AND POISONS *(continued)*

ANTIDOTE AND INDICATIONS	DOSAGE AND ADMINISTRATION	NURSING CONSIDERATIONS
methylene blue • Cyanide poisoning	• *Adults and children:* 1 to 2 mg/kg of 1% solution by direct I.V. injection over several minutes. May repeat dose in 1 hour.	• Contraindicated for patients with severe renal impairment or methylene blue hypersensitivity. • Use with caution in glucose-6-phosphate dehydrogenase deficiency because drug may cause hemolysis. • Avoid extravasation; S.C. injection may cause necrotic abscesses. • Warn patient that methylene blue will discolor his urine and stool and stain his skin. Hypochlorite solution rubbed on his skin will remove stains.
naloxone hydrochloride (Narcan) • Respiratory depression caused by opioids • Postoperative narcotic depression • Asphyxia neonatorum	***For respiratory depression caused by opioids*** • *Adults:* 0.4 to 2 mg I.V., I.M., or S.C. May repeat q 2 to 3 minutes p.r.n. If no response occurs after administering 10 mg, patient may not have narcotic-induced toxicity. ***For postoperative narcotic depression*** • *Adults:* 0.1 to 0.2 mg I.V. q 2 to 3 minutes p.r.n. • *Children:* 0.01 mg/kg I.V., I.M., or S.C. Repeat as necessary q 2 to 3 minutes. If patient doesn't improve with initial dose, he may need up to 10 times as much (0.1 mg/kg). ***For asphyxia neonatorum*** • *Neonates:* 0.01 mg/kg I.V. into umbilical vein. Repeat q 2 to 3 minutes for three doses if necessary.	• Use cautiously in patients with cardiac irritability or narcotic addiction. • Monitor respiratory depth and rate. Be prepared to provide oxygen, ventilation, and other resuscitative measures. • If neonatal concentration (0.02 mg/ml) isn't available, dilute adult concentration (0.4 mg) by mixing 0.5 ml with 9.5 ml of sterile water or saline solution for injection. • Respiratory rate increases in 1 to 2 minutes. Effects last 1 to 4 hours. • Duration of narcotic may exceed that of naloxone, causing patient to relapse into respiratory depression. • May administer by continuous I.V. infusion to control adverse effects of epidurally administered morphine. • May see "overshoot" effect—patient's respiratory rate after receiving drug exceeds his rate before respiratory depression occurred. • Safest drug to use when cause of respiratory depression is uncertain. • Doesn't reverse respiratory depression caused by diazepam. • Generally believed ineffective in treating respiratory depression caused by nonopioid drugs, but may reverse coma induced by alcohol intoxication.

ANTIDOTES TO DRUG OVERDOSES AND POISONS *(continued)*

ANTIDOTE AND INDICATIONS	DOSAGE AND ADMINISTRATION	NURSING CONSIDERATIONS
pralidoxime chloride (Protopam chloride) • Cholinergic drug overdose and organophosphate poisoning	• *Adults:* I.V. infusion of 1 to 2 g in 100 ml of 0.9% sodium chloride solution over 15 to 30 minutes. If patient has pulmonary edema, administer by slow I.V. push over 5 minutes. Repeat in 1 hour if muscle weakness persists. If patient needs additional doses, administer cautiously. If I.V. route isn't feasible, give I.M. or S.C., or 1 to 30 g P.O. q 5 h. • *Children:* 20 to 40 mg/kg I.V.	• Contraindicated for patients poisoned with carbayl (Sevin), a carbamate insecticide, because pralidoxime increases Sevin's toxicity. • Use with extreme caution in patients with renal insufficiency or myasthenia gravis because overdose may precipitate myasthenic crisis. • Use with caution in patients with asthma or peptic ulcer. • Use on hospitalized patients only; have respiratory and other supportive measures available. Before administering, suction secretions, make sure airway is patent, and provide artificial ventilation if needed. • Obtain accurate medical history and chronology of poisoning if possible. • Draw blood for cholinesterase levels. • Dilute drug with sterile water without preservatives. • Administer antidote as soon as possible after poisoning. Treatment is most effective if started within 24 hours of exposure. • Administer atropine along with pralidoxime. • For skin exposure to an organophosphate, remove patient's clothing and wash skin and hair with sodium bicarbonate, soap, water, and alcohol as soon as possible; a second washing may be needed. Wear protective gloves and clothes to avoid exposure. • Observe patient for 48 to 72 hours if he ingested poison. Delayed absorption may occur in lower bowel. • Caution patient to avoid contact with insecticides for several weeks. • Drug is not effective against poisoning with phosphorus, inorganic phosphates, or organophosphates with no anticholinesterase activity.
protamine sulfate • Heparin overdose	• *Adults:* usually 1 mg for each 78 to 95 units of heparin, based on venous blood coagulation studies. Dilute to 1% (10 mg/ml) and give by slow I.V. injection over 1 to 3 minutes. Don't exceed 50 mg in 10 minutes.	• Use cautiously after cardiac surgery. • Administer slowly to reduce adverse reactions. Have equipment available to treat shock. • Monitor patient continuously, and check vital signs frequently. • Watch for spontaneous bleeding (heparin rebound), especially in patients undergoing dialysis and those who have had cardiac surgery. • Protamine sulfate may act as an anticoagulant in very high doses.

INDEX

i refers to an illustration; *t* refers to a table.

i refers to an illustration; *t* refers to a table.

i refers to an illustration; *t* refers to a table.

i refers to an illustration; *t* refers to a table.